Sociological
Perspectives
on Community
Mental Health

Sociological Perspectives on Community Mental Health

Edited by

PAUL M. ROMAN

Associate Professor, Department of Sociology
Newcomb College, Tulane University
New Orleans, Louisiana

HARRISON M. TRICE

Professor, Department of Organizational Behavior
New York State School of Industrial and Labor Relations
Cornell University
Ithaca, New York

F. A. DAVIS COMPANY, PHILADELPHIA

Library of Congress Cataloging in Publication Data

Roman, Paul M
   Sociological perspectives on community mental health.
   Includes bibliographies.
   1. Community mental health services—United States.
2. Psychiatric social work—United States. I. Trice,
Harrison Miller, 1920-   joint author. II. Title.
[DNLM: 1. Psychiatry, Community. WM30 R758s 1974]
RA790.6.R65   362.2'0973   74-6168
ISBN 0-8036-7555-0

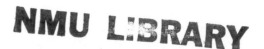

To

Hyman Rodman

for aid and encouragement

Preface

The delivery of quality health care services to the American people constitutes a major social problem as we move toward the final quarter of the twentieth century. This book is about an organization and mode of health care delivery that dramatically emerged on the American scene a decade ago—the community mental health center and the specialty of community psychiatry. In many ways, the issues surrounding this system and the problems toward which it is oriented sharply differ from those of other broader health care delivery systems. In the past decade, "anti-psychiatry" has gained some credence as a semi-ideological social movement which is actively supported by many sociologists. Thus, an assessment of the community health movement is necessarily framed within larger issues concerning the nature of "mental illness" and the role of psychiatry in modern society.

This book is neither a paean to the community mental health concept, a diatribe about psychiatry as a disguised form of social control, nor a handbook about how to implement a community mental health program. Instead it represents a well reasoned set of objective assessments of this social movement, prepared by sociologists. To our knowledge, this is the first attempt to focus a range of sociological viewpoints on the community mental health movement. As is evident in these chapters, sociological perspectives were largely neglected in the initial decade of the movement's development, but perhaps these analyses and assessments will be more useful by coming from outside "the action."

This volume and the companion volume, *Explorations in Psychiatric Sociology* (Philadelphia: F.A. Davis, 1974), are official projects of the Society for the Study of Social Problems, an organization of sociologists formed in the early 1950s to focus sociological expertise on the real-world issues of modern society. The project began when the editors were co-chairmen of the Society's Division on Psychiatric Sociology, when Division members agreed that these volumes would constitute a useful contribution consistent with the Society's objectives. All royalties from the sale of these volumes will go to the Society to support its activities.

All of the chapters were written especially for this volume. We are grateful to the contributors for making this project a rewarding experience for us, and their generosity in contributing their efforts for the benefit of the SSSP is deeply appreciated.

We are indebted to Hyman Rodman, past Chairperson of the SSSP Editorial and Publications Committee, who took many hours during a sabbatical leave to assure publication of the volume, and to Joe Witcher and Irma Agnew of the F. A. Davis Company for their considerable help in arranging the details of publication. The fine editorial hand of Donna Oberholtzer did a great deal to improve and polish the manuscript. Finally, as editors and friends, we owe a debt of gratitude to each other for the patience, flexibility, and optimism that have helped bring this project to fruition.

P. M. R.
H. M. T.

Contributors

SHIRLEY ANGRIST, Carnegie-Mellon University, Pittsburgh, Pennsylvania

NANCY BERAN, Ohio State University, Columbus, Ohio

ROSALIE COHEN, Temple University, Philadelphia, Pennsylvania

SIMON DINITZ, Ohio State University, Columbus, Ohio

H. WARREN DUNHAM, Wayne State University, Detroit, Michigan

DAVID L. ELLISON, Rensselaer Polytechnic Institute, Troy, New York

AUGUST B. HOLLINGSHEAD, Yale University, New Haven, Connecticut

DOROTHEA C. LEIGHTON, M.D., University of North Carolina, Chapel Hill, North Carolina

JOHN H. MARX, University of Pittsburgh, Pittsburgh, Pennsylvania

JAMES D. PRESTON, Memphis State University, Memphis, Tennessee

PATRICIA RIEKER, University of North Carolina, Chapel Hill, North Carolina

PAUL M. ROMAN, Tulane University, New Orleans, Louisiana

IRVING THOMAS STONE, State University of New York, College at Potsdam, Potsdam, New York

HARRISON M. TRICE, Cornell University, Ithaca, New York

Contents

Part I—Assumptions in Community Mental Health

Introduction 2

Chapter 1
The Sociology of Community Mental Health: Historical
     and Methodological Perspectives.............................9
       John H. Marx, Patricia Rieker, and David L. Ellison

Chapter 2
Community Psychiatry: Some Neglected Realities 41
       H. Warren Dunham

Chapter 3
The Meaning of "Community" in Community Psychiatry................51
       James D. Preston

Chapter 4
Neglected Legal Dilemmas in Community Psychiatry....................69
       Rosalie Cohen

Chapter 5
Private Rights versus Community Needs: The New Haven Experience 83
       August B. Hollingshead

Chapter 6
Strategies of Preventive Psychiatry and Social Reality: The Case of
     Alcoholism 95
       Paul M. Roman and Harrison M. Trice

Part II—Community Mental Health in Action

Introduction 114

Chapter 7
Dilemmas of Evaluation in Community Mental Health Organizations 119
        Harrison M. Trice and Paul M. Roman

Chapter 8
Organizational Adaptation to Community Mental Health: A Case Study . . 179
        David L. Ellison, Patricia Rieker, and John H. Marx

Chapter 9
Conflict and Cooperation in a Community Mental Health Program 195
        Nancy Beran and Simon Dinitz

Chapter 10
Community Development as a Therapeutic Force: A Case Study
      with Measurements 209
        Dorothea C. Leighton and Irving Thomas Stone

Chapter 11
Home Care for Psychiatric Disorders: Assessment of Effectiveness 233
        Shirley Angrist and Simon Dinitz

Part I

ASSUMPTIONS IN COMMUNITY MENTAL HEALTH

INTRODUCTION

The past decade has seen the innovation of new strategies for dealing with mental illness and its accompanying social problems, problems whose escalation in visibility produces a corresponding escalation of the need for active solutions. A new form of psychiatric practice called community psychiatry has been instituted to deliver services via community mental health centers now available in "catchment areas" across most of the United States. This perhaps unique phenomenon, a Federally funded social movement, has been dubbed "Psychiatry's Third Revolution" (the first being the recognition that madness is an illness, the second being the use of therapeutic techniques that made stereotypes of the madman obsolete). Now a decade after its inception, there is a need to chronicle the development of the community mental health concept and to critically examine this social movement which has materialized into buildings, massive payrolls, and a plethora of programs. Although new concepts of Federal funding, particularly revenue sharing with states and localities where allocation decisions may be made locally, have been perceived by many as a threat to community mental health systems as they are currently designed and funded, these systems in some form will most likely survive shifting priorities and alterations in decision-making control.

This book is written by sociologists. As a discipline, sociology has been minimally involved in the design of community mental health programs. Thus there is a temptation to watch with a cynical eye for a chance to exclaim, "I could have told you so." This, however, is not our intent; this book is neither a repudiation of the concept of community psychiatry nor a castigation of community mental health programs. Rather it is a series of observations of problem areas, at both the abstract and concrete levels, that we believe might be useful at this critical time in the development of the community mental health movement. The 1970s have been dubbed the "Era of Accountability." The effectiveness of publicly supported programs, especially those of a social nature, are headed for rigorous scrutiny. Most likely, revenue sharing will to some extent replace massive Federal nationwide funding. Furthermore, many community mental health programs were instituted as "demonstration projects," and received their Federal funding on a temporary basis with the assumption that those which proved valuable locally would eventually receive their support at the local level. Thus, the movement is at the point where analysis must replace paeans.

Rather than "psychiatry's third revolution," the community mental health center program may be psychiatry's first proliferation—one so vast that psychiatry itself may be diluted within it. Although cutbacks in Federal funding may blunt its spread, it is doubtful that it will change its nature. The rapid spawning of new dimensions of psychiatry began with the 1963 Community Mental Health Centers Act. This Act provided the basis for broadly widening the definition of (1) those people termed emotionally disturbed, (2) those qualified to treat the emotionally disturbed, (3) the therapeutic techniques that might be used, and (4) where treatment can be attempted. Proponents of the Act launched this expansion with a heavily-laden idealism compatible with basic American values, including the belief that anyone who is emotionally troubled has the *right* to treatment. Bold new programs were to bring to the unserviced, the poor, the dispossessed, and the uneducated those mental health services formerly available mainly to the middle and upper classes. Programs were to serve the *community*, to be open to all rather than specifically aimed at the poverty segment. The broad guidelines of the Act permitted almost any effort in the name of mental health. Paraprofessionals were to share treatment activities with professionals, while "selected" nonprofessionals from hard to reach rural areas and within urban ethnic groups were to receive training in adapting new ideas for delivering mental health care to their subcultures. Moreover, the community mental health center was to provide "comprehensive" care with a continuity of action that embraced a wide range of services, cutting across agencies and professions, and including both direct care for emotionally troubled people and indirect intervention into the pathological elements of community life through providing preventive, educational, and consultative services to pivotal community institutions. Innovations were encouraged. Perhaps the greatest promise was that the centers would move the care and treatment of the mentally ill into the community, avoiding the problems of public hospitalization, such as the allegedly huge hospital population, custodial norms, dehumanization, and the socially disruptive removal of the disturbed individual from his roles in the community.

The ideologies of the movement have tended to carry it beyond these worthy aims. In a sense, the role of the psychiatrist has been expanded. He has been given the freedom to become political in the basic sense of that word, manipulating community forces to reduce the emotional anxieties and troubles of its members. To do so, the community psychiatrist might intervene in community life by influencing legislation, mass media, and campaigns, altering personnel practices in work organizations, conducting marriage counseling, and giving guidance to community leaders. In a real sense, the community in its many facets could become his client.

Despite shortcomings and criticisms, psychiatry continues to occupy a position of great prestige in American society. Whether this is due to psychiatry's successful marketing of a need for happiness and self-actualization or to its tendency to replace religion as the source of values and standards for "the good life" remains debatable. What is clear, however, is that the survival of the community mental health movement may be in jeopardy because of the social powerlessness of its clientele. The future of the movement cannot be predicted, but it is safe to assume that changes are ahead that will probably include a reduction of available support. On the other hand, as established organizations, community mental health systems have a means for survival, i.e., the alteration of its activities to fit new national priorities, and it is likely that they will put up a fierce struggle to survive.

Without doubt, the community mental health movement offers a range of opportunities for involvement by psychiatric sociologists that have not been vigorously pursued in the past decade. Among the monies allocated for community mental health programs are funds for research, mainly under the rubric of evaluation, but dealing with both the operation of the existing centers as well as the exploration of new techniques for "the delivery of mental health care." Community mental health systems offer a range of opportunities for involvement in etiological research, perhaps more so now than in the past due to improvements in data collection. The increased involvement of nonpsychiatric professionals in community mental health has paved the way for sociological involvement. Furthermore, the numerous ambiguities within community mental health programs offer opportunities for sociologists to shape their own roles as they initiate their involvements.

To the uninformed observer, (the community mental health movement might appear to represent sociology's influence on psychiatry. Many of the concepts basic to community psychiatry appear to be direct reflections of sociological models, particularly the assumption that the removal of the individual from his community roles for the purpose of treatment may be a barrier to his return to these roles.)Writers such as Denzin[1] have gone so far as to imply that the community mental health movement reflects psychiatry's reaction to the sociological labeling perspective. As one of us has argued elsewhere,[3] however, it appears that the direct influence of sociology on the development of the community mental health movement has been random and incidental at best. Sociologists were only to a minor extent involved in the studies commissioned by the Joint Commission on Mental Health and Mental Illness. Many psychiatrists were aware of the findings of Hollingshead and Redlich[2] that mental health care for the poor was of generally low quality despite their evident need for such care. The genesis of the community mental health movement in the aforementioned legislative action of 1963 appears, however, to have been quite independent of sociological research results. To argue that psychiatric leadership has been unaware of research by psychiatric sociologists would be incorrect; but it would also be incorrect to argue that the community mental health movement stems from the data-based sociological critiques of psychiatry's care delivery systems. The changes in psychiatric practice reflected in the community mental health movement are responses to legislative action rather than the results of evaluative research. Sociological work has been freer than psychiatry of legislative influence, which may explain why it has tended to follow rather than to lead social movements.

The broadening of psychiatry's professional mandate via the community mental health movement raises many issues. The legislation requires a community mental health center to include preventive efforts. Such efforts frequently call for political acumen and manipulative skills not included in any part of the psychiatrist's training. Although the concept of preventive intervention is indeed laudatory, reflecting the American values of pragmatism and humanitarianism, the extent to which such efforts are possible or practical is quite another matter.

4

Instead of rejecting this broader mandate, however, psychiatry appears to have welcomed it, perhaps because an expansion of mandate usually means an expansion of power and resources. Unfortunately, the preventive goals of this expanded mandate do not lend themselves to rigorous evaluation.

While cautious about interpreting the community mental health movement as a consequence of sociological influence, the chapters of this book focus on the problems accompanying sociological involvement in the movement. There are many indications that the invitations for sociological involvement are based on a need for technical services rather than on the development of a partnership for theory construction. Because numerous assumptions of community mental health that constitute unresolved sociological questions have already found their way into specific programs, there is reason to question how sociology will grow from its involvement. Pressures to undertake specifically applied research roles in community mental health and other health delivery systems increase as university funds for research shrink, forcing many research sociologists to look to legislators and administrators for their research problem definitions. In terms of the advancement of sociology, the matter of integrating basic and applied research deserves comprehensive attention from sociologists as they become increasingly aware of the problems of their own goals as individuals and as sociologists. While the dictum that "purists need not apply" is indeed appropriate under these circumstances, the issues raised are particularly appropriate for the future development of psychiatric sociology.

In Chapter 1, Marx, Rieker, and Ellison provide an overview of several of the issues described above. They open with a historical perspective on the treatment of mental illness in the Western world, focusing upon developments in America. They view psychiatry as a social institution that has rapidly grown in prominence to become an essential part of what is loosely referred to as "the welfare state." They analyze how psychiatric projections and ideals blended with the design of "the great society" and perhaps foreshadow psychiatry's increasing importance in tomorrow's world. The authors are particularly concerned with sociology's research on contemporary forms of psychiatry and offer a fresh sociological perspective on the mental health field. The history of psychiatric sociology is one basically concerned with etiology, with a current shift toward the labeling perspective, i.e., viewing mental illness as partly or wholly a result of those formal institutions of psychiatry aimed at its treatment. Marx and his associates call for a refocus of research efforts away from individual behavior towards collective behavior in attempting to explain behavior disorders. In this sense, they call for research which probably should have preceded efforts to implement community mental health legislation. Yet since research on communities and other types of social collectivities should lead either to a reorientation or legitimization of the efforts of community psychiatry, the call of Marx and his associates for this type of sociological perspective is most appropriate. A sociological approach to the mental health field cannot be simply subsumed within a sociology of medicine, since mental health practice is quite different from other forms of medical practice. Psychiatry is also more directly involved in the public arena than the other branches of medicine. A basic understanding of what psychiatry is will become more pressing as community psychiatrists, following their broader mandates, become more involved with situations both empirically and conceptually distant from the mentally ill patient.

Throughout, Marx, Rieker, and Ellison emphasize the role of the medical model as establishing psychiatry's mandate, and urge further sociological scrutiny of both the validity and the relevance of this model. They thereby raise a significant dilemma for sociology in the mental health field: can sociologists reject the disease model of mental illness and still accept wide-scale psychiatric involvement in fulfilling the community mental health mandate? This issue is increasingly problematic at a time when many emphasize the need for sociological involvement in the problems of the real world. In short, sociologists attracted to employing labeling concepts in research may encounter head-on the difficulties of simultaneously (1) rejecting psychiatry's medical assumptions and (2) working with psychiatrists to improve their systems of practice.

In Chapter 2, Dunham introduces the issue of the theoretical social systems models on which community psychiatry rests. He describes community psychiatry as using both a rational systems model, i.e., one in which the separate parts can be manipulated individually, as well as a natural model, where interdependence produces a response of any part of the system to changes in any other part. Next he reminds community psychiatrists of what he regards as basic facts about mental illness derived from research that set limits within which their treatment objectives are necessarily contained; for example, schizophrenia, a disorder requiring a heavy increment of treatment resources, is present in all levels of all cultures, and evidence is accumulating that genetic influences may be operating in its etiology.

Dunham warns that community psychiatry may be tempted to unrealistically broaden the clinical labeling of deviant behaviors as mental illness in response to emerging middle-class, bureaucratic norms, thereby producing an expanded mandate for their professional authority. Furthermore, community psychiatry faces, in Dunham's opinion, several basic dilemmas. How can a psychiatrist maintain objectivity while involved in community organizations such as industry? Assuming that the ends of his efforts are commendable, what means is the community psychiatrist willing to embrace, and how might these infringe on personal liberties? Who, if anyone, does he represent, and to whom is he responsible? How does he retain his psychiatric identity while engaging in the political activity implied in many of the stated goals of the community mental health movement?

Dunham urges advocates of community psychiatry to think about some very basic questions generated by their proposed innovations. How will training for the community psychiatry specialization incorporate concepts and data from the social sciences? What forces will police the mandate of community psychiatrists so their labeling power will not be misused, i.e., what ethics apply to the community psychiatrist? Who else will define deviant behavior as community psychiatry attempts to expand into all areas of "problems of living"?

In Chapter 3, Preston outlines the interface between community sociology and community psychiatry. Preston's review clearly indicates that the question, "What is a community?" has received little attention in psychiatry's efforts to implement the community mental health movement. If preventive efforts are to locate community forces which exacerbate mental illness or which constitute barriers to successful rehabilitation, then an understanding of the community as a social system is essential. The concept of community, as Preston points out, includes numerous subconcepts, such as actors and associations. While community psychiatrists have generally ignored sociological contributions to the understanding of community structure, they have also paid little heed to sociological research on the nature of community functioning. Of particular importance are the dynamics of community involvement in decision-making and planning roles in programs implemented from outside the community. In the second part of this chapter, Preston cogently analyzes the aspects of community life that have been the subject of sociological research and that are relevant to the practice of community psychiatry. Research on community processes represents a long tradition in sociology—one which may be advanced by specific studies of the community mental health movement.

A related set of problems are described by Cohen in Chapter 4. Cohen's analysis of three significant areas of potential legal difficulties involved in community mental health programs demonstrate another aspect of social system analysis. To a considerable degree, the community mental health movement has been grafted onto existing community structures which include other agencies of social control. Particularly when involved in preventive activities, community mental health programs have political implications. Cohen's analysis of the problems of political and geographic jurisdiction when a mental health program delineates a "community" are directly related to Preston's review of the conceptual definition of community. Cohen reviews some of the potential difficulties between professionals that may arise when community psychiatrists attempt to carry out the broad mandate that has been provided for them through Federal legislation. She also explores significant research problems for the psychiatric sociologist: relationships among established agencies in the community and the new community mental health professionals and paraprofessionals, and the potential conflicts between mandated community mental health efforts and established individual civil rights.

Cohen's discussion of legal dilemmas surrounding civil rights sets the stage for Hollingshead's description in Chapter 5 of a specific research experience. Baseline data on individuals and ongoing data about patterns of treatment often prove essential for community mental health programs and to research efforts associated with these programs. Hollingshead outlines the rationale for such data collection and methods for its storage and use within the New Haven community. The unanticipated resistance to the data collection efforts he describes reflects a gap between the strategies of program planners and the values of community members. While Hollingshead illustrates how their dilemma was eventually resolved, there is no doubt that the resistance to collecting personal data that the researcher sees as essential is an escalating problem. The program planners' need for an understanding of the community may lead to efforts for broader community involvement in planning. It appears that most community mental health programs are instituted on the basis of the professional's judgement of community needs. Faulty professional judgement may cause community conflicts which eventually undermine original program goals.

In Chapter 6, Roman and Trice offer a sociological analysis of prevention, focusing upon specific strategies that have been set forth to deal with the problem of alcoholism. We suggest that while many of them appear to reflect ideals that are acceptable within the American value system, their effectiveness is questionable. The concept of prevention itself fits neatly with the American emphases on pragmatism and immediate action and the reluctance to devote all of our efforts to the complex treatment and often long-term rehabilitation of those already afflicted with disorders. It is clear, however, that the practical issues of realistic prevention must be faced before prevention can become more than a word. Given our experience with the problem of alcoholism, we are doubtful that successful prevention can occur without a cogent analysis of the effectiveness of specific strategies and a knowledge of what undesirable side effects preventive efforts may generate. This appears to be a particularly fruitful area for the involvement of psychiatric sociologists. But at present it appears that the most important use of "prevention" within the community mental health movement is as a slogan to reduce resistances and attract support.

REFERENCES

1. DENZIN, NORMAN: "Who Leads: Sociology or Society?" *American Sociologist* 5: 125-127, 1970.
2. HOLLINGSHEAD, A., AND REDLICH, F. C.: *Social Class and Mental Illness.* New York: John Wiley and Sons, 1958.
3. ROMAN, PAUL: "Labeling Theory and Community Psychiatry." *Psychiatry* 34: 378-390, 1971.

CHAPTER 1

The Sociology of Community Mental Health: Historical and Methodological Perspectives

JOHN H. MARX, PATRICIA RIEKER,
AND DAVID L. ELLISON

INTRODUCTION

The purpose of this chapter is to provide a new perspective for sociological involvement in the mental health field. This objective requires a historical review of the developments in public policy in the mental health field, a consideration of the consequences of this development for approaches to the problem of mental illness, and a consideration of traditional sociological involvement in the mental health field. Our assessment of the mental health field builds on the critiques of psychiatric sociology by such people as Manis, Schatzman, and Strauss. In addition, sociological efforts in the mental health field are assessed in light of Blau's critique of the objectives of sociology.

Our concern is neither exclusively restricted to psychiatry nor to psychiatric disorders and psychiatric patients. On the contrary, one of our central objectives is to broaden the heretofore parochial sociological preoccupation with psychiatry in order that sociological theory and research can encompass the full range of practitioners, behaviors, structures, and processes in the mental health field. The tendency to treat psychiatry as synonymous with all activities in the mental health field may have been partially justifiable in the past, at least until World War II, but since 1950, this identification has become increasingly unjustifiable. Yet some sociologists continue to talk exclusively about psychiatric sociology and the development of a sociology of psychiatry, to urge the examination of differences within psychiatry, and to suggest the fruitfulness of examining careers in psychiatry, paths available to psychiatrists, and the nature of professional psychiatric training. In contrast, this paper focuses upon the entire mental health field and its social context.

We illustrate the affinity between certain social structural characteristics and conceptions of mental health and illness by examining various historical periods in regard to how official policy and later public policy have emerged in the mental health field. Next, we argue that the medical disease model, which focuses exclusively upon individual intrapsychic processes, has been augmented by a social perspective that focuses on interactive processes in organized collectivities. In addition, we suggest that recent public policy has directed attention toward the community as the unit for research analysis and professional intervention. We assert that sociological research generally and investigations in the mental health field during the 1950s specifically have employed methodological strategies that focus on individual attributes as dependent variables. This enabled sociological research to complement the dominant psychotherapeutic perspective and to accept the meaningfulness and validity of psychiatric conceptions, categories, criteria, and diagnoses. It also gave sociologists access to individual treatment data, and provided acceptance and legitimacy for the place of sociology in the mental health field. These strategies, however, have resulted in the neglect of collectivity and a social system orientation.

Our analysis suggests that sociological involvement in the mental health field should:

(1) examine socially organized collectivities in the mental health field and treat them as dependent variables;

(2) eschew the individually oriented concepts of mental health and mental illness and replace them by the sociological perspective;

(3) establish meaningful operational measures and empirical indices of social system variables and community concepts that can be used for comparing various communities and community processes relevant to mental health.

The concluding section summarizes selected research in this tradition.

DEVELOPMENTS IN PUBLIC POLICY
IN THE MENTAL HEALTH FIELD

Rather than offer another history of psychiatric practices,* this review examines four aspects of past approaches to the phenomenon of mental illness in certain historical periods and thereby demonstrates the importance of viewing developments in the mental health field in their social context. Leifer[64] suggests that the "medical view of psychiatry has been firmly established as a habit of thinking, cemented by custom, convention and precedent and buttressed by huge financial commitments" [p. 18]. He further points out that the "medical model" view of psychiatry obscures the social functions of psychiatry and overlooks the

---

*The following give historical reviews of the development of psychiatric theories and practices from a medical perspective: Alexander and Selesnick,[2] Bromberg,[13] Schneck,[93] and Galdston.[37]

notion that developments in psychiatry, especially community psychiatry, are related to profound changes in modern social and political life—changes in national character, national purpose, and public policy [p. 214].

Our sociological focus also attempts to reduce the attention usually given to specific individuals as being responsible for critical changes in the mental health field and suggests[71] it is more correct to say that scientists merely further the thinking, perceiving, and denoting of other men before them.*

We will examine, first, the methods used to deal with the phenomenon of mental illness; second, the dominant conceptions of the etiology and nature of mental illness; third, the mode or form of public policy utilized (decrees, legislation, state and Federal policies); and finally, the significant aspects of social structure. These are examined in five historical periods: (1) the pre-seventeenth century, (2) the seventeenth and eighteenth centuries, (3) the nineteenth and early twentieth centuries, (4) 1920 to 1945, and (5) 1946 to the present. Our review will emphasize the contemporary period because of its relevance for the reorientation of sociological involvement in the mental health field.

In tracing developments in the mental health field within this framework, one discovers that the conception of the etiology and nature of mental illness varies in different historical periods. Thus it is necessary to offer an explanation of how the prevailing conception is socially determined. We utilize Weber's method of interpretation that emphasizes the affinity "between a concept and certain characteristics of a given social structure."† Thus, the focus of our analysis is the manner in which certain characteristics of the social structure of any given period "elect" or "select" out of the total range of conceptions a certain conception with which they have an affinity. We use the term "elective affinity" to designate an underlying compatibility between the dominant values and themes of an historical period and the particular conception of mental illness that is elected or selected. Generally, each period also develops an appropriate language reflecting its conceptual orientation.

Pre-Seventeenth Century

Until the seventeenth century, the method for dealing with lunatics was to isolate them from the community (as had been done previously with lepers) and

---

*For example, one could easily trace two of the principle features of dynamic psychiatry developed by Sigmund Freud back to Plato who suggested that one could write a psychological biography of a man from his earliest years to explain how he came to behave as an adult, and that the soul of man is divided into three parts: the rational (logistikon), the libidinal (epithumetikon), and the spirited (thumocides) portions, the latter a sort of half-way house, possessing certain animal qualities, but not entirely retrograde and deplorable. This division strikingly parallels Freud's concepts of id, ego, and superego.[17]

†For example, in Weber's studies of religion, he notes an affinity between the concept of God and certain very striking characteristics of the political community. Thus, the concept of the "Spirit of Heaven" "corresponds" to the early pacifism of the Chinese Empire; the ideas associated with Yaheve "reflect" the political and military history of the Jews, etc.[8]

treat them as not quite human, since they were subject to forces outside of human control.* Moreover, there was little attempt during this period to distinguish between lunatics and criminals; lunatics, therefore, were considered criminals. Wootton[113] points out that a complete reversal has taken place, i.e., criminals are now regarded as lunatics or, at least, as mentally disturbed.

In the dominant conception, lunacy was attributed to supernatural causes such as the gods, the devil, and the moon. The word *lunatic* (from *luna*, the moon) came into usage in the fifteenth century and referred to persons whose bizarre behavior was thought to be influenced by changes in the moon.[88]

Religious laws and royal decrees were the forms of official policy toward mental illness prevalent in this period. Religion set forth the rules of conduct, defined the objectives of life, and delineated right from wrong, good from evil, love of God from worship of the devil, and obedience from deviance. As with most critical societal decisions, the responsibility for lunatics belonged to both religious persons and royalty. Then, as now, lunacy was seen as a critical societal phenomenon because of its potential for disrupting the social order. The demonological conception of bizarre behavior had an affinity with the prevailing religious conception of the origin and purpose of man as created by one God to serve one God. Bizarre behavior was thought to be evil and disobedient, and lunatics (witches, paupers, criminals, etc.) were thought to be wrong-doers in league with the devil. The public attitude was one of fear and disgust.

Seventeenth and Eighteenth Centuries

The seventeenth and eighteenth centuries were times of considerable social unrest and economic depression. Pinel's act of freeing the "mentally ill" in 1793 reflected the spirit of the French Revolution.† Economic depression made it necessary for governments to assume responsibility for those who could not care

---

*Foucault[34] tells us that "Renaissance men developed a delightful, yet horrible way of dealing with their mad citizens: they were put on a ship and entrusted to mariners because folly, water, and sea, as everyone then 'knew', had an affinity for each other. Thus, 'Ship of Fools' crisscrossed the seas and canals of Europe with their comic and pathetic cargo of souls. Some of them found pleasure and even a cure in the changing surroundings, in the isolation of being cast off, while others withdrew further, became worse or died alone and away from their families. The cities and villages which had thus rid themselves of their crazed and crazy, could not take pleasure in watching the exciting sideshow when a ship full of foreign lunatics would dock at their harbors" [p. vi]. Foucault sees a connection between some of the attitudes toward madness and the disappearance between 1200 and 1400 of leprosy. In the middle of the 12th century, France had more than 2,000 leprosariums, and England and Scotland had 220 leprosariums with a total population of a million and a half. As leprosy vanished, in part because of segregation, a void was created, and the moral values attached to the leper had to find another scapegoat.

†A pleasant and romantic tradition has labeled Tuke and Pinel as saviors of the mentally ill, but this view obscures the complexity of the matter. "While the Quaker Tuke applied his religious principles, first to demented friends and later to foes also, partly to convert them, the great Pinel was not sure at times that he was dealing with sick people; he often cited the ability of schizophrenic women to sleep naked in subfreezing temperatures without suffering any ill effects. Were not these people more healthy, more resistant than ordinary human beings? Didn't they have too much animal spirit in them? [p. vii.]"[34] (Compare Mora[75] and Leifer.[64])

for themselves. The insane fit into this category. The custom of confining and persecuting the poor was replaced by the establishment of publicly supported social welfare programs. The asylums or houses of confinement, in which inmates were removed from society, punished, reformed, and pressed into labor, were redefined as hospitals to provide care and treatment for the mentally ill. Known as "moral treatment," this change consisted of social and rhetorical reforms rather than innovations in medical treatment or alterations of the basic social dynamics and functions of the asylum.[64, 86, 87] Basically, the inhuman way most patients had been treated and housed was changed.

During the seventeenth century, the supernatural or demonological conception of the causes of human behavior gave way to more rational ones.* In this "Age of Reason," much disputation revolved around whether man's behavior was to be understood on the basis of biology or environmental experience.

The word insane (in = not; sane = health) came into use and accompanied the assumption that insanity was an illness or disease of the mind. With the rise of the medical profession, insanity became part of the medical domain. The application of the medical "disease model" to mental illness received wide acceptance. Leifer[64] states that "the demonological model was under challenge; the medical . . . [disease] model prevailed as the preferred system for explaining and classifying the behavior of 'lunatics.' " The emergence of the medical profession with its scientific basis for judging the presence of disease had an affinity with the "scientific and reason revolution" of the Age of Reason.[82]

Political revolution brought different forms of government. Policy was now formulated mostly by legislation as governing became a matter of public election rather than inheritance. The ideas of social and public policy began to emerge along with elective forms of government.

In early colonial America, there were no psychiatrists, no mental hospitals, no public mental health policy or social welfare programs, and no provisions for the care of the insane or mentally ill as they came to be called. Insane persons were not differentiated from criminals and paupers. The term insanity was simply an informal epithet applied primarily to members of these two categories, depending upon their behavior.† As Deutsch[24] points out, "When insanity was publicly recognized, it was usually for the purpose of punishing or repressing the individual; when it was not, indifference to his fate was the dominating note. There was no uniform theory for dealing with the mentally ill" [p. 41]. As in Europe, prisons and poorhouses evolved into mental hospitals. As the idea of "moral treatment" spread from Europe, the inhuman manner of treatment of inmates was replaced by treatment centered around the principle of rehabili-

---

*The literary attitude toward madness, as in these lines by Dryden, illustrates the change in thinking during this period:

Great wits are sure to madness near alli'd,

And thin partitions do their bounds divide.

(Absolom and Achitophel)

†There is an increasing body of sociological and psychological literature which defines mental illness solely in terms of social deviancy.[97, 21, 58]

13

tation rather than just custodial care. However, it is safe to say that while "moral treatment" received wide recognition, its most durable and far reaching reforms had more impact on private than on public mental institutions. In America, the idea of social planning, public welfarism, or national public policy had not yet emerged as a course of action with respect to this problem.

Nineteenth and Early Twentieth Centuries

Confining the mentally ill in fortified custodial institutions and isolating them from the community continued into this period. However, the newly established United States brought with it systematic ways of dealing with societal phenomena such as mental illness, poverty, and crime. In earlier periods, housing and care for the mentally ill had been the responsibility of religious, wealthy, and charitable individuals. With the emergence of the state as the form of government, the mentally ill became a state or public responsibility. It is here that public policy and methods for dealing with the mentally ill begin to converge.

Before 1825 only two mental hospitals were completely supported by the states. From 1825 to 1865, the number of state mental hospitals increased to 62.[22] (Today there are approximately 280 such facilities.) The increase in the number of mental hospitals was related to the increase in the number of poor and indigent persons due to immigration and population growth. From 1840 to 1890, the population of the United States increased from 17 million to 63 million. During the same period, the population of mental hospitals increased from 2,500 to 74,000.[24] And as the inmate population increased, conditions deteriorated.

Physicians and psychiatrists were authorized to attend the mentally ill. However, since America had too few doctors to treat physical illnesses and hardly any psychiatrists, the mentally ill were treated by nonmedical personnel.

The conceptions of the etiology and nature of mental illness were neurological and organic, with the theory of hereditary insanity receiving considerable acceptance.* The development of psychiatry as a subspecialty of medicine was encouraged by the nosological work of Kraeplin, who systematized the practice of psychiatry with a new diagnostic scheme categorizing the symptomatology of the psychoses. As a result, psychiatry became acceptable as a real part of medicine, and included diagnosis and prognosis of circumscribed diseases and categorizable syndromes of symptoms. However, mental illness was generally looked upon as a degenerative process with little hope of recovery.

Prior to the mid-nineteenth century, the care and treatment of the mentally ill

---

*In response to public pressure, an Immigration Act was passed in the United States in 1903 which excluded those who had been mentally ill up to five years before the date of their attempted entry, and authorized deportation of those who broke down within three years of their arrival.

was not considered a state, Federal, or public responsibility in the sense of establishing a uniform policy. Nonetheless, public responsibility in this country has grown today to the point that about 70 per cent of the expenditures for mental health services are publicly financed, whereas only 20 per cent of all personal health expenditures are publicly financed[4] (a figure which must be changing in light of Medicare and Medicaid). Even though state responsibility was initiated in this period, it was not until the present century that a Federal public policy involving the states began to emerge. In order to suggest a possible explanation for this phenomenon, we must examine other aspects of American society.

By the late nineteenth and early twentieth centuries, Americans were still not particularly concerned with state hospitals or mental illness, despite the social reforms of Dorothea Dix and others. Folta and Schatzman[33] note that with the continued rise of industrialism, "America was concerned with material development—of land, mine and factory. Wealth was to be accumulated, concentrated, and invested, certainly not to be 'expended' for welfare services. Those who controlled wealth had no developed conception of a 'public sector' " [p.61]. Underlying the economic structure and subsequent public policy of the country was a philosophy of social Darwinism that dominated much of the intellectual and popular thought of the time.[46,72] Social Darwinism, the application of the principles of Darwin's biological evolutionary theory to society, was mainly the creation of Herbert Spencer. Spencer conceived of human society as a product of the struggle for existence and the survival of the fittest. He did not contend that social Darwinism operated in society, but that it ought to. Consequently, Spencer was opposed to every form of state intervention and ameliorative law, holding that these would interfere with the natural selection process.[46] Hofstadter[46] notes that:

> Spencer deplored not only poor laws, but also state supported education, sanitary supervision other than the suppression of nuisances, regulation of housing conditions, and even state protection of the ignorant from medical quacks. He likewise opposed tariffs, state banking, and government postal systems [p. 41].

Spencer's philosophy was amicably suited to the American scene and was inordinately popular, particularly among some business groups.

A practical and applied social Darwinism was presented in the work of William Graham Sumner, who is described by Hofstadter as "the most vigorous and influential social Darwinist in America." For Sumner, it is only a step from the struggle for existence to the permanent importance of property for civilization; the production of capital increases the fruitfulness of labor and makes possible the advance of civilization.[72] The theories of Spencer and Sumner led to the notion that the leaders of modern industry represent the fittest members of society* and to the assumption that social welfare, in aiding the socially under-privileged, destroys the biological potential of the race. Martindale[72] points out the notion that "The rich thus merited their wealth; the poor, by biological infe-riority, deserved their fate" [p. 174].

Thus, social Darwinism concluded that the positive functions of the state should be kept to the barest minimum. Hofstadter[46] sees an affinity between social Darwinism and "naturalistic Calvinism in which man's relation to nature is as hard and demanding as man's relation to God under the Calvinistic system" [p. 10]. This view found its expression in an economic ethic demanded by a growing industrial nation that needed all the capital and labor it could marshal to work on its vast unexploited resources. In Hofstadter's words, "Hard work and hard saving seemed to be called for, while leisure and waste were doubly suspect" [p. 10].

It was assumed that individual happiness and social justice would evolve from the initiative and hard work of each person and family. The United States had no philosophical or programmatic counterpart to the developing ideology and programs of social welfarism in Western Europe. America had yet to establish mass education, which was later thought to be the panacea to end all social ills through the socialization of large and varied immigrant populations. Within this social framework, Americans thought of mental illness or insanity mainly in terms of the medical disease model or as "manifestations of illness brought on by disease which attacked individuals. In general, it was understood that persons so afflicted must be sent away to an asylum for their own and society's protection" [p. 69].[33]

The convergence of method, policy and societal events can be illustrated by summarizing the discussion of this period. Although official policy was that the care and treatment of the mentally ill were a state responsibility, no specific federal public policy emerged concerning mental illness because the federal government made no distinction between physical and social problems. Before a national public policy could emerge, America had to develop a philosophy of social welfarism and to make a distinction between physical planning (in which they were already engaged) and social planning. Decisions about the mentally ill were not based on theoretical or clinical requirements, but mostly on humani-tarian and economic assumptions as well as an underlying philosophy of social Darwinism. Thus, although the state mental hospital was expected to provide

*Hofstadter[46] has assembled an interesting series of quotations to this effect from some of the business leaders of the time. James J. Hill, the railroad magnate, argued that "the fortunes of rail-road companies are determined by the law of the survival of the fittest." John D. Rockefeller identified the survival of the fittest with the law of God. "The growth of a large business is merely a survival of the fittest. . . . The American beauty rose can be produced in the splendor and fragrance which bring cheer to its beholder only by sacrificing the early buds which grow up around it. This is not an evil tendency in business. It is merely the working out of a law of nature and a law of God." Andrew Carnegie reports the reading of Darwin and Spencer to have been a source of great peace of mind. "I remember that light came as in flood and all was clear. Not only had I got rid of theology and the supernatural, but I had found the truth of evolution. 'All is well since all grows bet-ter' became my motto. . . ."

16

humane care and to function efficiently (i.e., at minimum cost), due to the social, political, philosophical and economic climate, it was unable to do either. Attention was primarily focused on protecting organized social life from the mentally ill, who could neither work nor contribute to the expanding nation's progress or well being.

1920 to the Present

The period between 1920 and 1970 contains what Bellak[6] refers to as the Second and Third Psychiatric Revolutions. The First Psychiatric Revolution consisted of the humanitarian and liberalizing reforms in the treatment of hospitalized mental patients and is associated with Pinel. The Second Psychiatric Revolution began in the early 1920s and consisted of the introduction, acceptance, popularization, and rise to professional dominance of psychoanalysis in American psychiatry, as well as the growth of "the Freudian Ethic"[62] in American society. The Third Psychiatric Revolution was the emergence and spread of the concepts of social psychiatry and community mental health institutionalized by the first Federal public policy dealing with mental illness, namely, the Community Mental Health Centers Act of 1963.

It would be naive and entirely inaccurate to suggest that social psychiatric and community mental health perspectives did not exist prior to the Community Mental Health Centers Act of 1963 or that the Third Psychiatric Revolution suddenly occurred in that year. Both the sociological and psychiatric literature clearly indicate that the intellectual perspectives, theoretical formulations, and substantive concerns subsumed under the labels of social psychiatry and community mental health had been developing for some time prior to 1963. Nevertheless, the legislation authorizing the federal government to launch a massive program for financing the construction and staffing of community mental health centers has frequently been used as a logical and convenient event for dating the marked innovation and transformation in the mental health field.

Our discussion of these two most recent historical periods is organized around two rather than four considerations, which reflects the major developments during this time. First, we examine how the dominant methods for dealing with the phenomenon of mental illness becomes increasingly related to the dominant conceptions of the etiology and nature of mental illness. Second, we examine the increasing interaction of societal events as well as social structure and philosophy with the mode, form, and scope of public policy in the mental health field. Because these periods have greater relevance for the current shape of the mental health field and for understanding sociological involvement in this field, our discussion of them is more extensive.

1920 to 1945

Methods and Conceptions: The introduction of psychoanalytic theory caused a shift in treatment modality from state mental hospital psychiatry to the one-to-one, psychodynamically oriented treatment in private practice settings. The pre-Freudian view that mental illness is a societal problem was replaced by the liberalizing and humanizing focus upon the disturbed or maladjusted individual. The Freudian theoretical framework evolved into a professional ideology, if not a national ethic.[62] By 1945, psychoanalytically oriented perspectives and methods were dominant in the mental health field.

Medical practitioners successfully established their claims to psychoanalysis as a medical subspecialty of psychiatry, with the corollary that psychoanalysis could legitimately be performed only by medically trained practitioners. A former President of the American Psychiatric Association noted:[10] "The only true specialty inside the general field of psychiatry is psychoanalysis. It has a body of knowledge, criteria for selection and training of its candidates, institutes to carry out training, and a method of certification" [p. 142]. The application of the medical disease model to the treatment of mental illness supported the claim that psychoanalysis was a medical subspecialty.

The term medical-disease model refers to the beliefs that evolved in the practice of physical medicine that were applied to mental disease by psychiatric professionals. Prior to the early 1960s, this model exercised a profound influence on mental health institutions, on the dominant public and professional conceptions of mental health and illness, and on the dominant therapeutic and research emphases of professionals dealing with mental illness. This belief system involved nosology, pathology, etiology, therapy, and professional authority and expertise.* The nosological beliefs assumed that symptom clusters could be discerned and recognized and that there were discrete disease entities or pathological processes underlying the symptoms. They assumed that an illness process produced mental "disease," that internal disease processes were responsible for an individual losing control of his behavior, and that each underlying disease produced a distinct symptomatology. The etiology assumed that a pernicious agent was the causal factor in a sequence leading to mental disease. The therapeutic beliefs included the assumption that pathological processes within the organism can be effectively treated.

Between 1920 and 1945, the entire range of disorders subsumed under the rubric of mental illness were viewed as "diseases," the underlying causes of which were to be sought within the individual "patient" and treated by a physician or, more specifically, by a medical specialist in the treatment of mental diseases. The medical disease model legitimated medical psychiatric dominance in the field, gave psychiatry influence over conceptions of human behavior and morality, and resulted in unprecedented authority and prestige for psychiatry as a professional specialty within medicine and American society generally.[†]

*Taber et al.[111] present an excellent discussion of the disease model as an ideology having important consequences for mental illness research and public policy.

†These assertions are not intended to be pejorative. Sociologists have devoted much attention to attacks on a psychiatric "devil" or straw man that probably never existed. Neither the foregoing remarks nor those that follow are intended as critical evaluations of American psychiatry. Quite the

Public Policy and Social Change: Although changes in the conception of mental illness had a significant impact on private psychiatry and private mental hospitals, they had little impact on state mental hospitals or national policy formulation. It was only after changes occurred in social philosophy that mental illness was redefined as one of the responsibilities of the Federal government. The depression of the 1930s provided the conditions for this important change. The consequences of the depression demanded a re-examination of the assumption of social Darwinism that social justice would occur without Federal intervention into socioeconomic processes and private life. Prior to the depression, most Americans thought of science as applicable mainly to the physical world. The depression ushered in an ideology of social welfarism which promoted thinking in terms of Federal intervention into national problems and the application of science to such socioeconomic problems as unemployment, housing, and child welfare for the formulation of social planning and public policy at the national level. During this time, the Federal government initiated the first of a continuing series of social planning efforts and programs, euphemistically termed the "New Deal."

Folta and Schatzman[33] note of this period that "With a welfare orientation and an educated and aggressive middle class, the country created needs as fast as it could define them, thereby creating the base for a human services industry" [p. 63]. Concomitantly, the search of the increasingly educated middle class for careers found an outlet in the nation's universities and professional schools. Careers in psychiatry were enhanced by the acceptance of Freudian psychology. The generation that accepted Freudian psychology was socialized into a new American tradition characterized by pragmatism, science, and the belief in material and human progress. The American belief that it could shape its own destiny and assure its material well-being through science and technology, found an affinity with the Freudian promise of shaping personality and altering human development. This hope was reflected by the Mental Hygiene Movement.[23,113]

During this period the population of state mental hospitals increased and conditions worsened. Despite the new social welfare ideology, mental illness had yet to be defined as a social problem requiring Federal intervention. Not until half a million servicemen were discharged in World War II because of emotional disabilities did the increasing mental health problem receive the attention of the Federal government.

1946 to the Present

Methods and Conceptions: The 1950s saw the emergence and acceptance of several competing conceptual formulations (such as Rogerian client-centered

---

contrary is true: it is our impression that almost all of the recent innovations and progressive approaches in the mental health field have been initiated by psychiatrists rather than by members of the other professional specialties with entry to this area. Psychiatrists have largely been responsible for breaking down the earlier psychiatric monopoly over the right to practice in the mental health field— a fact all too frequently overlooked by social (specifically sociological) observers and critics.

counseling and existential psychology) which were not based on or associated with the medical model, the increasing involvement of other professional treatment specialties (such as clinical psychology) in the mental health field, and a growing recognition of the importance of sociocultural factors in the etiology, nature, and consequences of mental disorders. This period also witnessed growing doubts about the efficacy of various traditional (psychoanalytically oriented) treatment modalities as a means of coping with the problem of mental illness in the entire society, the discovery and utilization of various pharmacological techniques, and a growing public concern over the prevalence and social costs of mental illness.

There were a number of reformulations in the 1950s of the concepts of mental health and mental illness that stressed the breakdown of social relationships, maladaptive interpersonal behaviors involving subjective discomfort due to unsatisfying human relationships, or more general "problems in living."* Taber and his associates[111] have suggested that the main definitions and conceptions of mental illness that emerged during this period converge on the common theme of:

> *behavior* on which a social *judgment* is passed. Recognition depends not upon expert diagnosis, but on social evaluation of specific behaviors. A second theme is that the phenomenon is clearly a property not of the individual but of the *interaction situation* [p. 354].

In addition, a large body of important sociological research began to develop and have considerable influence upon the perspectives of professional mental health practitioners, the lay public, and, finally, concerned legislators.

In marked contrast to the intrapersonal, individualistic emphasis associated with psychoanalytically oriented approaches, community mental health, social psychiatry and community psychiatry are oriented toward an interpersonal, sociocultural perspective that views individual behavior as intimately related to the sociocultural setting. Social and community perspectives involve the idea that in addition to organic or intrapsychic definitions, mental illness is also socially defined.

As the discussion moves into conceptually and semantically uncharted or ambiguously defined areas, it seems necessary to establish a common frame of reference and a consistent terminology. For purposes of this paper, then, "community mental health" refers to the social movement whose goals and objectives have multiple ramifications for public policy formulation, diverse service oriented professional groups, and the social organizational structure of various collectivities. The term "social psychiatry" refers to a field of theory and an area

---

*The term "problems in living" is associated with the writings of Szasz whose trenchant critique of psychiatry is explicitly based on a rejection of the medical disease model. Szasz[109] argues that psychiatrists should not be "concerned with mental illnesses and their treatment. In actual practice they deal with personal, social, and ethical problems in living" [p. 296].

20

of research that represents the intersection of dynamically oriented psychiatric theory and empirically oriented social scientific research. Finally, the term "community psychiatry" implies a set of services or practices operating as an intervention system in which the community is the operational unit as well as the unit of theoretical analysis.

Social and community perspectives preclude a clear-cut distinction between mental health and mental illness and view both as relative to the individual or collectivity to whom they are applied and their sociocultural context. Furthermore, this viewpoint emphasizes the need to focus on the role of various collectivities (such as the community, the hospital, and the society) in understanding and modifying human behavior. Social and community perspectives are based on and continue to underscore the prevention of mental illness and the promotion of mental health, rather than the treatment or containment of mental disease. Leifer[63] has summarized some of the objectives and characteristics of this new movement as follows:

> Community psychiatry programs have four distinguishable aims: (1) to minimize the separation and to facilitate the re-integration of the hospitalized mental patient into his family and community; (2) to obviate the need for hospitalization where possible and to reduce the incidences of re-hospitalization; (3) to reduce the incidences, duration, and disability due to mental disorder; and, (4) to promote the positive mental health of the community [p. 17].

With this "revolutionary" development in the mental health field, the previously exclusive concern with disease, intrapersonal problems, and *a priori* theoretically grounded diagnostic categories has been augmented by an interest in sociocultural factors that impair or support mental health and interpersonal functioning.

The shift in emphasis is from the individual toward organized collectivities; from disease-specific treatment to the prevention of functional, interpersonal disorders and the promotion of positive mental health; from hospital and private practice settings to organizations and communities. This shift has weakened the plausibility of arguments in favor of exclusive reliance on the medical disease model and psychiatric authority and, conversely, strengthened the claims of other, non-medical, professional specialties seeking authority in the mental health field. Thus, while social psychiatric and community mental health perspectives emerged and gained a significant measure of support, clinical psychology and psychiatric social case work began to make significant inroads into the mental health field.

Public Policy and Social Change: A new era and role for the Federal government in the mental health field began with the passage of the National Mental Health Act in 1946. Prior to this time, mental illness was considered to be a medical problem and left to state governments and the medical profession. World War II brought to light the growing number of individuals with emotional disorders. Mental illness became a focus and responsibility of the Federal government because it was now decreed to be in the *social domain*.

The 1946 National Mental Health Act led to the establishment of the National Institute of Mental Health to administer the funds for research and training provided by the act. The Institute started with an annual budget of $4 million, a figure which has increased today to about $230 million. Atwell[4] has stated that "It is worth noting that the NIMH today supports the training of two-thirds of the psychiatric residents in this country and a large proportion of the Ph.D. work in clinical psychology, and training in related mental health professions" [p. 5].

In response to the worsening state hospital system and the increasing recognition that mental illness is a *social* problem, Congress passed the Mental Health Study Act of 1955, which established the unprecedented Joint Commission on Mental Health and Illness. The specific mandate of the Joint Commission was "to survey the resources and to make recommendations for combating mental illness in the United States." The final report of the Joint Commission[51] was a searing indictment of national efforts in the mental health field and contained a particularly vigorous attack on state mental hospitals. The intensive Joint Commission studies were to provide the basis for a national mental health program.* Since the Commission was not a planning body in the executive branch, it could recommend policy and programs, but not enact them. In fact, its recommendations did not sharply define all alternatives or attempt to shape an exact national policy and left what proved to be serious ambiguities. Further difficulties resulted from the fact that it was a national committee mandated to make recommendations in an area which had been traditionally a state responsibility.

The expectations underlying the Joint Commission Study were the same as those underlying other Federal social planning programs such as the New Deal and the Great Society. The expectations behind the varied national *self-help* programs which centered on the cities were twofold: (1) that a just social order can be engineered, and (2) that every individual and group should share equally and fully in whatever the nation has to offer. Anything that appears to threaten the fulfillment of these expectations is considered a "social problem" requiring problem-solving policy and programs at the national level.

Hence, we "rehabilitate" and "integrate" into the production-consumption-service complex all the outgroups: school dropouts, delinquents, alcoholics, drug addicts, the job displaced, the unemployed, the aged, the retarded, the disturbed—in short, all the troubled and troublesome of the land [p. 67].[33]

---

*All volumes, except the last,[95] were published in New York by Basic Books in the years indicated. Each is a "report to the director" except for the final report, *Action for Mental Health*.[51] The latter was widely circulated in a paperback edition, but the other volumes had modest distribution. (See Jahoda,[50] Fein,[31] Albee,[1] Gurin *et al.*,[44] Robinson *et al.*,[84] Plunkett and Gordon,[81] Albinsmith and Goethals,[3] McCann,[73] and Schwartz and Schwartz.[95])

These efforts to reach all the disaffected are generally based on pragmatic, economic, political, and humanitarian concerns.

During this period, pharmacological methods of treatment began to be used widely. Custodial forms of treatment were discarded for "open door" and milieu therapy approaches, at least in most private mental institutions. For those who could afford it, one-to-one psychotherapy was still the treatment of choice offered by private psychiatry and the child guidance movement. For those who could not afford this treatment, including the vast majority of the severely mentally ill, the overcrowded, understaffed, and relatively unchanged state mental hospital was the only alternative.

In making its recommendations, the Joint Commission took into account the middle-class orientation of private psychiatry and the child guidance movement and focused its attention on the fact that adult psychiatric and child guidance clinics were absorbing large monetary and personnel commitments but, for the most part, were not reaching the most severely ill, those in state hospitals.[52] The primary emphasis of the final report of the Joint Commission[51] is reflected in these often quoted statements:

[M]ajor mental illness is the core problem and unfinished business of the mental health movement and . . . the intensive treatment of patients with prolonged mental breakdowns should have first call on fully trained members of the mental health professions [p. xiv].

[T]he bias of this report gives a little discomfort to some . . . who have a strong commitment toward practices and programs aimed at the promotion of positive mental health in children and adults . . . . We have assumed that the mental hygiene movement has diverted attention from the core problem of major mental illness [p. 242].

Furthermore, the Joint Commission was aware (from its own studies and other sociological research) that there were many existing community treatment resources, but that each facility had its own channeling mechanisms reflecting class, ethnic, educational, and cultural preferences and biases.[52]

In its 1960 recommendations, the Joint Commission decided "to redirect attention to the possibilities of improving the mental health of the mentally ill." Essentially, this referred to the state hospital population, and the Commission proposed a massive outlay of Federal and state funds to increase expenditures on the state hospital system over a period of ten years from the one billion dollars being spent at that time to three billion dollars, one-half of the increment to come from the Federal government. The funds were to be used primarily to strengthen the state hospital system by improving the quality of services available and reducing the number of patients in individual institutions.

The Joint Commission report came out at about the time President John F. Kennedy took office. The President appointed a cabinet level committee to study the report and to develop alternative courses of action for the Federal government. Kennedy, however, proposed a totally different approach to that recommended by the Joint Commission. In his February, 1963 message to Congress, he proposed "a national mental health program to assist in the inauguration of a wholly new emphasis and approach to care for the mentally ill." Specifically, he called for the creation of comprehensive community mental health centers that would make it possible for most of the "mentally ill to be successfully and quickly treated in their own communities and [to] *return to a useful place in society.*" Congress responded in October, 1963, with the passage of the Community Mental Health Centers Act, which provided funds for construction of facilities, and with an amendment in 1965, which provided funds for staffing the centers. The centers envisioned by this legislation were to include in-patient and out-patient facilities, day and night care services, halfway houses and foster home placement services, 24-hour emergency services, and consultation and educational programs.

The national mental health program was compatible with the social planning of other social welfare self-help programs such as urban renewal, Medicare, Medicaid, and the Poverty Program. In all of these national programs, the Federal government channeled funds directly to the cities or to organizations within the cities, as the units of government closest to the individual. Generally, and often after the fact, some method of integrating these programs with existing state efforts was worked out, but for the most part the Federal government communicated directly with the cities.

Some of the explicit and implicit assumptions underlying the community mental health centers program were the following:

1. If a volume of community services were developed, it might be possible to eliminate the state mental hospital as it now exists within a generation or two. The act was sold to the Congress on the basis of this economic reasoning.[41]
2. Every citizen has a "right to treatment" for physical and mental problems regardless of age, race, or ability to pay.
3. The Federal government has a responsibility to those providing care as well as those needing care. Provisions in the health program make it possible for private physicians and psychiatrists to be involved without upsetting the one-to-one fee for service principle.
4. Communities within cities are the unit for organizing and distributing mental health services.

SOCIOLOGICAL IMPLICATIONS OF COMMUNITY ORIENTED PUBLIC POLICY

The 1963 Act initiated the influence of national public policy—presumably representing the views and concerns of the American public as a whole—on the mental health field. The Act squarely placed the issues of the nature, treatment, prevention, and socioeconomic costs of mental illness within the public domain;

24

mental illness was seen as a national problem. This reflected and supported the view that mental health and mental illness are defined in sociocultural and normative rather than universal, ideal-typical terms. In addition, the 1963 Act provided massive economic support for the implementation of a collectivity-oriented approach to mental illness.

The public policy which established comprehensive community mental health centers was not based on any significant theoretical innovations or specific therapeutic techniques and approaches which were not extant prior to 1960. The Act did, however, legitimate and place public support as well as financial backing behind the creation of social psychiatric and community alternatives to the state hospital system that involved a shift away from the heretofore fragmented network of services toward a more integrated continuity of care within the community. The ideas of continuity of care and integrated services included within the concept of comprehensive community mental health services brought into the open the previously ignored relationship between mental health treatment services and social planning. But even more importantly, by making community programs the operational focus for the provision, development, and distribution of mental health treatment services in metropolitan areas, the Federal legislation established the community as the strategic conceptual, methodological, and programmatic unit of analysis and focus of planning in the mental health field.

The legislation contained a provision requiring that a single community mental health center serve a population of not less than 75,000 and not more than 200,000 people. It explicitly recognized the extent to which differences in community characteristics within metropolitan areas created differences in needs for services and facilities, and it attempted to make socioculturally meaningful collectivities the strategic unit of analysis, rather than the more arbitrarily defined demographic, ecological, or legislative district units. This meant an emphasis on considerations of patterns of communication, social control, socialization, cohesion, differentiation, conflict, and integration within the community for purposes of Federal legislation.

This public policy reinforced and legitimatized the trend toward concentrating mental health services, facilities, and professionals in major metropolitan areas and underscored the relationship between mental illness and urban problems. Folta and Schatzman [pp. 60-73][33] have predicted that the mental health field will be almost exclusively "urban-based and urban-oriented" and that various currently disparate mental health services will have been integrated into a larger "psycho-social life support system" by the end of this century.

The 1963 legislation was part of the more general body of Federal legislation dealing with urban problems that emerged during the 1950s and gained impetus during the 1960s. Folta and Schatzman[33] note:

However we may characterize the roles of the cities, states, and the Federal government, all three of these organizations are today increasingly caught up in an identical problem: social order in the major cities [p. 66].

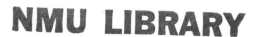

Urban problems involving the issues of socialization, social welfare, and social control have become *the* national problems in the second half of the 20th century. Moreover, insofar as the treatment of mental illness is viewed as a form of resocialization and/or social control, the 1963 legislation may be seen as an attempt to bolster the apparently faltering mechanisms of socialization and social control in metropolitan areas. And like a considerable body of domestic legislation enacted during this period, it intimately links these mechanisms to psychosocial welfare and social services.

In brief, the 1963 Act provided formal impetus for a basic reorientation of a considerable segment of the mental health field. As a reflection of national policy, the 1963 Federal legislation created an explicit connection between the mental health field and social planning. More specifically, the Act emphasized the linkage of the mental health field with urban based social planning which took socioculturally defined communities as its strategic unit of analysis. This focus on collectivities opened the way for an examination of the application of mental health approaches and treatment techniques to urban systems and subsystems. The emphasis on community-based urban collectivities converged with the increasing tendency to view mental health treatment services as part of the more general welfare apparatus.

SOCIOLOGICAL PERSPECTIVES AND OBJECTIVES IN THE MENTAL HEALTH FIELD

In regard to the objectives of sociology, Blau[11] has suggested a basic distinction between a focus on the determinants and a focus on the consequences of social organization.

> In the first case, various social conditions are treated as independent variables to account for patterns of behavior and attitudes of individuals. In the second case, the characteristics of social structures are considered dependent variables to be explained by antecedent factors. The difference lies in what is taken as given and what is defined as the problem under investigation [p. 49].

Blau argues that in contrast to the earlier, classical sociological theorists, recent theory and (particularly) research has focused attention on the problem of "how varying conditions in the social structure affect the attitudes and behavior of individuals." His explanation for this shift in sociological emphasis warrants inclusion in its entirety:

> An important reason for the predominant concern with the consequences of social conditions for individual behavior, rather than the factors governing how these conditions themselves became organized, is the extensive use of interviewing surveys in empirical studies. Interviewing surveys make the individual the unit of analysis, particularly, though not only, if samples are used in

which each respondent represents many other individuals with similar characteristics. With individuals as units of analysis, it is possible to investigate variations in the behavior and attitudes of individuals and how these are related to variations in the social conditions to which these individuals are exposed, but it is not possible to study variations in social structure and their determinants. To do the latter requires that the collectivities whose social structures are under examination be made the units of analysis in order to be able to compare structures with different characteristics and search for related variations in antecedents that may account for the differences. As sociology became transformed into an empirical science from the social philosophy in which it originated, methods of research had to be devised, and these methods altered the dominant problem focus of the discipline. . . . As a result, the structure of social conditions in organized collectivities, originally conceived as the dependent variable to be explained by sociologists, became increasingly the independent variable in the study of variations in individual behavior [p. 51].

Blau's observations were intended to describe one among several alternative emphases for sociology generally. Our objective in this section of this paper is to indicate some of the underlying factors that generated this focus on the consequences of social conditions for individual attitudes and behaviors rather than the factors influencing how these social organizational conditions themselves came into being. We will also describe the kinds of sociological research that resulted from this focus and examine some of the reasons developments in sociology have not kept pace with changes in the mental health field.

The general tendency of sociological research in the mental health field to focus on individual attributes as consequences of structural conditions, which, in turn, are treated as independent variables, was eminently compatible with the dominant theoretical perspective and therapeutic approach in the mental health field until the early 1960s. The resulting relationship between sociology and the mental health field involved a considerable amount of intellectual exchange and empirical research which had value to and impact on the mental health field. Sociological research was at least partially responsible for the gradual emergence of an increasingly important alternative set of theoretical, therapeutic, and professional perspectives and models that have been termed social psychiatric and community mental health approaches.

The very research methods that transformed sociology into an empirical science and that altered the dominant concerns of the discipline during the period between 1920 and 1950 also gave sociologists access to the veritable bounty of fascinating and behaviorally-relevant materials in the mental health field. In spite of findings that have yet to be rivaled in their substantive and theoretical significance, the early demographic and ecological analyses were slow to generate excitement and interest among mental health professionals or sociologists.[25] On the other hand, mass interviews, survey techniques, and opinion studies undertaken in the 1940s and 1950s had a resounding impact. The "New

Haven Studies" of Hollingshead and Redlich,[47] the "Midtown Manhattan Studies" of Srole and his associates,[101] and the studies of Levinson[67] at the Massachusetts General Hospital are only some of the better examples. All of these studies were remarkably compatible with and complementary to the dynamic, individually oriented, intrapersonal approach pre-eminent among professional psychotherapists until the early 1960s. This common perspective of psychotherapists and sociological researchers served a number of extremely useful functions for both parties. It in no way threatened the medical disease model, but legitimated the intensive treatment of specific mental "diseases" on a one-to-one, fee-for-service, private practice basis. On the other hand, sociological research could proceed, empirical findings could be obtained and reported, and sociology could legitimate its claims to scientific status. Its research could be of considerable pragmatic value to professional mental health practitioners, and it was increasingly accepted. This focus, however, enabled sociologists to avoid confronting the difficult tasks of analysis and the creation of operational measures and empirical indices of the characteristics of collectivities and social systems.

Blau[11] describes the prerequisites and difficulties in studying the characteristics of collectivities or social structures as the dependent variables to be explained by antecedent factors:

> To investigate the characteristics of social structure as the dependent variables to be accounted for by various antecedents, including other aspects of the social structure, necessitates (1) that different organized collectivities be examined rather than individual differences within one . . . ; (2) that organized collectivities be treated as units of comparative analysis; (3) that the empirical data, though usually referring to an observed conduct of individuals, be converted into measures of social structure . . . ; and ideally, (4) that a large sample of collectivities be studied because . . . only multivariate analysis of many cases can hope to distinguish causal connections from correlated biases [p. 52].

TYPES OF SOCIOLOGICAL RESEARCH APPROACHES

The emphasis on individual attributes that has characterized most sociological studies in the mental health field is reflected the three types of research approaches that gained prominence in the postwar period. These were: first, community surveys of the incidence, prevalence, social and psychological correlates of, and attitudes toward mental health and illness; second, descriptive studies of psychiatric hospitals; and, third, dynamically oriented studies of ideology and personality among psychiatric staff personnel.

The leading community survey studies of this period were concerned with demonstrating the importance of sociocultural and socioeconomic variables in the etiology, correlates, manifestations, and treatment of mental illness. Exam-

28

ples of these studies are those done by Srole and his associates,[101] Hollingshead and Redlich,[47] Leighton,[65] Hughes and his associates,[48] and Eaton and Weil.[26] These studies received widespread attention in both sociological and psychiatric circles and have tended to be used as models for most subsequent community survey research on mental health and illness. Common to all of these studies was a reliance on the logic or specific techniques of survey analysis. As a result, the focus was not on the community as an organized social collectivity, but on the community as an aggregate of individual characteristics that were presumed to be additive. This focus on the demographic, behavioral, and attitudinal attributes of individuals emphasized the importance of case identification and diagnosis of individual "diseases." This in turn had important consequences. It led community researchers to turn to the established psychiatric diagnostic criteria and categories as authoritative and legitimate for defining, conceptualizing, and diagnosing mental illness* and treated these concepts and definitions as beyond the scope of sociological inquiry.[68] The studies emphasized the role of psychiatry as *the* profession responsible for dealing with mental illness, and, finally, they generated a body of empirical findings that were of considerable theoretical and pragmatic value to therapists precisely because these findings emerged from a compatible perspective. In every respect, then, these community studies complemented and legitimated the dominant orientation in the mental health field prior to the 1960s. It is important to acknowledge, however, that their findings did challenge the assumptions underlying the organization and delivery of treatment.

The second prominent type of sociological research in the mental health field during the postwar period, particularly during the 1950s, comprised descriptive studies of psychiatric hospitals by researchers such as Stanton and Schwartz,[102] Belknap,[5] Goffman,[42] Caudill,[16] and others. These studies differed enormously among themselves in their research style, objectives, methods, and settings. This was partly due to the fact that various investigators belonged to and used the distinctive methods of different behavioral sciences, but it was also because the hospital settings they studied were frequently very different. However, these studies shared one basic characteristic: all of them tended to focus on the *consequences* of the structure, functions, professional composition and relationships, or institutional environment of a particular facility for individual patients. Like the community studies, these investigations focused on individual attributes as dependent variables to be explained by various structural characteristics of organizations and were frequently critical of the institutions they examined. They focused their criticism on the evils of "custodialism" and the monolithic, autocratic structure of "total institutions"; they presented unequivocal evidence of the deleterious effect of various interpersonal conflicts and relationships among the professional

*For example, the study by Srole and his associates utilized actual psychiatric diagnostic interviews; Hollingshead and Redlich employed psychiatric records and utilized the American Psychiatric Association categories of mental illnesses for its analysis. For an excellent discussion of the role of the psychiatrist as the "ultimate criterion" for defining and diagnosing mental illness, see Blum.[12]

staff on the welfare of the patients; and they raised a humanitarian cry against organizations or institutional arrangements that, in the absence or inadequacy of personnel and resources, provided little or no treatment for the mentally ill and, frequently, only exacerbated problems. Such criticism was particularly explicit in regard to state mental hospitals. Most of these criticisms represented viewpoints with which mental health practitioners could readily agree. The explicit thrust of these studies was for more and better treatment—specifically, for more humane conditions in which to provide more comprehensive and extensive one-to-one dynamic, psychoanalytically oriented therapy which was generally seen as the preferred mode of treatment. Moreover, none of these studies explicitly or systematically challenged the medical model nor its implication that mental health hospitals are analogous to general hospitals in that they require medical authority and supervision.

The third general type of study is best represented by the work of Levinson and his associates at Massachusetts General Hospital. Specifically, the studies of Gilbert and Levinson,[38, 40] Sharaf and Levinson,[96] and Pine and Levinson[80] dealt with custodialism and humanism in mental hospital structure and in staff ideology, psychotherapeutic and sociotherapeutic orientations among psychiatric residents, and relationships between role conceptions and treatment ideologies among psychiatric aides and professionals.

The dominant focus of these studies was on relationships between individual personality characteristics (authoritarianism and egalitarianism), mental health treatment ideology, and "modal institutional policy." Even more explicitly than the investigations already discussed, these researches reflect the methodological biases, emphases, and limitations that accompany a focus on individual personality attributes; they utilize dynamic, psychoanalytically oriented concepts and definitions; and they reduce the emergent properties of collective social phenomena to psychological characteristics. In fact, it is possible to argue that they represent an almost remarkable illustration of the thesis presented in this section.

We have attempted to demonstrate that the period prior to the early 1960s witnessed the emergence of a methodologically-based complementary relationship between sociological research and the dominant psychotherapeutic perspectives. This compatability has not been without its liabilities. A number of sociologists have begun to question the sociological relevance and usefulness of much of the recent research in the mental health field and to suggest that the principle beneficiaries of this research have been professional practitioners rather than sociologists. Implicit in these questions is the suggestion that much of what passes for sociological research in the mental health field actually constitutes a subtle form of applied sociological "service research," rather than basic sociological investigation whose objective is developing general conceptions about social interaction. Schatzman and Strauss,[92] in an earlier attempt to suggest an appropriate "perspective and some organizing foci" for "a sociology of psychiatry," question the benefits accruing to sociology from its association with, and application to, professional practice and service fields. . . . [M]uch work being done constitutes a service to these practice fields, answering to practical problems suggested by practitioners rather than to problems of fundamental importance to social science itself. In psychiatry, much of what goes by the name of sociological research contributes little toward developing theory essential to an exclusive sociological position—a position which carries no notable concern for the legitimacy, efficacy, efficency, or morality of psychiatric practice. For several decades now, sociologists have dealt with problems of mental illness, psychiatric practice, and psychiatric institutions. Many, and perhaps most of them, have come to accept both the legitimacy of psychiatric practice and its supporting assumptions, though not necessarily its underlying theories. They tend to accept the "facts" of mental illness, and concern themselves with applying their expertise to "problems" of etiology, ecology, treatment, administrative structures and processes. . . . Many of these sociologists want to help psychiatrists understand how social events impinge upon psychiatric events or, intrigued with mental illness as a phenomenon, want to learn for themselves how "it" occurs. Some have collaborated with psychiatrists on such matters and have come to share concepts—indeed, whole frameworks—with them. . . . [I]t would be much more fruitful for sociology if more research were done about psychiatry than in it or for it. . . . [A] more sociologically oriented model forces a much larger range of relevant questions about the field of study [pp. 3-4].

The mental health field began a series of marked reorientations in the early 1960s. The subtle and complex changes involved the shift from a uni-causal, psychoanalytically oriented preoccupation with individual pathology toward more multi-causal approaches that emphasize sociocultural factors in the home and community as well as the shift from a uni-professional perspective based on the medical model to more multi-professional approaches based on the diverse skills and perspectives of a treatment team. Thus, interest and concern began to shift from the genesis of individual psychopathology to various institutional arrangements that affect behavior patterns and social functions.

A NEW SOCIOLOGICAL PERSPECTIVE
ON THE MENTAL HEALTH FIELD

This section will suggest some of the directions in which sociology must move in order to keep pace with and contribute to developments in the mental health field, on one hand, and to make significant, innovative contributions to the development of sociological theory and research, on the other. At the most general level, we will be concerned with the task of developing a truly sociologically oriented (Durkheimian) design for sociological participation in the mental health field.

The proposals and suggestions contained in the following pages offer an alternative to the social-psychologically oriented perspective of Schatzman and Strauss.[92] The two approaches are complementary rather than incompatible. Schatzman and Strauss, in their development of a "sociology of psychiatry," describe their perspective as that of "sociologically-oriented social psychology" which takes the point of view of the actor and his social worlds. This perspective, reflecting that of most sociologists approaching the mental health field, is entirely legitimate and highly fruitful.* The following proposals, then, may be seen as a sociological alternative to this essentially social psychological perspective for behavioral science research in the mental health field.

Our first proposal is that sociologists must begin to examine socially organized collectivities in the mental health field as dependent variables explained by antecedent factors, including other aspects of social structure and social organization. We have alluded to some of the prerequisites for and difficulties in carrying out this proposal. Development of operational measures of social system variables that treat the characteristics of collectivities as dependent variables, rather than as aggregates of individual characteristics, is necessary for most sociological research. However, there are a number of characteristics of sociological research in the mental health field which require more explicit attention.

The methodological bias in sociology and the dominant mental health field model have complemented each other in such a way that sociologists have been unable or unwilling to undertake studies of communities in terms of group-level variables. Manis[68] notes:

> The concept of community mental health usually refers to an aggregate of *individual* characteristics. Thus, the findings of community mental health research are reported in the form of population statistics, rather than social system characteristics [p. 493].

Sociologists must develop their own socioculturally and socioeconomically based models of mental health and illness.

If sociologists are to reject the medical disease model, psychiatric diagnostic definitions and categories as standards for defining and appraising mental illness, and the preoccupation with individual attributes as dependent variables, what are the models, perspectives, concepts and methods that sociologists can use to contribute both to their own discipline and to the mental health field? The answer would clearly seem to lie in the following directions: the development of group-level variables and concepts that refer to the emergent characteristics of socially organized collectivities (treated as the dependent variable in analysis); the use of sociologically derived, socioculturally defined conceptions of mental

---

*We must repeatedly acknowledge the extent to which the present paper is indebted to the ideas and perspectives contained in the Schatzman and Strauss discussion. In fact, the very idea of attempting to propose a new sociological perspective on the mental health field comes from their paper.

health and illness based upon community-specific models; the critical evaluation of the impact of national and local policies and institutional patterns on specific socially organized collectivities (such as the community); and the evaluation of particular techniques and services related to various social categories.

A basic prerequisite for reorienting sociological inquiry is to establish meaningful operational measures of social system concepts that can be utilized for comparing communities and community processes relevant to mental health and illness. Measures of "community" and "community mental health and illness" as group-level variables must be developed. A shift toward socio-culturally defined, community-based conceptions of mental health and illness has begun to emerge in the mental health field, spurred on by the 1963 Federal legislation. Such a shift does not imply a rejection of the assumptions underlying the medical disease model that have been unquestionably useful in dealing with the problems of mental illness. Our point is that sociologists need not, and, indeed, should not base their formulations and investigations on these assumptions. By moving away from the medical disease model, sociologists should be able to develop a truly social and collective equivalent of the concept of community mental health and illness. Such an emphasis is needed to complement (not substitute for) existing individual approaches that are becoming less fruitful.

An increasing body of literature is questioning the methodological validity of psychiatric rating scales[117] and the reliability of diagnoses.[83] Syme[107] is one of the few to argue for the environmental management of disease affecting collectivities. This emphasis also emerged from the Stirling County Studied. Leighton[66] studied several Nova Scotia communities that were highly "disintegrated" and had high rates of mental disorder. While both the measure of disintegration and of mental disorder were based on the individual, these were generalized to describe a relationship between the social structure and the rates of mental disorder. Leighton and his colleagues encouraged change in the collectivity rather than treatment of individuals. Selecting one particularly disintegrated neighborhood of 118 people known as "the Road," they attempted to strengthen social organization through the development of leadership, education, and improved economic opportunity. In 1962, when Leighton and his colleagues re-investigated rates of mental disorder, "the Road" had a significantly lower rate of illness than other similar communities used as controls. (The components and consequences of this intervention are described in detail in Chapter 10 of this volume.) The collectivity approach used here raised interesting questions about the relation of social organization to the prevention of mental disorder.

Ecological studies provide yet another example of the collectivity approach. Faris and Dunham's findings[29] regarding the ecological distribution of rates of mental disorders raised important sociological questions about the nature of social organization in various zones of a city. One ecological finding with important collectivity implications has not yet been thoroughly investigated. In 1939, Faris and Dunham[29] stated:

33

It is significant that although the rate for the Negroes in Area 9, the apartment house (Negro) district, is extremely low as compared to the rates for Negroes in other areas of the city, the rates for the native white of native parentage and the foreign-born white for this area are the highest rates within these classifications as compared to any other areas of the city. It is apparent that the schizophrenic rate is significantly higher for those races residing in areas not primarily populated by members of their own groups [pp. 54-56].

Additional factors are necessary to explain these patterns that are the same no matter which race or nationality inhabits the area. This finding begged for more sociological studies of the relationship between majorities and minorities and for studies of structural effects and residential congruence. Few such studies emerged.

Migration studies focusing on collectivities have produced results with similar implications. A study by Murphy[77] focused upon Chinese immigrants to Canada. Immigrants to Vancouver, where there is a large Chinese settlement, had low rates of mental disorder; immigrants to Ontario, where there are only a few isolated Chinese citizens, had high rates of mental disorder. The author concluded that the characteristics of the "receiving population" were crucial for the successful adjustment of immigrants. In this research the significant factor is at the collectivity level.

The social psychiatric-community mental health movement generated new opportunities for collectivity level research. For example, the concept of the therapeutic community can apply to various collectivity levels, such as an entire community, a specific hospital, or a hospital ward.[115] We would suggest developing comparative studies of matched wards or hospitals to test the effect of this new treatment approach against more traditional approaches. Though such studies are professionally and politically sensitive, they provide a basis for relating the properties of collectivities to mental disorder.

The Community Mental Health Centers Act required that each center assume responsibility for a geographically and demographically defined catchment area. The diversity of approaches among the centers makes available natural experiments which permit comparative studies evaluating contrasting methods of organizing and delivering services (similar to floridation experiments in Newburgh and Kingston, New York). In some catchment areas, populations are stable enough to permit studies of collectivities or cohorts of all people born in a given time period. In this way, an unbiased sample or denominator can be obtained for epidemiological studies of groups.[83] Finally, the development of community mental health centers encourages studies of the resultant changes in institutional patterns. Such studies require a collectivity emphasis.

CONCLUSION: "CIVILIZATION AND ITS DISCONTENTS"

Freud's famous study of man in relation to his culture[36] viewed both specific neurotic symptoms and general social problems as the price of man's renuncia-

34

tion of sexual and aggressive instincts on behalf of civilization. These renunciations constituted both the source and the cost of civilization: without them, civilization could not exist; yet the problems thereby created were beyond the means of man's psychological coping mechanisms. Thus, the individual became the victim of the very civilization he created.

The professional treatment orientation that grew out of Freud's formulation emphasized the task of treating the individual who had been wounded or abused by the external demands and pressures of his culture or civilization. The civilized collectivity was viewed as an inescapable (and in some ways ineluctable) cause of individual discontent. Thus, despite this collectivity emphasis, specialized professional intervention was directed at assisting individual victims of civilization.

The social psychiatric-community mental health orientation represents an antithetical perspective on "troubled and troublesome" or "discontented" individuals, emphasizing direct social intervention and modification of "civilization" as represented by those sociogeographically defined collectivities referred to as communities. This attempt to modify communal life is based on the presumption that the nature of social organization and community life (civilization) significantly affects, if not determines, the focus and extent of individual discontent. Thus, social and community psychiatry attempts to alter community processes in order to promote collective mental health (or psychosocial well-being), rather than attempting to treat the discontented victims of organized social life.

Sociology is part and product of the cultural context from which it springs. Thus, most sociological attention in this century has reflected a humanistic concern with the problem of reintegrating discontented individuals and groups into the civilized collectivity. This has led to an interest in deviance, socialization, minority group relationships, assimilation, and acculturation. More generally, sociological research has focused on problems surrounding the maintenance and improvement of the existing social order by revealing the social causes, correlates, and consequences of particular "discontents." These humanistic concerns with the plight of individuals at the hands of inexorable social processes have overshadowed the critical *sui generis* function of sociology, which is to analyze collective social phenomena. The recent emergence of social and community psychiatric orientations provides a new opportunity for sociology to return to its concern with the nature and functions of collectivities and their interdependence.

REFERENCES

1. ALBEE, GEORGE W.: *Mental Health Manpower Trends.* New York: Basic Books, 1959.
2. ALEXANDER, FRANZ, AND SELESNICK, SHELDON: *The History of Psychiatry.* New York: Harper and Row, 1966.
3. ALBINSMITH, WESLEY, AND GOETHALS, GEORGE W.: *The Role of Schools in Mental Health.* New York: Basic Books, 1962.
4. ATWELL, ROBERT: "Recent Trends and Current Problems in Mental Health Services." *Inquiry* 11: 3-12, 1965.

5. BELKNAP, I.: *Human Problems of the State Mental Hospital*. New York: McGraw Hill, 1956.
6. BELLAK, LEOPOLD: "Community Psychiatry: The Third Psychiatric Revolution," in Bellak, Leopold (ed.): *Handbook of Community Psychiatry and Community Mental Health*. New York: Grune and Stratton, 1963, pp. 1-11.
7. BELLAK, LEOPOLD (ed.): *Handbook of Community Psychiatry and Community Mental Health*. New York: Grune and Stratton, 1963.
8. BENDIX, REINHARD: *Max Weber: An Intellectual Portrait*. New York: Doubleday and Company, Inc., 1960.
9. BIERSTEDT, ROBERT: *A Design for Sociology: Objectives, Scope and Methods*. Philadelphia: The American Academy of Political and Social Science, Monograph 9, 1969.
10. BLAIN, DANIEL: "Private Practice in Psychiatry." *The Annals of the American Academy of Political and Social Science* 286: 136-149, 1953.
11. BLAU, PETER M.: "Objectives of Sociology," in Bierstedt, Robert: *A Design for Sociology: Objectives, Scope and Methods, op. cit.*, pp. 43-72.
12. BLUM, RICHARD H.: "Case Identification in Psychiatric Epidemiology: Methods and Problems." *Milbank Memorial Fund Quarterly* 40:253-288, 1962.
13. BROMBERG, W.: *The Mind of Man: The History of Psychotherapy and Psychoanalysis*. New York: Harper and Brothers, 1959.
14. CAPLAN, GERALD: "Comments on Leifer's 'Community Psychiatry and Social Power.' " *Social Problems* 14: 23-25, 1966.
15. CAPLAN, GERALD, AND CAPLAN, RUTH: "Development of Community Psychiatry Concepts in the United States," in Freedman and Kaplan (eds.): *Comprehensive Textbook of Psychiatry*. Baltimore: Williams and Wilkins Company, 1967, pp. 1499-1516.
16. CAUDILL, WILLIAM: *The Psychiatric Hospital as a Small Society*. Cambridge: Harvard University Press, 1958.
17. CHARTON, MAURICE: "Psychiatry and Ancient Medicine." in Galdston, I. (ed.): *Historic Derivations of Modern Psychiatry*. New York: McGraw Hill, 1967, pp. 9-16.
18. CLAUSEN, JOHN A.: *Sociology and the Field of Mental Health*. New York: Russell Sage Foundation, 1965.
19. COHEN, E.J., GARDNER, E.A., AND ZAX, M.: *Emergent Approaches to Mental Health Problems*. New York: Appleton-Century-Crofts, 1967.
20. COLEMAN, JULES V.: "Workers in the Field of Mental Health." *The Annals of the American Academy of Political and Social Science* 286:81-91, 1953.
21. CUMMING, ELAINE: *Systems of Social Regulation*. New York: Atherton Press, 1968.
22. DAIN, NORMAN: *Concepts of Insanity in the United States, 1789-1865*. New Jersey: Rutgers University Press, 1964.
23. DAVIS, KINGSLEY: "Mental Hygiene and the Class Structure." *Psychiatry* 1:55-65, 1938.
24. DEUTSCH, ALBERT: *The Mentally Ill in America: A History of Their Care and Treatment from Colonial Times*. New York: Columbia University Press, 2nd rev. ed., 1937.
25. DUNHAM, H. WARREN: *Community and Schizophrenia*. Detroit: Wayne State University Press, 1965.
26. EATON, JOSEPH W., AND WEIL, ROBERT J.: *Culture and Mental Disorders*. New York: Free Press, 1965.
27. EHRLICH, DANUTA, AND SABSHIN, MELVIN: "Psychiatrists' Ideologies and Psychotherapeutic Function for Other Helping Professions." Paper presented at 72nd Annual Convention of the American Psychological Association, Los Angeles, California, (September) 1966.
28. EHRLICH, DANUTA, AND SABSHIN, MELVIN: "A Study of Sociotherapeutically Oriented Psychiatrists." *American Journal of Orthopsychiatry* 33:469-480, 1964.
29. FARIS, ROBERT E.L., AND DUNHAM, WARREN H.: *Mental Disorders in Urban Areas*. Chicago: University of Chicago Press, 1939.
30. FARNSWORTH, P.R., McNEMAR, O., AND McNEMAR, Q.: *Annual Review of Psychology*. California: Annual Reviews, Inc., 1962.
31. FEIN, RASHI: *Economics of Mental Illness*. New York: Basic Books, 1958.
32. FELIX, ROBERT H.: "The Image of the Psychiatrist: Past, Present and Future." *American Journal of Psychiatry* 121:318-322, 1964.
33. FOLTA, JEANNETTE R., AND SCHATZMAN, LEONARD: "Trends in Public Urban Psychiatry in the United States." *Social Problems* 16:60-73, 1968.

34. FOUCAULT, MICHAEL: *Madness and Civilization: A History of Insanity in the Age of Reason.* New York: Vintage Books, Random House, 1973.

35. FREEDMAN, ALFRED, AND KAPLAN, HAROLD (eds.): *Comprehensive Textbook of Psychiatry.* Baltimore: Williams and Wilkins Company, 1967.

36. FREUD, SIGMUND: *Civilization and its Discontents.* New York: W.W. Norton and Company, 1962.

37. GALDSTON, IAGO (ed.): *Historic Derivations of Modern Psychiatry.* New York: McGraw Hill, 1967.

38. GILBERT, DORIS C., AND LEVINSON, DANIEL J.: "Ideology, Personality and Institutional Policy in the Mental Hospital." *Journal of Abnormal and Social Psychology* 53:263-271, 1956.

39. GILBERT, DORIS C., AND LEVINSON, DANIEL J.: "Custodialism and Humanism in Mental Hospital Structure and in Staff Ideology," in Greenblatt, Levinson, and Williams (eds.): *The Patient and the Mental Hospital.* Glencoe: The Free Press, 1957, pp. 20-35.

40. GILBERT, DORIS C., AND LEVINSON, DANIEL J.: "Role Performance, Ideology and Personality in Mental Hospital Aides," in Greenblatt *et al., ibid.,* pp. 197-203.

41. GLASSCOTE, R., SUSSEX, J., CUMMING, E. AND SMITH L.: *The Community Mental Health Center: An Interim Appraisal.* Baltimore: Garamond/Pridemark Press (Joint Information Service of the American Psychiatric Association and the National Association for Mental Health), 1969.

42. GOFFMAN, ERVING: *Asylums.* New York: Doubleday & Company, Inc., 1961.

43. GREENBLATT, M., LEVINSON, D.J., AND WILLIAMS, R.H. (eds.): *The Patient and the Mental Hospital.* Glencoe: The Free Press, 1957.

44. GURIN, GERALD, VEROFF, JOSEPH, AND FELD, SHEILA: *Americans View Their Mental Health.* New York: Basic Books, 1960.

45. HAWKINS, DAVID R.: "The Gap Between the Psychiatrist and Other Physicians." *Psychosomatic Medicine* 24:94-102, 1962.

46. HOFSTADTER, RICHARD: *Social Darwinism in American Thought.* New York: Braziller, rev. ed., 1954.

47. HOLLINGSHEAD, AUGUST B., AND REDLICH, FREDRICK C.: *Social Class and Mental Illness: A Community Study.* New York: Wiley and Sons, 1958.

48. HUGHES, CHARLES H., TREMBLAY, M.A., RAPOPORT, R., AND LEIGHTON, A.H.: *People of Cove and Woodlot.* New York: Basic Books, 1960.

49. HYDE, ROBERT W., AND WILLIAMS, RICHARD H.: "What is Therapy and Who Does It?" in Greenblatt *et al., op. cit.,* pp. 173-199.

50. JAHODA, MARIE: *Current Concepts of Positive Mental Health.* New York: Basic Books, 1958.

51. JOINT COMMISSION ON MENTAL HEALTH AND ILLNESS: *Action for Mental Health.* New York: Basic Books, 1961.

52. KAHN, ALFRED J.: *Studies in Social Policy and Planning.* New York: Russell Sage Foundation, 1969.

53. KAHN, ALFRED J.: *Theory and Practice of Social Planning.* New York: Russell Sage Foundation, 1969.

54. KANTOR, MILDRED (ed.): *Mobility and Mental Health.* Illinois: C.C. Thomas, 1965.

55. KARTUS, IRVING, AND SCHLESINGER, HERBERT J.: "The Psychiatric Hospital Physician and His Patient," in Greenblatt *et al., op. cit.,* pp. 286-299.

56. KENNARD, EDWARD A.: "Psychiatry, Administrative Psychiatry, Administration: A Study of a Veterans Hospital," in Greenblatt *et al., op. cit.,* pp. 36-45.

57. KENNEDY, JOHN F.: "Message from the President of the United States Relative to Mental Illness and Mental Retardation." 88th Congress 58, February, 1963.

58. KENNISTON, KENNETH: "How Community Mental Health Stamped Out the Riots (1968-78)." *Transaction,* June, 1968, pp. 21-29.

59. KLERMAN, GERALD L., *et al.*: "Sociopsychological Characteristics of Resident Psychiatrists and Their Use of Drug Therapy." *American Journal of Psychiatry* 117:111-117, 1960.

60. KRUGMAN, MORRIS, *et al.*: "A Study of Current Trends in the Use and Coordination of Professional Services of Psychiatrists, Psychologists and Social Workers in Mental Hygiene Clinics and Other Psychiatric Agencies and Institutions." *American Journal of Orthopsychiatry* 20:1-62, 1950.

61. LANGNER, THOMAS S., AND MICHAEL, S.T.: *Life Stress and Mental Health*. New York: The Free Press, 1963.
62. LAPIERE, RICHARD: *The Freudian Ethic*. New York: Duell Sloan and Pearce, 1959.
63. LEIFER, RONALD: "Community Psychiatry and Social Power." *Social Problems* 14:16-22, 1966.
64. LEIFER, RONALD: *In the Name of Mental Health*. New York: Science House, 1969.
65. LEIGHTON, ALEXANDER H.: *My Name is Legion*. New York: Basic Books, 1959.
66. LEIGHTON, ALEXANDER H.: "Poverty and Social Change." *Scientific American* 212:21-27, 1965.
67. LEVINSON, DANIEL J.: "The Mental Hospital as a Research Setting: A Critical Appraisal," in Greenblatt *et al., op. cit.,* pp. 633-649.
68. MANIS, JEROME G.: "The Sociology of Knowledge and Community Mental Health Research." *Social Problems* 15:488-502, 1968.
69. MANIS, JEROME G., BRAWER, M.J., HUNT, C.L., AND KERCHER, L.C.: "Validating a Mental Health Scale." *American Sociological Review* 28:108-116, 1963.
70. MANIS, JEROME G., BRAWER, M.J., HUNT, C.L., AND KERCHER, L.C.: "Estimating the Prevalence of Mental Illness." *American Sociological Review* 29:84-89, 1964.
71. MANNHEIM, KARL: *Ideology and Utopia: An Introduction to the Sociology of Knowledge*. New York: Harcourt, Brace and World, 1936.
72. MARTINDALE, DON: *The Nature and Types of Sociological Theory*. Boston: Houghton Mifflin Company, 1960.
73. McCANN, RICHARD V.: *The Churches and Mental Health*. New York: Basic Books, 1962.
74. MILLS, C.W.: "The Professional Ideology of Social Pathologists." *American Journal of Sociology* 49:165-180, 1943.
75. MORA, GEORGE: "From Demonology to the Narrenturm," in Galdston, I., *op. cit.,* pp. 41-74.
76. MUNCIE, W., AND BILLINGS, E.G.: "A Survey of Conditions of Private Psychiatric Practice Throughout the United States and Canada." *American Journal of Psychiatry* 108:171-172, 1951.
77. MURPHY, H.B.M.: "Migration and the Major Mental Disorders: A Reappraisal," in Kantor, M., *op. cit.,* pp. 5-29.
78. MYERS, JEROME K., AND SHAFER, LESLIE: "Social Stratification and Psychiatric Practice: A Study of an Out-Patient Clinic." *American Sociological Review* 19:307-310, 1954.
79. PARSONS, TALCOTT: "The Mental Hospital as a Type of Organization," in Greenblatt *et al., op. cit.,* pp. 108-129.
80. PINE, FRED, AND LEVINSON, DANIEL J.: "Two Patterns of Ideology, Role Conception and Personality Among Mental Hospital Aides," in Greenblatt *et al., op. cit.,* pp. 208-217.
81. PLUNKETT, RICHARD J., AND GORDON, JOHN E.: *Epidemiology and Mental Illness*. New York: Basic Books, 1960.
82. RIESE, WALTER: "The Neuropsychologic Phase in the History of Psychiatric Thought," in Galdston, I., *op. cit.,* pp. 75-138.
83. ROBINS, LEE N.: "Social Correlates of Psychiatric Disorders: Can We Tell Causes from Consequences?" *Journal of Health and Social Behavior* 10:95-104, 1969.
84. ROBINSON, REGINALD, DEMARCHE, DAVID, F., AND WAGLE, MILDRED K.: *Community Resources in Mental Health*. New York: Basic Books, 1960.
85. ROMANO, JOHN: "Basic Contributions to Medicine by Research in Psychiatry." *American Journal of Psychiatry* 118:1147-1150, 1961.
86. ROSEN, GEORGE: "Hospital, Medical Care and Social Policy in the French Revolution." *Bulletin of the History of Medicine* 30:124-149, 1956.
87. ROSEN, GEORGE: "Social Attitudes to Irrationality and Madness in 17th and 18th Century Europe." *Journal of the History of Medicine and Allied Sciences,* 18:220-240, 1963.
88. ROSEN, GEORGE: *Madness in Society: Chapters in the Historical Sociology of Mental Illness*. New York: Harper and Row, 1968.
89. RUSHING, WILLIAM A.: *The Psychiatric Professions: Power, Conflict, and Adaptation in a Psychiatric Hospital Staff*. North Carolina: The University of North Carolina Press, 1964.
90. SCHATZMAN, LEONARD, AND BUCHER, RUE: "The Logic of the State Mental Hospital." *Social Problems* 9:337-349, 1962.
91. SCHATZMAN, LEONARD, AND BUCHER, RUE: "Negotiating a Division of Labor Among Professionals in the State Mental Hospital." *Psychiatry* 27:266-277, 1964.

92. SCHATZMAN, LEONARD, AND STRAUSS, ANSELM: "A Sociology of Psychiatry: A Perspective and Some Organizing Foci." *Social Problems* 14:3-16, 1966.
93. SCHNECK, J.: *History of Psychiatry.* Illinois: C.C. Thomas, 1960.
94. SCHWARTZ, MORRIS S.: "What is a Therapeutic Milieu?" in Greenblatt *et al., op. cit.,* pp. 130-144.
95. SCHWARTZ, MORRIS S., AND SCHWARTZ, CHARLOTTE, G.: *Social Approaches to Mental Patient Care.* New York: Columbia University Press, 1964.
96. SHARAF, MYRON R., AND LEVINSON, DANIEL J.: "Patterns of Ideology and Role Definition Among Psychiatric Residents," in Greenblatt *et al., op. cit.,* pp. 263-285.
97. SCHEFF, THOMAS F.: *Being Mentally Ill: A Sociological Theory.* Chicago: Aldine, 1966.
98. SMITH, HARVEY L.: "Psychiatry: A Social Institution in Process." *Social Forces* 33:310-316, 1955.
99. SMITH, HARVEY L.: "Psychiatry in Medicine: Intra or Inter Professional Relationships." *American Journal of Sociology* 63:285-289, 1957.
100. SMITH, HARVEY L., AND LEVINSON, DANIEL J.: "The Major Aims and Organizational Characteristics of Mental Hospitals," in Greenblatt *et. al., op. cit.,* pp. 3-8.
101. SROLE, LEO, LANGNER, THOMAS S., MICHAEL, STANLEY T., OPLER, MARVIN K., AND RENNIE, THOMAS A. C.: *Mental Health in the Metropolis.* New York: McGraw-Hill, 1962.
102. STANTON, A.H., AND SCHWARTZ, MORRIS S.: *The Mental Hospital.* New York: Basic Books, 1954.
103. STRAUSS, A., SCHATZMAN, L., BUCHER, RUE, EHRLICH, D., AND SABSHIN, M.: *Psychiatric Ideologies and Institutions.* New York: The Free Press, 1964.
104. STRUPP, HANS H.: "Psychotherapy," in Farnsworth *et al., op. cit.,* pp. 445-478.
105. SUCHMAN, EDWARD A.: *Sociology and the Field of Public Health.* New York: Russell Sage Foundation, 1963.
106. SUNDLAND, DONALD M., AND BARKER, EDWIN N.: "The Orientations of Psychotherapists." *Journal of Consulting Psychology* 26:201-212, 1962.
107. SYME, LEONARD S.: "Clinical Biases in Social Epidemiology." Paper read at the American Sociological Association Meeting, Miami, 1966.
108. SZASZ, THOMAS S.: *Pain and Pleasure.* New York: Basic Books, 1957.
109. SZASZ, THOMAS S.: *The Myth of Mental Illness.* New York: Paul B. Hoeber, 1961.
110. SZASZ, THOMAS S.: *The Manufacture of Madness.* New York: Harper and Row, 1970.
111. TABER, MERLIN, QUAY, HERBERT, MARK, HAROLD, AND NEALEY, VICKI: "Disease Ideology and Mental Health Research." *Social Problems* 16:349-357, 1969.
112. WILLIAMS, RICHARD H.: "Implications for Theory," in Greenblatt *et al., op. cit.,* pp. 620-632.
113. WOOTTON, BARBARA: *Social Science and Social Pathology.* London: George Allen and Unwin, Limited, 1959.
114. ZANDER, ALVIN, COHEN, ARTHUR R., AND STOTLAND, EZRA: *Role Relations in Mental Health Professions.* Michigan: University of Michigan Research Center for Group Dynamics, Institute for Social Research, 1957.
115. ZEITLYN, B.B.: "The Therapeutic Community—Fact or Fantasy?" *British Journal of Psychiatry* 113:1083-1086, 1967.
116. ZINBERG, NORMAN E.: "Psychiatry: A Professional Dilemma." *Daedelus* 92, Fall, 1963.
117. DOHRENWEND, B.P., AND DOHRENWEND, B.S.: "The Problem of Validity in Field Studies of Psychological Disorder." *Journal of Abnormal Psychology* 70:52-69, 1965.

39

CHAPTER 2

Community Psychiatry: Some Neglected Realities

H. WARREN DUNHAM

The increasing prominence of the psychiatric profession in all areas of our national life suggests the necessity to explore the implications of such ubiquity. One possible course of exploration is to take a fresh look at community psychiatry, the new subspecialty of general psychiatry, by analyzing the theoretical model upon which it has been grafted, by examining some of the facts of mental illness seemingly forgotten by its advocates, and, finally, by discussing some problems in the political process in which the new community psychiatrists will be and are being involved.[13]

This new psychiatric specialty taking shape is, in great measure, attributed to the pioneering work of Duhl[7, 8, 9] and to the several symposia on community psychiatry that have taken place in various parts of the country during the past decade. A report of a committee of the Group for the Advancement of Psychiatry[28] attempts to deal with the kind of education a community psychiatrist should receive, but it fails to clearly focus on how the subspecialty is to be described and delimited. This particular committee has naturally been concerned with the possible relationships between community psychiatry and clinical and psychoanalytically oriented psychiatry. As might be expected, the committee recognized that there is not an "either/or" relationship, and that dynamic psychiatry is being enriched, not replaced. And finally, after stating that "the proper role of social psychiatry is to treat the community and not the individual patient," the report states that "community psychiatry is considered as supplementary to the psychiatrists' core skill, his one-to-one clinical approach" [p. 3].

In spite of these apologetics, the report attempts to spell out the proper training for a third, fourth, or fifth year resident aiming to become a community psychiatrist. The committee advocates knowledge of human ecology, epidemiology of mental illness, and social system theory, along with several weeks of field work in various agencies, such as courts, industrial organizations, family agencies, schools, public health departments, and health departments of labor unions. At the same time, various ongoing training programs in departments of psychiatry offer other special courses, such as the design and conduct of surveys, community organization, mental health planning, experimental design, principles of preventive psychiatry, community processes, legal aspects of community mental health, and advanced statistics. Training that has been developed for community psychiatrists in schools of medicine and public health attempts to cover this spectrum in its curriculum. However, the theoretical underpinnings for community psychiatry are to be found in contemporary sociology, specifically in the structural-functional or social system theory.

SYSTEM MODELS IN COMMUNITY PSYCHIATRY

The various attempts to delineate the subject matter of community psychiatry point to the necessity of examining the theoretical models upon which this new subspecialty is based. One such model of the social system, the rational type, projects an organized structure of separate parts, each of which can be individually manipulated and modified with a view toward an increased efficiency of the total structure. In contrast, a natural system model projects a structure also made up of different parts, but stresses the interdependence of the parts, in that any change introduced with respect to any one part will have ramifications throughout the entire organized system. These structures can be regarded as having evolved from simpler social structures and often are viewed as the most complex type of organization in nature. In the hands of sociologists, these models have been used to point up researchable hypotheses, to guide empirical studies, and to foster more meaningful interpretations of empirical findings. While recent sociological theory has developed a greater precision in the intellectual construction of these models, their roots are deeply embedded in the history of Western social thought.

From the perspective of these models, if the evolving system develops too much disequilibrium, it can generate types of mental and behavioral pathology among the various individuals composing it. On the other hand, these models also imply the possibility of social engineering. In other words, they seem to hold out the promise that if social knowledge can be developed in one area of the social system, represented by, for example, the social class structure, then it would seem to follow that the application of such knowledge might bring about changes in the class structure that would enhance the functional utility of the entire system. This possibility is particularly attractive to Western man, especially in the United States, where the ideal is man's mastery of his environment, if not his own soul. While I do not intend to negate the possibility of social engineering based on a body of tested social knowledge, I do intend to challenge any social engineering effort when our knowledge about social intervention is vague, uncertain, and untested.[24,25]

The position has been taken that the theoretical models upon which community psychiatry is based lend themselves to various kinds of empirical investigation which in turn lead to the output of transmittable objective and verifiable knowledge. The model is from the natural sciences where objective and verifiable knowledge forms the basis of our developing technology. In this case the objective and verifiable knowledge of the social sciences can be transmitted to the scientifically trained psychiatrist who can apply such knowledge in his work in the community or in various institutional structures to bring about a more healthy functioning of the total social system which, in turn, will develop more harmonious and healthy personalities.

The work of the community psychiatrist has been envisioned not only through these theoretical models, but also by the *GAP Report* and the numerous papers by Duhl. The following paragraph[10] not only describes the work of the community psychiatrist but also gives implicit support to our rational model of a social system:

> The psychiatrist's investment of himself in the organization increases and he becomes interested in personnel not referred to him. These personnel may be characterized by low productivity, absenteeism or other discernably aberrant behavior traceable to personality or situational disorders. Soon his attention is drawn to all members of the organization who may not be functioning optimally. As his relationship with administrative personnel becomes closer he is asked to help with problems of selection, placement and promotion. Now the psychiatrist is making judgments about relatively healthy persons and, through his screening techniques, is influencing the quality of persons that make up the organization. Increasing demands within this relatively stable system require modifications of his initial model of functioning. He begins to realize that when mental disorder occurs there are a variety of possibilities available for modifying interpersonal relationships and re-establishing a healthier equilibrium [p. 67].

Three aspects of this statement are noteworthy. First, the community psychiatrist will work closely with the administrative personnel of an organization in order to achieve the optimal functioning of individuals. However, key questions have not been raised; namely, how is optimal functioning to be measured, and what standards are to be employed? Secondly, the statement implies that by modifying interpersonal relationships and reestablishing a healthier equilibrium within the organization, it may be possible to prevent mental disorder. Finally, the community psychiatrist is assigned the task of screening personnel and, thus, influencing the quality of persons who make up the organization. One can only wonder if the committee was aware of the implications of its requirements of the community psychiatrist. Will the function of the community psychiatrist supplant the ordinary selection process that goes on in the organization? In dealing with so-called healthy personalities, what kind of criteria will the psychiatrist utilize? Finally, what about the relatively healthy persons who are eliminated from the organization by the psychiatrist's screening techniques? What is likely to happen when these persons discover that they were refused employment because a psychiatrist decided that they were unfit? I am, of course, referring here only to the psychiatrist selecting employees and not to his already established role of treating those persons in the organization for some emotional problem.

There are already objections to the wide use of tests developed and utilized by psychologists in personnel selection. These tests, however, at least have some objective character to them and thus do not have the stigma attached to them that a psychiatrist's screening does. These tests have also proven valuable in such large scale undertakings as military induction when judgments of many people have to be made in a short period of time.

In much the same vein as the screening proposal, Duhl[10] has projected some of the new tasks for the community psychiatrist:

> As I view it, there are six levels of preventive measures which can be taken: 1. The general promotion of mental health by increasing the strength and toleration to stress of individuals and communities in a non-specific manner. . . . 2. The elimination of deprivations. . . . 3. The interruption of the pathogenic trains of events by diminishing or eliminating stress which lead to disaster. . . . 4. The prevention of major mental illness, delinquency, drug addiction, and so forth, by early detection and referral to available community resources. . . . 5. The arrest of illness by treatment, and the subsequent rehabilitation of the ill through coordinated activities of private practitioners, institutions, clinics, and the community. . . . 6. The prevention of permanent disability by the treatment of psychological disturbance. . . .
>
> We are becoming increasingly aware of the changed world in which we live. . . . For example, we can look at adolescence not only as a period of psycho-social growth, but as an economic market to be catered to and developed, thus leading to tremendous pressures on the individual to conform. . . . The psychiatrist, too, must look at the total ecology of man and decide where are the best points of intervention. . . . A simple awareness of the impact of community decisions on people can often be the key to maintaining or replacing these supports. . . . The psychiatrist must truly be a political personage in the best sense of the word. He must play a role in *controlling* the environment which man has created [pp. 72-73].

While recognizing Duhl's attempt to delineate some of the needs of our emerging social order, I cannot help but point out the big gap between the theory underlying his proposals and the realities of some community mental health problems. For example, Duhl's six levels of preventive measures have been reiterated from time to time in various contexts by numerous professionals. But does the psychiatric profession possess the techniques and the skills necessary to achieve these preventive measures? How is the psychiatrist to go about increasing the individual's strength and toleration of stress? What evidence exists to show that major mental illness, delinquency, or drug addiction can be arrested by early detection and referral? For example, delinquency, by its very nature, is often detected early. But early identification has hardly helped us to achieve prevention. What evidence exists that permanent disabilities are necessarily eliminated by the treatment of psychological disturbance? How is the psychiatrist going to eliminate the cultural and economic deprivations that are so tightly interwoven into the fabric of our society? Finally, note Duhl's concluding remark that the psychiatrist "must play a role in *controlling* the environment which man has created." At the risk of being facetious, I might point out that apparently the American psychiatrist is here being asked to usurp the role of the political partisans on the radical left.

In sum, these and numerous other papers and remarks support my contention that it is the rational model of the social system that is providing the theoretical underpinnings for community psychiatry.

FACTS OF MENTAL ILLNESS

If the community psychiatrist is a skilled professional utilizing his knowledge to detect, diagnose, treat, and prevent mental disorders in the community by working both with individuals and in institutions, then he must take cognizance of certain known facts about mental illness. If he ignores these facts in the design of community mental health programs, there is a good probability that he will be frustrated with the results of community psychiatric practices.

Relevant facts about mental illness include the following:

(1) Evidence has been increasing that the psychoses of the central age groups have not increased in the United States over the past two or three generations.[18,15]

(2) There is mounting evidence that the major mental disease, schizophrenia, is found in every culture of the world and at every social level within those cultures.[5,3,22,27,17]

(3) Individuals with manic-depressive psychosis have, for the most part, been removed from hospitals and are being managed in the community due to the increase of office psychiatric practice.[12]

(4) There is some fairly reliable evidence that some kind of genetic defect is operative in the etiology of the psychoses, certain types of mental deficiency, and certain psychophysiological disorders.[19,20,4]

(5) Epidemiological evidence shows that psychopathic, situational, and personality disturbances are highly concentrated in the culturally and economically impoverished areas of our communities.[21,12]

(6) It is clearly recognized that certain types of environment reinforce various kinds of mental symptoms.[21,15,26]

45

(7) Mounting evidence indicates that the outcome the various psychotherapeutic techniques is extremely uncertain.[16]

(8) The detection and treatment of schizophrenia during childhood has not
prevented this disorder from reoccurring or continuing into adulthood.[1,2]

In its attempt to develop a new role and function for the psychiatrist, community psychiatry often seems to ignore these realities about mental health and
illness. These are stubborn realities, and it is difficult to see how the new theory
and new techniques with which the community psychiatrist is to be equipped
will eliminate or change these facts.

Therefore, in all likelihood, the big opportunity for a community psychiatry
will come through the increase in various kinds of nonconforming behavior accompanied by a corresponding decrease in tolerance of nonconformity, both of
which may be consequences of forces operating in contemporary middle-class,
urbanized, bureaucratic society. Such a situation has been foreshadowed by
Duhl, and it is now a standard contention in community psychiatry that the reduction of these kinds of deviancy can be obtained by strengthening our basic
social institutions: family, school, and church. But, of course, herein lies a great
dilemma: how do we strengthen these institutions without enhancing and rein-
forcing those institutional social values which have proved so unrealistic for
contemporary society?

Judgments regarding nonconforming behavior can be diagrammed by showing
the relationships between clinical and societal judgments as to who is to be defined as mentally ill (see Table I). There are, of course, four possibilities.[11] A
person can be: (A) defined as mentally ill by his significant others who act as society's representatives and also judged mentally ill on clinical examination; (B)
defined as mentally ill by significant others but judged not mentally ill on clinical
examination; (C) defined as not mentally ill by significant others but judged
mentally ill on clinical examination; (D) defined as not mentally ill by significant
others and not mentally ill on clinical examination. Cell A, where the two judgments coincide, includes all psychotics; cell B includes individuals with behavioral and character disturbances; cell C, psychoneurotics; and cell D, so-
called normals. Our primary concern is with cells B and C because these indicate
the areas where societal and clinical judgments are moving closer together as a
reflection of the continuing and growing pressure to eliminate all types of
nonconformity from our increasingly middle-class society.

TABLE I—Relationship between Societal and Clinical Judgments

Social Judgment	Clinical Judgment	
	Mentally Ill	Not Mentally Ill
Mentally Ill	(A) Psychotics	(B) Character Disturbances
Not Mentally Ill	(C) Psychoneurotics	(D) Normals

The social and clinical judgments represented in cells B and C are very loose. This fact is supported by the great variations in rates of nonconforming behavior reported in epidemiological studies conducted in various parts of the world. There are marked variations in total rates reported from surveys of all psychiatric disorders. However, these variations are reduced considerably when only rates for total psychoses are considered. The variations in rates between different cultures and nations are further reduced when only the rates for schizophrenia are considered.[12] These findings clearly point to the fact that the fluctuations between social and clinical judgments are greatest in the areas indicated by cells B and C.

The growing number of cases which fall in cells B and C reflect an expansiveness of judgments about mental illness or what I have termed in various contexts the widening definition of mental illness. Symptom criteria, both social and clinical, for who is to be categorized within these two cells will continue to be distorted by social values and preferences.[22]

Given the difficulties implicit in arriving at valid clinical judgments, it staggers the imagination to attempt to envision how the community psychiatrist will operate when faced in various institutions with numerous persons and cliques presently regarded to fall within a normal range. As I interpret it, the community psychiatrist is to play a role in restructuring organizations so that they function more harmoniously and provide environments that facilitate more healthy personal development and behavior of its members. His goal is to increase societal competence in carrying out the socialization process of mentally healthy personalities. This goal creates a range of implications and problems that the community psychiatrist must face.

THE POLITICS OF COMMUNITY PSYCHIATRY

First, the community psychiatrist faces the problem of how to be involved in an organization and yet still maintain enough distance and detachment to view the operation objectively and to advise accordingly. The psychiatrist encounters an acute methodological difficulty often apparent in sociological and anthropological research. The anthropologist, in his studies of various cultures, attempts to solve the involvement-detachment problem by going into a given culture for a short time, making observations, securing data from informants, and then immediately leaving the culture in order to conceptualize the manner in which it is organized and functions. At this point, he is nearly always struck with the doubt that he never got deep enough into the culture to gain real comprehension and understanding. Consequently, he sometimes chooses to make a second attempt, living within the culture for a long time, acquiring the language, adopting the customs, participating in the ceremonies, and maybe even taking a native wife. At this point, he may have become so immersed in the new cultural world that upon his departure he finds it difficult to report exactly what he has found out about the society.

47

The community psychiatrist may find himself in such a dilemma when he seriously attempts to become involved in an organization. His situation may be particularly difficult if his involvement reaches the level of entering the political arena, competing for public office, and committing himself to numerous reciprocal promises and obligations. It is noteworthy that a similar dilemma is often encountered by the clinical psychiatrist involved in psychotherapy: there is always the danger that emotional involvement with the patient will result in an inability to unravel various emotional strands or effectively treat the patient. (There have been a few cases where analysts have married their patients.)

A second problem for the community psychiatrist centers around the ends to be achieved by working through various organizations and institutions within the community. As he becomes involved in urban renewal, community planning, industrial strife, poverty programs, retraining programs, family groups, and university conflicts, the community psychiatrist faces this most acute problem: What is the correspondence between the ends toward which he is working and those toward which he wants to work? The goals of many of these programs and organizations are amorphous, general, and uncertain, although typically regarded as "progressive." And, in fact, the goals are modified, changed, and redirected as they grow out of the collective life of the organization. Many of the goals of communities and institutions center upon such specifics as better housing, more private and public health facilities, improved schools, up-to-date technology, better roads, and increased profits. While there is little controversy over such aspirations, conflicts typically emerge over how best to achieve them. A question of equal significance is whether these goals really constitute improvements over past situations. How does the community psychiatrist work within these existing goal structures, not of his own making? Should he direct his energy in a business organization, for example, toward improving the general mental health of the personnel, increasing their total efficiency, reducing the tensions in interpersonal relationships, improving morale, clarifying the employee's relationship to organizational conformity, increasing workmen's compensation, or lowering the retirement age? Or should he attempt to do all of these things? Are there not inherent conflicts among these goals?

I am not attempting to throw obstacles in the path of the community psychiatrist but only to indicate that our knowledge and skill with respect to intervention in the life of a community, an institution, or a society, particularly with reference to general goals, is extremely minimal. Involvement in such real world situations is a far more complex business than a limited residency training in the theory and techniques of the social sciences might indicate.

A final problem facing the community psychiatrist in his complex undertaking is: Whose agent is he? Does he function as an independent consultant on a fee basis, spelling out alternatives for an organization's accomplishment of certain goals, or does he function as a salaried member of the organization, accepting its goals and then determining how they can best be achieved? Does the community psychiatrist see himself as the agent for some governmental structure, advising, consulting, and planning to bring about social conditions that will lead to a decline of behavioral deviancy and social dysfunction? Under these circumstances, does he regard himself as an official of a government unit, utilizing his skills to obtain social controls that will favor the interests of certain personalities and groups?

When the psychiatrist leaves the clinic, hospital, or private office to enter into the community, he will indeed find himself in a world he never made, a land of psychiatric limbo. If he proceeds cautiously and sympathetically, he will be tolerated by his new colleagues, but his anxieties and frustrations will mount with respect to the three problems discussed above. On the other hand, if he proceeds with authority and conviction, spelling out answers with a quick and confident tongue, he will be regarded as a threat by some and a fanatic by others.

To summarize, community psychiatry must directly face the issue of whether it possesses adequate knowledge of organizational functioning for its intervention to have significant and positive consequences. Likewise, in efforts where they take a part in controlling the sociocultural environment, community psychiatrists must not only have goals clearly in mind, but also must face the issue of whether their intervention will actually lead to more harmonious development of individual personalities. Will controls inaugurated by a community psychiatrist constitute an improvement over the existing controls now operating? Finally, when the psychiatrist moves from his traditional role as agent of a patient or hospital and becomes the agent of some larger community based organization, either public or private, how will he retain his true identity and function? Is it not likely that he will find himself serving ends that he only dimly comprehends? Might he not promote controls that will serve certain persons and groups to the disadvantage of others?

I have been intentionally critical in order to highlight these issues as sharply as possible. Large sums of money have been, are, and probably will continue to be available to treat mental illness as adequately as we possibly can and to bring about those social and economic conditions that will enhance mental health. We must face these issues and dilemmas forthrightly if we are to use the available monies effectively to achieve the highest possible level of mental health and welfare for our people.

REFERENCES

1. BENDER, L.: "The Origin and Evolution of the Gestalt Function, the Body, Image and Delusional Thoughts in Schizophrenia." *Recent Advances in Biological Psychiatry,* Vol. 5. New York: Plenum Press, Inc., 1963.
2. BENDER, L.: "Schizophrenia in Childhood—Its Recognition, Description and Treatment." *American Journal of Orthopsychiatry* 26:499, 1956.
3. BENEDICT, P. K., AND JACKS, I.: "Mental Illness in Primitive Societies." *Psychiatry* 17:377, 1954.
4. BOOK, J.: "A Genetic and Neuropsychiatric Investigation of a North Swedish Population." *Acta Genetica et Statistica Medica* 4:1-100, 1958.
5. DEMERATH, N. J.: "Schizophrenia among Primitives." *American Journal of Psychiatry* 98:703, 1942.

6. DUHL, L. J.: "Mental Health and the Urban World." Paper presented at White House Conference on Health, November, 1965.
7. DUHL, L. J.: "New Directions in Mental Health Planning." *Archives of General Psychiatry* 13:403-410, 1965.
8. DUHL, L. J.: "The Psychiatric Evolution," in *Concepts of Community Psychiatry, A Framework for Training,* pp. 19-32. Washington: Department of Health, Education and Welfare, 1965.
9. DUHL, L. J.: "The Psychiatrist in Urban Social Planning." Paper presented at Brandeis University, March, 1965.
10. DUHL, L. J.: "The Changing Face of Mental Health." Paper presented at the Detroit Regional Meeting of the American Psychiatric Association, October, 1959.
11. DUNHAM, H. W.: "Epidemiology of Psychiatric Disorders as a Contribution to Medical Ecology." *Archives of General Psychiatry* 14:1-19, 1966.
12. DUNHAM, H. W.: *Community and Schizophrenia: An Epidemiological Analysis.* Detroit: Wayne State University Press, 1965.
13. DUNHAM, H. W.: "Community Psychiatry: The Newest Therapeutic Bandwagon." *Archives of General Psychiatry* 12:303-13, 1965.
14. DUNHAM, H. W.: *Sociological Theory and Mental Disorder,* Chapter 6. Detroit: Wayne University Press, 1959.
15. DUNHAM, H. W., AND WEINBERG, K.: *The Culture of the State Mental Hospital.* Detroit: Wayne State University Press, 1960.
16. EYSENCK, H. J.: "The Effects of Psychotherapy." *International Journal of Psychiatry* 1:317, 1965.
17. FORESTER, E. F. B.: "Schizophrenia as Seen in Ghana." Congress Report of the Second International Congress for Psychiatry 1:151, 1959.
18. GOLDHAMMER, H., AND MARSHALL, A.: *Psychosis and Civilization.* Glencoe, Ill.: The Free Press, 1953.
19. KALLMAN, F. J.: *Heredity in Health and Mental Disorder.* New York: W. W. Norton, 1953.
20. KALLMANN, F. J.: "The Genetic Theory of Schizophrenia." *American Journal of Psychiatry* 103:309, 1946.
21. LEIGHTON, D. C., *et al.: The Character of Danger.* New York: Basic Books, Inc., 1963.
22. LIN, T.: "The Epidemiological Study of Mental Disorders." *World Health Organization Chronical* 21:509-516, 1967.
23. LIN, T.: "A Study of the Incidence of Mental Disorder in Chinese and Other Cultures." *Psychiatry* 16:313, 1953.
24. POPPER, K. R.: *Poverty of Historicism.* New York: Harper and Row Publishers, Inc., 1964.
25. POPPER, K. R.: *The Open Society and Its Enemies,* Vols. I and II. New York: Harper and Row Publishers, Inc., 1963.
26. STANTON, A. H., AND SCHWARTZ, M. S.: *The Mental Hospital—A Study of Institutional Participation in Psychiatric Illness and Treatment.* New York: Basic Books, Inc., 1954.
27. YAP, P. M.: "A Diagnostic and Prognostic Study of Schizophrenia in Southern Chinese." Congress Report of the Second International Congress for Psychiatry 1:354, 1959.
28. "Education for Community Psychiatry." Group for the Advancement of Psychiatry, Circular Letter No. 344, 1965.

CHAPTER 3

The Meaning of "Community" in Community Psychiatry

JAMES D. PRESTON

The concept of community has historical centrality in sociological theory and research. Along with the group and the family, the community was a major theoretical focus in American sociology until World War II. Thereafter, community sociology declined in importance due to the widely accepted idea that regional and community differences in attitudes and behavior among the members of American society were diminishing through a process of "massification."[30,14,46] In recent years, however, there has been a resurgence of interest in community as a planning concept in the instigation of various "community oriented" action programs in fields such as anti-poverty, health and mental health, adult and vocational education, and natural resource planning. In the formulation of each of these programs, practitioners have been faced with crucial decisions concerning the desirability and consequences of local involvement. Especially crucial has been the development of strategies that would lead to a level of local involvement consistent with program needs.[62]

This chapter will: (1) review the literature concerning traditions in community theory and research; (2) present a theoretical framework of community and examine the community psychiatry movement within this framework; and (3) suggest possible implications of community sociology for those interested in research in and the practice of community psychiatry. The principal focus of this chapter is community as a concept. Community psychiatry is dealt with extensively and critically elsewhere in this volume. The contributions of community sociology are logical antecedents to a consideration of the variety of practices subsumed under the rubric of community psychiatry.

Researchers in the area of community have defined their subject in various ways. Hillery's classic review of community literature[18] revealed 94 definitions of community. He concluded that ". . . most students were in basic agreement that community consists of persons in social interaction within a geographical area and having one or more additional common ties." Few researchers would object to the inclusion of these factors at a very abstract level; however, finding agreement among community sociologists concerning the nature of interaction, common ties, and boundaries of localities is more difficult. Some of the more popular usages of the term are discussed below.

In the minds of most laymen and unfortunately many sociologists, community is viewed simply as a *place*.[63, 23] This definition does not go beyond giving community a definite geographical referent. In the sociological literature, the concept community is used most often to refer to the total *local society*. This usage denotes a society or social system existing within a delimitable locality. Hiller[17] has given a similar definition, viewing community as a *social group* or that group which remains in a local society after all other groups have been factored out. In many sociological studies, community traditionally has been viewed as a smaller, representative *segment of the larger society*.[4, 6, 3] Community has been defined as a psychological, nonterritorial entity or a *way of life*[33]; thus one may speak of ethnic or religious communities. Also, the term community is used by political scientists to identify local *governmental units*. In summary, an examination of any specific locality group probably would yield a different set of boundaries, depending upon which of the above definitions is utilized.

There have been many attempts to classify communities according to some specific criteria. Indeed, one of the main reasons for disagreement about definition of the concept of community arises from the variability among communities themselves.[8] Communities have been classified according to such varying criteria as size, historical development based on cycles of growth and decay, location, economic activity or function, and form of settlement.[8, 55] The various definitions of community and the criteria used in categorizing types of communities provide the background for the major theoretical perspectives in community study.

TRADITIONS IN COMMUNITY THEORY AND RESEARCH

Traditions in community theory and research generally parallel the nontechnical definitions of community presented above. The various ways social scientists have utilized the concept of community in theoretical discussions and in empirical research can be classified into the following types: (1) ecological, (2) structural-functional, (3) cultural-ethnographic, (4) monographical, and (5) typological.

The Ecological Approach

The oldest, most systematic, and best articulated approach to community is the ecological perspective. The study of human ecology has a long tradition in

American sociology[16, 47, 64, 13, 10, 41] and focuses on the interdependence of people within a given area as they deal with problems of adapting to their natural environment. The basic foci have been sustenance and residence. According to Hawley,[16] human life revolves around two axes: (1) corporate groups, which develop from symbiotic relationships—that is, from the interdependent relationship of unlike forms, and (2) categoric groups, which develop from commensalistic relationships—that is, from the co-action of like forms. The balance of symbiotic and commensalistic relations thus determines the character of a community. Competition is viewed as the basic process in both the biological and social realms. Ecologists, usually viewing community as a whole, have studied extensively many variables within this context, such as crime and delinquency rates, participation in voluntary organizations, and ethnic stratification. However, ecologists have made perhaps their major contribution in urban sociology, focusing on the basic ecological processes (concentration, segregation, invasion, and succession) and also on the spatial patterning of urban growth (ecological zones). The major criticisms of the classical ecological perspective are: (1) the concepts of biotic and economic factors are inadequate because men are motivated not only by physical but also by socially and culturally determined drives and values; (2) many advocates of the ecological approach make it so all-inclusive that it is too broad and abstract to be useful in community research; and (3) many ecologists appear to have superimposed biological concepts on social data, whereas critics question the existence of biotic and symbiotic forces.[37, 2]

There is a basic division within the ecological "school." What we have described above is classical and neo-orthodox ecology; since 1950 an extensive trend toward sociocultural ecology has emerged. This trend emerged as an attempt to incorporate social, cultural, and psychological forces within the ecological framework in order to avoid the criticisms of classical ecology. For example, Alihan[2] and Firey[11] challenged the traditional ecological assumption that subsocial (biotic) competition was the main determinant of urban spatial structure. Likewise, the concentric ecological zone pattern of urban growth was attacked by Sjoberg,[54] who showed that urban patterning varies greatly in foreign and preindustrial cities. Duncan and Schnore[10] have attempted to make ecology an overall approach in sociology, in contrast to cultural, behavioral, social psychological and social organizational approaches. An implication of their work is that all variables (e.g., social, psychological, and cultural) other than the demographic and ecological can be inferred from the ecological variables.

The Social System Perspective

The most prominent theoretical perspective in sociology since World War II has been the structural-functional or social system perspective;[42, 43, 28, 34] the community has frequently been analyzed as a social system.[57, 52] Functional analysis emphasizes the systematic organization of society and the operation of various

53

subsystems to fulfill functions that are prerequisites for the maintenance of society. Within this approach, community is viewed as ". . . that combination of social units and systems which perform the major social functions having locality relevance."[57] Those functions having locality relevance are: (1) production, distribution, and consumption, (2) socialization, (3) social control, (4) social participation, and (5) mutual support. The function of production, distribution, and consumption of goods and services in a locality is met by the economy. The socialization function has traditionally been met by the family and other primary groups. The function of social control within the community is provided formally by government and police through law enforcement, and informally by family, other primary groups, and religious groups. Social participation is expressed through voluntary associations, business and welfare organizations, the family, kinship and recreational groups, and religious groups. The function of mutual support has traditionally been met by familial and kinship groupings and other primary groups (e.g., neighborhood, friendship, and religious groups). This systemic definition of community refers to the organization of social activities and groups to afford people daily access to those broad areas of activity that are necessary in day-to-day living in a specific locality. Emphasis is principally on locality relevant functions and less on the particular social structures or institutions which are designed to meet these functions. Functional analysis is most valuable in analyzing a community or society at a given time; it is weakest when attempting to explain social change within a community or society. In order to overcome this problem of time boundedness, some functionalists (e.g., Loomis[29]) have advocated the study of a social system at two or more periods in time and a subsequent measurement of the extent of change. Others[22] have drawn parallels between "open systems theory" in the biological sciences and in sociology. Critics maintain that the concepts of equilibrium and balance are dominant in systems models and that no provision is made for change. However, Reiss[50] has suggested that systems models should not be criticized for failing to do what they are not constructed to do, that is, explain social change.

The Cultural-Ethnographic Approach

This approach generally corresponds to the view of community as the "total local society" mentioned earlier. It is the study of the organization of the "full round of life" of people in a given area. This approach is in the anthropological tradition and has yielded many valuable case studies of communities. The Lynds' studies of Middletown[30, 31] and Redfield's work[48] are excellent examples. Although at one time "social completeness" and economic self-sufficiency were important community components studied in such an approach, few communities today would meet these criteria. Nevertheless, community as used in this sense emphasizes primary group relations and active participation by community residents in community institutions. The most obvious limitation of such studies is that they can be made only in relatively small communities, where only a small proportion of our present population lives. Even so, this approach can be utilized to some advantage in smaller subcommunities within metropolitan areas. A more significant limitation is that valid generalizations cannot be based on case studies, although valuable insights may be gained.

Monographical Studies

Many studies undertaken within a community setting have not actually dealt with community as such but with problems in the larger overall society represented there. Within such a "monographical" approach, frequently used in social anthropology, the community is merely a convenient research site or a miniature representative of the larger society. The pioneering study by Hollingshead and Redlich[19] of the relationships of social class and mental illness illustrates this approach.* In contrast to the cultural-ethnographic approach, monographical studies disregard the uniqueness of the particular community and instead regard it as a cross section of the larger society.

The Typological Tradition

A major tradition in sociology in general and in community studies in particular has been the effort to explain a wide range of behavior on the basis of typologies or relatively simple classification schemes.[53] The dimensional approach, including traditional community-society typologies, fits this category. The focus is on integrative factors as key variables in defining community and society, such as Maine's "status and contract relations," Tonnies' *"Gemeinschaft* and *Gesellschaft,"* Cooley's "primary and secondary groups," Durkheim's "mechanical and organic societies," Redfield's "folk-urban continuum," and Becker's "sacred-secular" typology. All emphasize regulative forces integrating the society or community. Attempts to classify communities and to develop typologies along other lines focus upon the variables of size, historical development,[38] location,[7] and economic activity or function.[40] A recent effort to provide a basis for the classification of community dimensions has been the work of Bonjean and his associates[8] utilizing factor analysis.

The basic shortcoming of this tradition has been a tendency to exaggerate the facts on which typologies are based and thus to oversimplify reality. In many instances, research has indicated that distortion by exaggeration has been extreme.†

---

*It is interesting to note that even though the subtitle of the book is "A Community Study," nowhere in the volume is community defined.

†Perhaps the most striking critique of the typological tradition is Oscar Lewis's attack[27] on Redfield's work in the Mexican community of Tepoztlan.

A FIELD THEORY OF COMMUNITY

The Field Concept

The dominance of systems theory has overshadowed what appears to be a promising attempt at developing a social psychological or "interaction field" perspective of community.[23, 59, 61, 62] The purpose of this section is to present a field framework for community analysis as an alternative to the various approaches discussed above. Community psychiatry will then be examined within this framework.

The concept of field has a long history in various disciplines, such as physics (the electromagnetic field), biology (the dynamic interaction between organism and environment), and psychology (the Gestalt tradition that the individual experiences his environment in terms of "wholes" or complete, meaningful patterns). Wilkinson[61] points out that in its various usages, the concept of field has four common characteristics, regardless of discipline:

1. *A field is a holistic interaction nexus,* meaning that the parts influence one another and include both causes and consequences of focal objects or events.

2. *A field is unbounded* in any strict sense, but is distinguishable from other fields by its characteristic focus or core of field-relevant properties.

3. *A field is dynamic* in the sense that it is in a continuous state of change. Change in both structure and process is such that the field exists through time with elements continually realigning themselves with one another and with elements entering and leaving what is operationally defined as the field at a given moment.

4. *A field is emergent,* meaning that its character is not governed entirely by the collective properties of its parts, but is the outcome of the interaction of the parts and is thus novel [pp. 313-314].

Community as a Field

Although the community has frequently been conceptualized as a social system,[57, 52] the conceptualization of community as a social field is very recent. There are two important distinctions between systemic and field conceptualizations. First, the concept of system implies an inherent maintenance tendency while the field concept makes social and psychological concomitants to change its central focus. Second, boundary maintenance and the notion of a closed system is emphasized in the system model, whereas the field perspective emphasizes community as an *emergent* social field. In the latter notion, boundaries are limited only as one moves outward from the center of the interactional core of activity and, consequently, into other fields. The interactional field perspective draws emphasis on the physical size, shape, and location of the community from the ecological approach and an interest in the arrangement and interrelation of locality groups and institutions from the systemic and cultural approaches.[63] Taken together, these factors provide the setting or background in which community action takes place. In other words, analysis begins with place, people, and institutions, but moves quickly to the interaction process. Community is thus viewed as a behavioral phenomenon having an essentially sociopsychological nature, existing within the context of spatial and institutional considerations, but having a distinct existence of its own.[62] In applying the interactional perspective to the analysis of specific community action programs, the action process is traced through a set of phases, beginning with the awareness of a problem and continuing through the application of some solution. Coordination of interest fields is always a major focus. Analysis of community begins by identifying problems or issues within a local society and then traces the action that arises to deal with these problems. Various types of leaders and associations and various types and degrees of resident participation become important during different phases of the community action process. The major advantage of the interactional approach is that it is specifically change oriented. Also, because community actors and associations are an integral part of the perspective, the vagueness possible in process theory is largely avoided.

Interest Areas

Within any local society, numerous social fields coexist. With the decline of primary communities and the corresponding growth of urban areas, there has been a marked increase in the number and types of interest groups. Interactional processes and institutional structures reflect all the major interest areas within a community (e.g., religion, recreation, government, and economics). For the purpose of analysis from the field perspective, key elements within the community are *actors* or individuals participating in various interest area programs and activities; *associations* or community groups, which may be either formal, such as voluntary associations, or informal, such as coffee cliques; and *actions,* the major unit of analysis, which consist of the interrelated activities of actors (individuals) and associations (groups) as they participate in programs and projects within various interest areas. Consequently, a behavioral pattern of community structure (i.e., the relationships among actors and associations within a community action process) is revealed. The essence of community from the interactional viewpoint thus becomes the "generalizing process." Generalization occurs as actions representing different interest areas are coordinated. Generalizing actions, those which comprise the community field, are distinguished from limited interest actions or actions in other local fields because (1) they express comprehensive interests and thereby meet a variety of local needs; (2) the action is identified with the locality; (3) many local residents are involved as either participants or beneficiaries or both; (4) the action is conducted through local associations; (5) the action is oriented toward changing or maintaining the local

57

society; (6) the action is organized; and (7) coordination of activities among various interest fields is a major objective.[23, 61]

Levels of Analysis

Various levels of analysis are possible when conceptualizing community as a social field. Four distinct levels are (1) the ecological and demographic, (2) the cultural-institutional, (3) the social, and (4) the psychological or individual. The ecological and demographic level of analysis focuses on place and people and is concerned with identification and delineation of community boundaries. Some assessment of the viability of the local society in ecological terms can be given. Major characteristics of the local society at this level of analysis include the physical clustering of people, population size and location, population characteristics, and ecological functioning of the community. The cultural-institutional level of analysis focuses on the institutional wholeness or completeness of the community.[32, 26] Relevant considerations include relations among institutions, dominant value complexes existing within the local society (achievement themes, orientation to action, collective action, consensus or conflict), and related variables concerning ethnicity and social class. The social level is distinctly sociological, in contrast to the other three, and includes group and associational structures through which action occurs, informal relational structures, action potentiality (e.g., coordinating structures with or without gaps in communication), prevailing action styles (cooperation or conflict), and external linkages and relationships (largely autonomous or working in coordination with external agencies). The fourth level, the psychological or individual, focuses on the orientation of the individual (actor) to the community field and includes at least three sub-levels: (1) cognition or knowledge; i.e., what the individual knows about the community field, (2) attitudes as a result of his knowledge and inclinations, either favorable or unfavorable, and (3) behavior or actual participation in activities within various interest areas.

Types of Community Fields

Community fields may be categorized according to their leadership structure (pluralist-elitist), prevailing action styles (autonomous-coordinative), type of coordinating association (limited interest-multi-interest), and linkages and relationships to the larger society (interventive-collaborative). Utilizing these four dimensions, two pure types or polar extremes may be delineated. One extreme, the segmented community, would have a diffuse leadership structure, perhaps factional, autonomous action style, a minimum of coordination among the various interest areas, and a largely interventional relationship to the larger society, that is, relating to external agencies directly, with local values and social structures altered as necessary to provide the necessary infrastructure for project accomplishment. Such a segmented field is perhaps characteristic of contemporary metropolitan areas. Dahrendorf[9] suggests that an urban community is a network of conflicting interest groups. The other extreme, the consensual community, would have an elitist or monolithic leadership, coordinative action style, a maximum of coordination among the various interest areas, and a largely collaborative relationship to the larger society, that is, incorporating resources of external agencies into comprehensive integrated plans of development. Such a field is the rare exception today. Obviously many other types of community fields exist in empirical reality. For example, a pluralistic leadership structure need not automatically lead to an autonomous action style. However, these two ideal types serve for illustrative purposes.

Project Accomplishment and Community Consequences

In the process of intervention by an external agency into the community field, how the program is conducted is crucial. Every community action program has both structural and project accomplishment dimensions. Project accomplishment is defined as achieving the stated or implied objectives of the program. The structural dimension refers to *how* project accomplishment is performed, i.e., the structure and conduct of its program. Is, for example, the action program well integrated in the community field or is it relatively isolated and on the periphery? Has the program promoted a community better prepared to solve similar problems in the future? If the program has aroused hostility and animosity by its intervention, the community may be less capable of solving future problems even though the stated objectives of the agency program have been achieved. The capability of the community to solve problems may be as important as, or even more important than specific program objectives. Each community and agency must approach the process of problem solving on a "benefits and costs" basis. Local participation or control has certain costs, such as possible decreased efficiency and loss of agency autonomy in controlling resources. On the other hand, the benefits, such as local acceptance of the program, may overshadow the costs.

The Community Field and Community Psychiatry

Community psychiatry,* or the entire community mental health program spawned by Federal funding in the 1960s, may be viewed as one action program

*No elaborate definition of community psychiatry will be presented in this chapter. The reader is referred to the definitions presented elsewhere in this volume. This author uses the term community psychiatry to refer to the movement towards helping larger numbers of people restore appropriate social and interpersonal functioning, which departs from the traditional psychiatric practice of treating patients in the one-to-one, patient-doctor clinical setting, and to the efforts designed to prevent mental illness. It involves a commitment by the psychiatrist to work in cooperation with fellow professionals (e.g., medical doctors, social workers, psychologists, and ministers) in providing mental health services to the broadest segment of society, namely, the community. As used here, such endeavors as the broad educational programs and the treatment and prevention of mental illness, including walk-in clinics, etc., are all subsumed under the rubric of community psychiatry.

within the community field. Each of the four levels of analysis, the ecological, institutional, social, and psychological dimensions, have potential value in the development of community psychiatry. In planning a program, one must begin with a basic knowledge of the ecological factors in the community; that is, the territory to be served by the mental health program must be delineated and the population determined. This does not imply that mental health practitioners should become involved in an elaborate attempt either to define community in the sociological sense or to delineate boundaries precisely. However, a distinct implication of viewing community psychiatry as part of the community field is that community (or, more precisely, the community field) is defined for operational purposes, and it can be defined and redefined as new mental health programs and projects are undertaken. Ecological processes influence community mental health programs, but these are considered extraneous to the development of the program itself.

An institutional-cultural analysis can provide a basis for making predictions. Many writers have viewed the community as a system of integrated institutional structures.[24, 25] Once the researcher or community practitioner has delineated these institutional structures and their functions, he should be in a relatively favorable position for planning his mental health program in relation to the functional interrelationships of the community institutional structures.

The social level focus is upon the operation of groups, associations, organizations, and action structures within the community field. The formal structure of community mental health programs is similar in all communities. An external (Federal) agency usually develops a plan, perhaps after taking an inventory of local problems, facilities, and interests. However, the mode of entry into each community field is unique. In regard to the type of community field (the segmented-consensual continuum), the entry of a community mental health program into the field immediately raises two significant questions. First, what should be the extent of local decision-making in the planning and implementation of the program? Second, since mental health is only one of many interests within the community field, to what extent should this interest be coordinated with others? Obviously communities vary drastically with regard to the ability of their citizens to carry on planning and decision-making, particularly in highly technical areas; thus each entry is unique. In the consensual type of community field, the mental health agency becomes a resource offering technical expertise to the community. Mental health interests are meshed and coordinated with various other community interests. In the segmented type of community field, power, functions, and authority remain largely with the outside agency. Thus the community merely serves as a convenient locale with community boundaries for the mental health program. In both fields, a local program delivery organization is needed within each community. The key distinction is that in the consensual community, integration of the program is stressed, while in the segmented community, a "line" type of organization is followed.

Key research questions, with their inherent applied ramifications, become:

Which type of entry is best in terms of costs and benefits to both project accomplishment and structural consequences? What is the optimum level of local input into decision-making possible in a highly technical program such as community mental health? The question of local values is also important. Is the consensual notion desirable? Many specialists[35, 36] would argue that the effectiveness of the organization is enhanced by autonomy. Thus an hypothesis for empirical research becomes: Community mental health programs should be autonomous, with a minimum amount of local input into policy-making. The needed local support can be generated from a single interest area. Because of the highly technical nature of the program, the need for agency control is strong. The uniqueness of the conceptualization of community mental health as an action program introduced into the community field lies in the synergistic, cumulative resource mobilization through the community action process which can tap all interest fields as needed.

At the psychological level, the interactional field concept has relevance for individual mental health. For example, the development of a mental disorder within the individual may be viewed as a quite normal adjustment from the field perspective. Within any interactional field, the individual attempts facilitative adjustments to continue functioning at least a minimum level of psychosocial competence. In so doing, he may develop a mode of adjustment that is generally considered abnormal, but that is entirely appropriate when considering the field in which he must interact. Examples of fields fostering such behavior include families where one or both parents are severely neurotic or where children are subject to improper mothering practices (e.g., overprotection, denial of affection, rejection). In such interactional fields, the development of neuroses or other mental aberrations may be necessary or helpful for the children to continue functioning. Although it is not within the scope of this chapter to elaborate on the individual field concept, it is readily apparent that the individual field differs from the community field. The individual exists and interacts within a variety of social fields that overlap and converge eventually into the community field. Both the community field and the total sphere within which the individual is involved have meaning for the individual's mental health. The approach in community psychiatry that sees the patient's maladjustment as a symptom of a "sick" family and the method of treating the whole family appears to be valid. A related and quite critical factor is the level and degree of individual involvement in the community. One might hypothesize that, in terms of his orientation to the community field, the individual's cognitive, affective, and behavioral dimensions are cumulative.[61] One may distinguish between the community as an interactional field and the interactional fields of the individual in the search for the cause of mental illness. At the community level, all fields have inequities and injustices, great or small, intended or unintended, that can contribute to psychosocial distress. At the individual level, the search for causes can focus around such variables as family, social class, and occupation. Treatment or helping techniques can also occur on at least two levels—the environmental, including the biological, physical, and social variables within the community field, and the individual, including the prognosis of the case and the appropriate treatment. Change may occur at the community level, the individual level, at both, or at neither.

IMPLICATIONS OF COMMUNITY SOCIOLOGY
FOR COMMUNITY PSYCHIATRY

Several potential contributions of community sociology for community psychiatry have not yet been realized. In general, these contributions do not take the form of theoretical propositions, concepts, and models as such, but are substantive areas within community sociology that have practical utility for community psychiatry. In addition to a discussion of these areas, several research hypotheses will be suggested here.

Sociologists can take some pride in the fact that psychiatrists and mental health practitioners have finally "discovered" the community, a social unit we have long studied. However, the writings and theories of community sociology have been largely ignored by the community psychiatry movement. This is probably due to the fact that sociologists are considered marginal contributors at best to knowledge about mental health practice. Community mental health has been the domain primarily of psychiatrists, social workers, and psychologists. However, some sociological expertise can benefit community psychiatry.

With regard to the acceptance and support of the mental health program within the community field, several relevant issues arise. Many Federal programs—anti-poverty, model cities, urban renewal, public housing—require effective community action. A great deal of sociological research has been devoted to studying the conditions under which these programs are most likely to succeed. A major condition, for example, is the support of the program by the community power structure. Belknap and Steinle[5] demonstrated convincingly that the quality of community hospitals is related to the support of the community power structure. Similarly, Nix[39] concluded that the acceptance of community action programs by the power structure greatly enhanced their chances for success. The same is probably true for community mental health programs. In a similar vein, Hawley[15] has hypothesized that communities with a centralized or monolithic power structure are most likely to mobilize for effective action, and he has used the adoption of urban renewal programs as a measure of his contention. Fowler, in a study of 30 New York communities,[12] found that the communities with more concentrated power structures had higher welfare levels. Based on these studies, a plausible hypothesis for empirical research is that communities with monolithic or concentrated power structures are more likely to effectively mobilize and support a community mental health program. Sociological research on leadership and planning of community mental health programs[21] and on techniques of leadership identification[44, 45] also make distinct but as yet unused contributions to community psychiatry. All of these studies indicate that the community mental health practitioner would be well advised to identify the relevant power structure in the community and to gain its support before proceeding in his planning. Obviously, this procedure will not guarantee the acceptance of the program by the community as a whole, but the community will tend to be more receptive to the program if it has the support, or at least not the active opposition, of the relevant power structure.

The fact that community mental health programs are largely innovations arising from outside the community rather than from local initiative or community felt needs makes local acceptance more difficult. When pressures have originated internally, such as when rural communities undertake specific initiatives to obtain physicians, acceptance of a program is usually routine. However, one would expect that programs imposed from the outside and set up to comply with Federal guidelines in order to gain construction and staffing assistance would have difficulty in gaining local acceptance. Research is needed that would compare the success of programs in communities that seek outside help by responding to local initiative with communities that merely comply with Federal guidelines for assistance.

The choice of a leader of the community mental health team upon its entry into the community raises some problems. Howe[20] has pointed out that a psychiatrist may not be the best choice. There are indications that gaining community support may be particularly difficult if the mental health team leader is a psychiatrist. Moreover, preparation for a community leadership role, including knowledge of establishing rapport with community groups, is not part of a psychiatrist's training. Howe makes the good point that it is unfair to expect the psychiatrist to learn a new set of professional skills after he has spent many years establishing a practice. It may be that a social worker, a professional mental health administrator, or a sociologist would be a better choice for the major leadership position in a multidisciplinary mental health team. However, even though he may not be the best qualified, the psychiatrist is so accustomed to the leader role that he will not easily relinquish his position, and it may be difficult for him to relate to other community mental health professionals as equals. "Deconditioning the doctor" is probably one of the biggest challenges for future training. Perhaps the psychiatrist can best be utilized not as the leader of a multidisciplinary team, but as a consultant or specialist to work in his more accustomed role with the individual patient.

One problem of community psychiatry is to design programs and services appropriate and beneficial to all classes within the community. Indeed, perhaps the overriding goal of the community mental health movement is to reach people from all income levels, something traditional psychotherapy has failed to do. An excellent example of this concern is the introduction of the "walk-in clinic." Ideally, such facilities remain open on a 24-hour basis and provide mental health services to groups that cannot seek assistance on a nine-to-five basis. This clinic facilitates case finding and early intervention. Discrepancies between community mental health purposes and actual practice are another problem. For example, as Reiff[49] has pointed out, the walk-in clinics were originally intended to deal with the obstacles of waiting lists and referrals and to provide immediate service. But in many cases, these clinics have in effect become small-scale psychotherapy clinics because psychotherapy is what the staff knows how to do. Other program problems include relating to people from low-income and various minority ethnic groups and the high costs of services. Titmus,[53] for example, has estimated that treating patients in the community may be just as expensive as treating them in hospitals. There is also the problem of the stigma attached by community members to individuals who participate in a community psychiatry program. One hypothesis to test would be that the stigma attached to participants is greater in rural than in urban communities because of the lesser anonymity of individuals. If so, the acceptance of the community mental health concept would be greater in urban than rural areas.

The question of how to delineate the geographical boundaries within which the community mental health program must operate must also be considered. The Federal government's concept of the geographic catchment area of no less than 75,000 and no more than 200,000 population has not proven to be a workable solution. Whittington[58] has demonstrated that in Denver a rigid adherence to the Federal prescription of a maximum population of 200,000 per catchment area would have denied mental health services to 340,000 people within a geographically contiguous area. Adrian[1] has suggested that community boundaries be delineated in a functional rather than a geographical manner. Such an approach is consistent with the notion of field presented above (although the semantics differ), namely, that participation within a field is the significant factor in determining community. With today's rapid means of communication and transportation, this approach to delineating community boundaries seems most appropriate. While the Federal delineation of catchment areas may not be problematic for treatment purposes, this delineation may offer potential difficulties for the prevention arm of community mental health services. It is naive to assume that the boundaries for these two distinct purposes should necessarily coincide. Future research should focus on the hypothesis that different catchment area boundaries should be used for the purposes of treatment and prevention. But until more precise indicators of the concept of prevention have been specified, this hypothesis will be difficult to test empirically. However, the community literature suggests that a broader geographical area should be utilized for prevention (as, for example, through mass education programs) than for treatment.[51]

Responsibility for the failure to utilize sociological studies of the community in the planning and implementation of community mental health programs does not rest solely on mental health practitioners. Sociologists are just now considering how to integrate community theory into a meaningful set of related propositions that can be applied to community psychiatry. This chapter has attempted to conceptualize community and community psychiatry, to demonstrate the potential utility of community theory, and to suggest hypotheses for research in the community mental health movement. This framework should be regarded as subject to the reflection, critiques, and suggestions of other interested researchers, and is hopefully a step in the right direction.

REFERENCES

1. ADRIAN, CHARLES R., ROSSI, PETER H., DAHL, ROBERT A., AND RODWIN, LLOYD: *Social Science and Community Action*. East Lansing: Michigan State University Press, 1960.
2. ALIHAN, MILLA A.: *Social Ecology*. New York: Columbia University Press, 1938.
3. ARENSBERG, CONRAD M.: "The Community as Object and Sample." *American Anthropologist* 63:246-264, 1961.
4. AXELROD, MORRIS: "Urban Structure and Social Participation." *American Sociological Review* 21:13-18, 1956.
5. BELKNAP, IVAN, AND STEINLE, JOHN G.: *The Community and Its Hospitals: A Comparative Analysis*. Syracuse: Syracuse University Press, 1963.
6. BELL, WENDELL, AND FORCE, MARYANNE T.: "Urban Neighborhood Types and Participation in Formal Associations." *American Sociological Review* 21:25-34, 1956.
7. BOGUE, DONALD J.: *The Structure of the Metropolitan Community: A Study of Dominance and Subdominance*. Ann Arbor: Horace H. Rackham School of Graduate Studies, University of Michigan, 1949.
8. BONJEAN, CHARLES M.: "The Community as Research Site and Object of Inquiry," in Charles M. Bonjean *et al.* (eds.), *Community Politics: A Behavioral Approach*. New York: Free Press, 1971.
9. DAHRENDORF, RALF: *Class and Class Conflict in Industrial Society*. Stanford, California: Stanford University Press, 1964.
10. DUNCAN, OTIS D., AND SCHNORE, LEO F.: "Cultural, Behavioral and Ecological Perspectives in the Study of Social Organization." *American Journal of Sociology* 65:132-153, 1959.
11. FIREY, WALTER: *Land Use in Central Boston*. Cambridge, Massachusetts: Harvard University Press, 1947.
12. FOWLER, IRVING A.: "Local Industrial Structures, Economic Power and Community Welfare." *Social Problems* 6:41-51, 1958.
13. GALPIN, CHARLES J.: "The Social Anatomy of a Rural Community." Research Bulletin No. 34. Madison: University of Wisconsin, Agricultural Research Station, 1915.
14. GLENN, NORVAL D.: "Massification versus Differentiation: Some Trend Data from National Surveys." *Social Forces* 46:172-180, 1967.
15. HAWLEY, AMOS H.: "Community Power and Urban Renewal Success." *American Journal of Sociology* 68:422-431, 1963.
16. HAWLEY, AMOS H.: *Human Ecology: A Theory of Community Structure*. New York: Ronald Press, 1950.
17. HILLER, E. T.: "The Community as a Social Group." *American Sociological Review* 6:189-202, 1941.
18. HILLERY, GEORGE A., JR.: "Definitions of Community: Areas of Agreement." *Rural Sociology* 20:111-123, 1955.
19. HOLLINGSHEAD, AUGUST B., AND REDLICH, FREDRICK C.: *Social Class and Mental Illness*. New York: Wiley & Sons, Inc., 1958.
20. HOWE, LOUISA P.: "The Concept of the Community: Some Implications for the Development of Community Psychiatry," in Leopold Bellak (ed.), *Handbook of Community Psychiatry and Community Mental Health*. New York: Grune and Stratton, 1964.
21. JAMES, GEORGE, AND MICO, PAUL: "Community Study and Leadership: Keys to Effective Health Action." *Journal of Public Health* 54:1957-1963, 1964.
22. KATZ, DANIEL, AND KAHN, ROBERT L.: *The Social Psychology of Organizations*. New York: Wiley Press, 1966.
23. KAUFMAN, HAROLD F.: "Toward an Interactional Conception of Community." *Social Forces* 38:8-17, 1959.
24. KLEIN, DONALD C.: *Community Dynamics and Mental Health*. New York: John Wiley and Sons, 1968.

25. KLEIN, DONALD C.: "The Community and Mental Health: An Attempt at a Conceptual Framework." *Community Mental Health Journal* 1:301-308, 1965.
26. KONIG, RENE: *The Community* (Edward Fitzgerald, trans.). New York: Schocken Books, 1968.
27. LEWIS, OSCAR: *Life in a Mexican Village: Tepoztlan Revisited.* Urbana: University of Illinois Press, 1951.
28. LOOMIS, CHARLES P.: *Social Systems: Essays on Their Persistence and Change.* Princeton, New Jersey: D. Van Nostrand Company, Inc., 1960.
29. LOOMIS, CHARLES P.: *Turrialba: Social Systems and the Introduction of Change.* Glencoe: The Free Press, 1952.
30. LYND, ROBERT S., AND LYND, HELEN MERRELL: *Middletown in Transition: A Study in Cultural Conflicts.* New York: Harcourt, Brace and Co., 1937.
31. LYND, ROBERT S., AND LYND, HELEN MERRELL: *Middletown: A Study in Contemporary American Culture.* New York: Harcourt, Brace and Co., 1929.
32. MACIVER, ROBERT M., AND PAGE, CHARLES H.: *Society: An Introductory Analysis.* New York: Rinehart, 1949.
33. MARTINDALE, DON: *American Society.* Princeton, New Jersey: D. Van Nostrand Company, Inc., 1960.
34. MERTON, ROBERT K.: *Social Theory and Social Structure.* New York: The Free Press, 1968.
35. MORRIS, ROBERT: "Basic Factors in Planning for the Coordination of Health Services." *American Journal of Public Health* 53:248-259 and 462-472, 1963.
36. MORRIS, ROBERT, AND BINSTOCK, ROBERT H.: *Feasible Planning for Social Change.* New York: Columbia University Press, 1966.
37. MYERS, JEROME K.: "Assimilation to the Ecological and Social Systems of a Community." *American Sociological Review* 15:367-372, 1950.
38. MUMFORD, LEWIS: *The Culture of Cities.* New York: Harcourt, Brace and Co., 1938.
39. NIX, HAROLD L.: "Concepts of Community and Community Leadership." *Sociology and Social Research* 53:500-510, 1969.
40. OGBURN, WILLIAM F.: *Social Characteristics of Cities.* Chicago: The International City Managers' Association, 1937.
41. PARK, ROBERT E.: "Human Ecology." *American Journal of Sociology* 42:1-15, 1936.
42. PARSONS, TALCOTT: *The Social System.* Glencoe: The Free Press, 1951.
43. PARSONS, TALCOTT, BALES, ROBERT F., AND SHILS, EDWARD A.: *Working Papers in the Theory of Action.* Glencoe: The Free Press, 1953.
44. PRESTON, JAMES D.: "The Identification of Community Leaders." *Sociology and Social Research* 53:204-216, 1969.
45. PRESTON, JAMES D.: "The Search for Community Leaders." *Sociological Inquiry* 39:39-47, 1969.
46. PRESTON, JAMES D.: "Community Norms and Adolescent Drinking Behavior: A Comparative Study." *Social Science Quarterly* 49:350-359, 1968.
47. QUINN, JAMES A.: *Human Ecology.* New York: Prentice-Hall, 1950.
48. REDFIELD, ROBERT: *The Little Community: Viewpoints for the Study of a Human Whole.* Chicago: University of Chicago Press, 1955.
49. REIFF, ROBERT: "The Ideological and Technological Implications of Clinical Psychology," in *Community Psychology,* a Report of the Boston Conference on the Education of Psychologists for Community Mental Health, pp. 51-64. Boston, 1966.
50. REISS, ALBERT J., JR.: "Some Logical and Methodological Problems in Community Research." *Social Forces* 33:51-57, 1954.
51. ROGERS, EVERETT M.: *Diffusion of Innovations.* Glencoe, Illinois: The Free Press, 1962.
52. SANDERS, IRWIN T.: *The Community: An Introduction to a Social System.* New York: Ronald Press, 1966.
53. SIMPSON, RICHARD L.: "Sociology of the Community: Current Status and Prospects." *Rural Sociology,* June:127-149, 1965.
54. SJOBERG, GIDEON: *The Preindustrial City.* Glencoe: The Free Press, 1960.
55. SMITH, T. LYNN, AND ZOPF, PAUL E., JR.: *Principles of Inductive Rural Sociology.* Philadelphia: F. A. Davis Company, 1970.
56. TITMUSS, RICHARD M.: "Community Care—Fact or Fiction?" in Hugh L. Freeman and James Farndale (eds.), *Trends in Mental Health Services,* pp. 221-225. Oxford, New York: Pergamon Press, 1963.

57. WARREN, ROLAND L.: *The Community in America*. Chicago: Rand McNally Company, 1963.
58. WHITTINGTON, HORACE G.: "The Development of an Urban Comprehensive Community Mental Health Program," in Milton F. Shore and Fortune V. Mannino (eds.), *Mental Health and the Community: Problems, Programs, and Strategies*. New York: Behavioral Publications, 1969.
59. WILKINSON, KENNETH P.: "Phases and Roles in Community Action." *Rural Sociology* 35:54-68, 1970.
60. WILKINSON, KENNETH P.: "Population and Community Characteristics of Multi-County Development Regions." Outline of remarks made at the Rural Sociological Society annual meetings in Washington, D. C., August 27, 1970.
61. WILKINSON, KENNETH D.: "The Community as a Social Field." *Social Forces* 48:311-322, 1970.
62. WILKINSON, KENNETH P.: "Special Agency Program Accomplishment and Community Action Styles: The Care of Watershed Development." *Rural Sociology* 34:29-42, 1969.
63. WILKINSON, KENNETH P.: "Identification with Community: A Review of Literature." State College: Mississippi State University, Social Science Research Center, Preliminary Report No. 1, 1963.
64. WIRTH, LOUIS: "Human Ecology." *American Journal of Sociology* 50:484-488, 1945.

CHAPTER 4

Neglected Legal Dilemmas in Community Psychiatry

ROSALIE COHEN*

The report of the Joint Commission on Mental Illness and Health (1960) led to a national program presented to Congress in 1963 which proposed changing the locus of publicly supported psychiatric treatment from state mental hospitals to community mental health centers. Later in 1963, Congress passed the Mental Retardation Facilities and Community Mental Health Centers Construction Act providing the means to shift treatment into the patients' communities.

In presenting the notion of community psychiatry, its advocates cited four major concerns. A first concern was for the effective treatment of the mentally ill. In the new frame of reference, the patient's social environment was viewed as a potential "therapeutic community"; an understanding of this principle on the part of mental health staffs could be expected to promote recovery. Second was concern about how to use the patients' family, social, and neighborhood relationships both to prevent illness and to enhance treatment. A third issue was how to organize and finance the centers so that groups and individuals in the community could be involved in the policy direction of the centers. The final concern was for a reduction in the "load factor" of existing treatment facilities. Many proponents believed that by providing prompt service and 24-hour care, community mental health centers could reduce the pressure on state facilities.[4]

Despite the attempt to provide readily accessible, effective mental health care to the population, a number of problems in implementation appeared very early. The earliest of these was the basic issue of definitions. Neither the 1963 legislation nor the Federal agencies responsible for the new program provided a clear interpretation of "community" or "mental health." The term "community

---

*Assisted by Anita M. Cohen, J.D.

mental health center" is similarly vague. As a result, many view the centers as consisting of a single building even though the intent was an administrative coordination of services which might be separately housed. Other problems have been inherent in the reorganization plan itself. The attempt to plan rationally for the development of needed services set in motion a massive restructuring of the service delivery system. Restructuring is apparent in the definition of a superstructure of service populations for the centers over existing service facilities. Restructuring is also apparent in the development of the necessary multidiscipline professional staffs, many of whose preparatory requirements and scopes of practice are defined by statute. The focus on prevention and the concern with normal processes of growth and development have produced new interinstitutional links and created new kinds of decision makers. The notion of community causality has also produced a subtle transformation in the belief systems of treatment personnel by focusing on social as well as individual causation. Invasion of privacy issues became apparent when efforts were made to have readily accessible medical and social histories in central data banks, as is described by Hollingshead in the following chapter. Conversely, the right of the community to be free from the threat of potentially disruptive individuals has also surfaced as a problem of the new program.

All of these issues represent legal dilemmas of community psychiatry that may take considerable time to resolve. This chapter does not attempt to deal with all of the issues which appear in relevant literature. Several problems have been selected that are common to all states and that have been discussed most frequently in the medical and legal literature. These have been cast into three categories of "jurisdictional problems": 1) the political, 2) the interprofessional, and 3) those dealing with individual rights and the public interest. Although regional service administration agencies have been developed as an attempt to bring some coherence to the field, it is noteworthy that in none of the three areas have any definitive directions been drawn either legally or administratively. It is hoped that this brief overview may place these areas in some perspective so that the developments of the next few decades may be more meaningful.

POLITICAL JURISDICTIONAL PROBLEMS

The 1963 Community Mental Health Centers Act was a commitment to easily accessible, locally supported, comprehensive mental health centers. Interpretation of this commitment, however, has varied problems. A mental health facility that is accessible to its clientele and able to provide continuous comprehensive care has one set of implications; an agency that not only provides referral and support services but that is also locally controlled and financed carries a different set of implications. Already existing agencies could have provided more accessible facilities by placing them in metropolitan centers, but many supporters of the community mental health movement believe that its success requires responsible local involvement, i.e., that the centers must be controlled and financed by the community.[28] Such involvement presents the questions of how to define the center's community and how to determine who within it will implement the program.[4]

What is a community? Communities have been both geographically and socially defined, as broadly as national interest groups or as narrowly as neighborhoods. Older sources view community in bounded terms as consisting of a large commercial center and interdependent hinterland;[8] newer concepts see communities as multiple overlapping patterns of concerted activities.[9] In this view, a citizen is likely to belong to different communities for the purposes of schooling, water supply, recreation, mail service, and so forth.[1] Whether geographically or socially defined, planners are faced with shifting populations and the dissolution and reforming of interest groups. (See Preston, Chapter 3.)

Deep community involvement in the new mental health program was obviously intended by the legislation, but the logistics of implementation impelled an administrative definition of community. That is, the language of the legislation presented the unresolvable impasse of implying a common social identity in the communities to be served, yet it described them as geographical catchment areas. Regulations governing the administration of the program required that each state plan provide for mental health centers to serve populations consisting of from 75,000 to 200,000 individuals "so located as to be near and readily accessible to the populations to be served, taking into account both political and geographical boundaries."[7]

The geographical definition of community may have appeared to be administratively viable, but even this objective is not easily accomplished, especially in high density urban centers. Within these areas there are many overlapping geographical unities defined and described by state law as political jurisdictions with specific powers and responsibilities. They are the basic units for the design and control of all public functions, and they are legitimated both by public sanction and public usage. With the national government's requirement that they be stratified or subsumed within new mental health center boundaries, intergovernmental relationships became problematic, especially in metropolitan centers where jurisdictions are most numerous and populations most dense.

Connery[4] calls attention to this dilemma with the following statistics: In 1960, metropolitan centers contained two thirds of the nation's population, and they accounted for four fifths of the population growth between 1950 and 1960. This two thirds of the population lived within 212 standard metropolitan statistical areas, but not within the jurisdiction of 212 local governments [p. 65]. In 1962, there were 91,185 local governments such as counties, townships, municipalities, school districts, and the like. Of that total, 12,387 fell within the 75 largest metropolitan areas [p. 69], yet in no metropolitan area with as many as 300,000 inhabitants was there one political unit which bore sole responsibility for all phases of local government activity [p. 65].

71

Metropolitan areas are literally mazes of political jurisdictions. The boundaries of parks, sewage and water districts, and health, welfare, and correctional areas are superimposed upon the boundaries of counties, cities, and school districts. Some urban areas extend over states or national boundaries. These jurisdictions consist of many more or less independent authorities with legally defined duties and powers, and they are administered by legitimately appointed or elected boards, councils, and commissions. In some way, they are all involved with mental health program activity. Unlike agencies concerned only with mental illness, mental health programs involve activities concerned with normal growth and development related to school, recreation, public health and welfare programs, and even housing. These related services may be provided by hundreds of separate jurisdictions. This fragmentation appears to be typical of metropolitan areas, and although the number of local governments in the country as a whole has been decreasing, the reverse has occurred in urban areas.[4] Where boundaries overlap, a number of authorities may compete for the same tax dollar. In regard to mental health programming, this fragmentation presents the problem of what governmental unit should assume responsibility for local decision making and financial participation.[4,3]

In order to comply with the 1963 legislation, various efforts were made to fit existing units of government into the required population limits. Consolidation of small units, stratification of larger ones, changes in administration, and establishment of new districts of the necessary size were early adaptations. It is apparent, however, that no common plan or design has been generally useful, and the maze of governments is not fully responsible for sluggish implementation. Some highly fragmented centers have been slow and others more rapid in developing their services.[4]

It appears that size and population density are the only characteristics that urban areas have in common. These similarities are overpowered by regional and local differences. Within cities, some sections are growing rapidly, others are declining in population density, and the character of their populations is shifting in different areas. Some sub-communities within cities press for local control and for their statutory definition as "service communities," while others appear less concerned with the concept of community than with the variety of services provided.

There are also great variations among states in the types of mental health services available and in the kinds of public and private agencies that administer their programs. There is a health authority in every state, but the responsibility for program design and implementation is distributed among departments of health, education, and welfare, hospitals, and so forth. Locally, many private agencies administer their own program, have their own service populations, and their own sources of management and funding. Each unit is responsible to its own governing agencies, and they frequently compete for patients, service personnel, and funding. In general, each policy making body acts independently of others. This fragmentation is not only a problem to coordinate, but it is also a constraint on innovation. Both private and public agencies have preferred to assign new duties to already existing departments, to create a new department to serve the same clientele as are receiving their other services, and, in general, to accommodate their clientele within their current program structure.[4]

Whether the new government structure will complicate or simplify the task, however, it not the only problem involved. Connery[4] notes that:

> With hundreds and thousands of inmates, state mental institutions have had bigger budgets and more employees than most other state programs. The location of a mental hospital in a community brings jobs and money to the area in which it is located. . . . On the surface the concern might have seemed to be solely with programs, but real battles were often fought over power, dollars, and jobs. . . . The financial rewards of vastly larger federal appropriations will make the political stakes more attractive. . . . Political prestige, the rewards of public office, the control of public funds, profit from construction contracts and indirect economic advantages—all will be involved in the new mental health center program [pp. 9-10].

The question of who will make decisions in mental health programming has thus become more important. The emergence of new social identities, especially among those populations which have not been well served in the past, makes salient the need for a widely accepted definition of community, a problem which, in the early phases of implementation, had remained dormant.

Despite the clear definition of catchment area, rankling differences in the concept of community are still apparent. In sparsely settled locales outside of metropolitan centers, large geographical areas are required to provide minimal populations for mental health centers. Although they present singular problems, such as transportation difficulty, the availability of new or broader services may be sufficient reason for participation in the center's programs and for support among its service populations. In heavily urbanized areas, however, where it is not difficult to demark sections with the required populations, the sociological notion of community may become an important force in the determination of programming. Supporters of community control argue that the catchment area concept leads one to ignore community involvement as central to service delivery and to deny the view that the variations within the catchment areas are the substance of community identity.*

The problem of intergovernmental relations within states is also reflected in interstate relations. Given the enormity of the jurisdictional tangle described above and the presence of generalized hazards to mental health, such as air and

---

*However, defining community along racial lines may be a violation of civil rights legislation. Also where Federal funds are dispensed directly to center units, Federal legislation (e.g., the Hatch Act) which prohibits political activity by Federal employees may preclude efforts of low income communities to actively engage in activities to develop viable decision making potential in community mental health.

water pollution, interstate regional administrative agencies have been developed to attempt to bring coherence to the field. The problems of the sociological notions of community assume a larger scale when a community is also a state with constitutionally based functions and when jurisdictional disputes are cast in the light of state and Federal duties.

In broad perspective, planners are left with many unresolved questions. Can community be defined as a geographical catchment area, or does it refer to a group of people who share a common social identity? If a potential therapeutic community can be identified, will it remain sufficiently stable in size and character to justify a comprehensive program? What proportion of its community is needed to support the centers? Who will represent the community and how will representatives be selected? Does community use alone reflect acceptance of the centers, or must communities finance and control them? Will regional administration affect the state's traditional role in administering mental health services? Will the new service system result in the coordination of services, or will it merely add to existing fragmentation? The long term impact of the legislation may thus require statutory revisions and/or a lengthy process of judicial clarification of the powers and responsibilities of the jurisdictions which, in the process of coordination, have been stratified or subsumed as service districts.

PROFESSIONAL JURISDICTIONAL PROBLEMS

The 1963 Community Mental Health Centers Act designated certain target populations as especially important in its implementation and directed that each state construct a plan based on "an inventory of facilities and a survey of need . . . furnishing needed services to persons unable to pay therefor. . . ."[19] The regulations specified that in addition to concern with the total number and the proportions of people with mental disorders, centers must consider such related factors as "the existence of low per capita income, chronic unemployment and sub-standard housing; the extent of . . . alcoholism, drug abuse, crime and delinquency; and the special needs of certain groups, especially the mentally handicapped, the aged and the children. . . ."[5] Thus, in specifying a concern with social and environmental conditions external to the individual, the regulations reflected a subtle shift from a focus on intraindividual conditions related to mental health to a concern with "salient causes" and the "control of disability"[16] within a multicausal framework.

This shift in the restructuring of professional service delivery systems is apparent where services are offered by multidisciplinary professional teams and decision makers. Although this new focus on a multifactor framework appears appropriate to the social scientist, it brings to the fore new issues of professional accountability that are not entirely consistent with existing practice statutes. For some professions, practice statutes delineate professional jurisdictions with their attendant rights and responsibilities, in a fashion similar to the definition of political jurisdictions described earlier. These statutes are not easily revamped to include innovative practices which, it is felt, may reduce quality or dissipate accountability in treatment. Some of the restructuring involves existing types of medical teams with medical, allied, or auxilary practice statutes, while others, less definitive in the problems which they will involve, have to do with interinstitutional linkages between medical professionals and other types of licensed and unlicensed professionals.

Public efforts to insure accountability in the treatment of the ill have been made since the Code of Hammurabi. They arose to protect the public from exploitation by physicians, to compensate individuals for losses they might sustain in treatment, and to assure the public that minimum standards in the quality of services would be maintained.[22] With the development of a highly sophisticated medical technology, many specialized tasks were differentiated out of generic medical practice, defined by statute, and clarified by judicial decisions. These tasks were designated, along with related rights and responsibilities, as the unique areas of practice of particular professions (e.g., nurses, technicians, etc.). Since the opportunity to practice is viewed as a privilege and not a natural right,[25,10] performance and quality standards of professional participation have been carefully guarded and controlled.

As this privilege is embodied in state statutes, it provides for (1) a "contract" between a physician and a "patient"[26] who is generically defined;* (2) a broad scale responsibility for patient welfare on the part of the physician, whether treatment involves only himself or includes auxiliary workers (some of whom may be adequately trained professionals whose concerns are not specifically medical in nature and whose goals in treatment may be distinct and different from his own); and (3) legal culpability of the physician for negligence or wrongs committed in the treatment procedure, whether or not this culpability is shared with others or with the treatment center.[27,29] If statutory functions are not responsibly carried out, the profession as a whole may bear the brunt of the withdrawal or limitation of this privilege. If the individual practitioner does not comply with the practice regulations, his privilege to practice may be withdrawn and he may also be subject to legal penalties. The limited specifications as to which functions may be delegated, the quality standards for the profession which are specified in practice statutes, and the possibility of civil or criminal liability for the individual practitioner have acted as constraints on innovative collaborative practices.[30] For this reason, the licensure of many allied and auxiliary personnel has been made possible only by clarification of the medical practice acts in court. Because many possible methods for more effectively dealing with growing complexities in practice have not been adequately covered by licensure statutes or court decisions, the possibility of litigation has made licensed health personnel reluctant to share the performance of any task outside of their conventional scope of practice. For physicians with unlimited licenses to

---

*Any individual "with any pain, disorder, or human ailment, deformity, infirmity or disease, whether physical or mental, whether real or imaginary, or one with any departure from complete health and proper condition." Federation of State Medical Boards.[10]

perform all activities, the critical questions concern what functions they may delegate, to what personnel, and under what conditions. Other personnel are limited by what services they may and may not perform. Both medical and nonmedical professionals receive little guidance from the statutes as to how to modify their collaborative activities without subjecting themselves to penalties for violation of the practice statutes.

One common avenue for development is through the mechanism of the "supervised delegation," i.e., organized groups of nonmedical professionals who function semi-autonomously in medical settings under general medical supervision. The utility of this mechanism is characterized by the absence of licensure of such professionals in all but a few states.[23] In cases where supervised delegations function at some distance geographically from the supervisor or in highly visible settings with greater discretionary judgement in the control of patients, however, there is concern as to whether this delegation of responsibility will be sanctioned by the courts and whether the supervising medical personnel will be willing to share culpability with them.

A number of links are envisioned between mental health centers and other major institutions of society, including schools, churches, businesses, labor unions, and recreational facilities. All of these are regulated in some way by law. To the extent that their functions can be carried out as contingent therapeutic communities within the framework of existing statutes governing accountability and quality standards, no conflict is anticipated. However, where their definitions of normal growth and development are in conflict with those of supportive medical systems, some failures of communication and difficulties in collaboration can be expected.

Much of the problem of interprofessional and interdisciplinary collaboration lies in the undefined notion of mental health. Some disciplines define mental health negatively as the absence of disease while others see it more positively as the presence of certain identifiable psychological characteristics.[13,14] These different views call for different intervention strategies. Traditional methods based in the first view focus on the individual and on therapy and rehabilitation. The second view directs both research and intervention toward the social contexts of family and community.[6] Defining mental health is further complicated by the view of some sociologists and anthropologists that many aspects of psychotic behavior are culturally, rather than universally, deviant. So varied are the conceptions of the term community mental health that some refer to it as "all activities carried out in the community in the name of mental health."[20]

The community psychiatry concept as legislated provides no definition of mental illness. It leaves communities and states to define their own mentally ill populations using whatever definition their publics will sanction. But it also gives recognition to state mental health agencies, to the private practice of psychiatry, and to the separate professions, again providing a plethora of legitimate agencies with conflicting jurisdictional claims. Some observers feel that the process of restructuring will be sufficiently slow as to obviate anticipatable legal problems. However, much depends upon the process of contextual social change. In many cases, the centers may select the most easily treated clients in the communities to be served, leaving societal "rejects" to other institutions such as the courts.[18] Much of its future direction may thus be determined by the emergence of "communities of interest" within the population and by judicial decision as to whether their demands are within the public interest.

In brief, then, existing practice statutes define professional jurisdictions and their rights, responsibilities, and relevant interaction patterns. As such, they act as constraints on innovative collaborative treatment activities. Where multidisciplinary practitioners are involved, differences in critical definitions among them (e.g., of mental health) also emerge as constraints on interinstitutional coordination. They pose differences both in theory and in related intervention strategies, and they involve questions of confidentiality and depersonalization of information and the ethics of research and practice. In addition, the relocation of accountability in treatment remains to be judicially confirmed or clarified in future years.

INDIVIDUAL RIGHTS AND THE PUBLIC INTEREST

In addition to those jurisdictional problems of overlapping political units and service districts and of the vague yet restrictive scope of practice statutes, certain dilemmas have arisen concerning the relationship of the individual and the public. Some of these issues involve the privacy of the individual, privileged information, the ability of the individual to control his own destiny, and the desire of the public to remain free from hazards related to mental illness.

Perhaps the most common concern of the layman involves the collection of information about individuals and its storage for retrieval in central data banks or psychiatric case registers.[2] Despite the apparent need for the easy retrieval of such information in order to study patterns of illness in an area and to plan for the coordination of services, people in the United States have been reluctant over the years to participate in the assembling of "dossiers" of any type, seeing this as an invasion of their Constitutional right to privacy or, in special cases, as an infringement on their right to protection from giving evidence against themselves.

The Community Mental Health Centers Act requires an assessment of need as a prerequisite to the planning and coordination of services. Assurances of continuity of care, service evaluation, and efforts toward prevention have required the development of biostatistical research and a shift in its focus from the collecting of purely descriptive statistics with inferences of causality to the collecting of analytic statistics with the identification and testing of causal relationships. Coordinated services that provide for a free flow of patients among public and private agencies and private practitioners require a similar flow of information about individuals. Long term information about each individual, coordinated on the county, state, and national levels, is viewed as necessary to achieve the objectives of the new program. Coordinated services require data not only on the number of facilities in the area, the nature of their services, and the characteristics of their patients, but also on the extent to which each patient has used more than one facility and on the patterns of patient flow among the facilities. Such services also require personal statistics such as data on social identifications and psychiatric assessment, marital status and sexual habits, household composition, fertility, eating habits, school and work histories, and so forth.[15] Although the present intent is to use this data to develop, evaluate, and plan an effective service delivery system, there is some concern as to how this collection of intimate details about the individual will affect his life. This concern is expressed by those who argue the need for legislation to control input into community case registers and its use by the community at large. Moreover, the relative weighting of such data as, for example, cumulative school records compiled by persons untrained in psychiatric assessment is at issue. Questions regarding who has access to such information, how much information will be released, whether it will be raw or interpreted data, and if the latter, who will interpret it, are all unresolved. These questions are of special concern where the extension of credit, employment, or higher education of the individuals are involved. Some observers argue that in addition to the danger of possible error in data collection and handling, there is the possibility that the early identification of an individual as prementally ill may limit available life opportunities from which he may choose.[15]

Secondly, there are statutes in many states that prevent a physician from releasing privileged information that a patient might believe is damaging to him. That is, information given to the individual psychiatrist or medical practitioner by a patient as part of a treatment process is considered "privileged," and it may not be released to others without the patient's consent.[11] At certain times, the issue of public interest arises. The release of certain types of information may be viewed as in the public interest for various institutional reasons, including the planning of facilities, in spite of the protests of the individuals involved. Legal precedent has controlled the use of data in the possession of the physician; no precedents control the use of these new banks of information. There is, therefore, concern with the planning of relevant legislation to do so. Individuals may find at some time that in order to use the extended service facility, they may be required to give up some measure of their privacy.*

The legal status of the mentally ill as a category of individuals in our society is antiquated. In early law, the madman *(furioses)* was not distinguished from the criminal; both were subjected to police restraint. The source of our current laws

---

*Social class differences are expected as they reflect differential ability to use existing provisions in the law for the protection of privacy. For instance, those who are familiar with contracts may be aware that if the condition of confidentiality is placed on the use of the service at its outset, information obtained by treatment personnel in the care of a patient may not be disclosed, except for those reasons detailed in the conditions. Where individuals are less familiar with the protection which may be provided, this may not be the case. It is forseeable, though, that individuals may lose their ability to contract for the limited dispersal of personal information. For example, a standard form contract may be designed, similar to standard form leases, in which the tenant (or in the medical contract, the patient) has little or no bargaining power.

is found in 13th century English law which dealt primarily with the property, rather than the person, of the mentally ill.[17] The indigent at that time, left to care for themselves and designated as rogues, vagrants, beggars, the idle, the disorderly, and the lewd, all were subject to police control. It was not until 1845 that detention for therapeutic purposes was envisioned.[21] In the late 19th century, all states enacted laws governing hospitalization. These provisions focused on wrongful commitment and on the disposition of the property of the hospitalized. Although these laws varied greatly from state to state, they all reflected the notion that the mentally ill are as dangerous as the criminal and that mental disability is a social deviance requiring social control, rather than an illness. Roche[21] says,

> In all of the state laws affecting hospitalization, mental disability is defined either specifically or by implication as a change in behavior beyond community norms, amounting to social disability at variance with common sense values and carrying the threat of unpredictable danger. In no law is there a use of scientific labelling, specifying a category of mental disease, except for broad categories as drug addiction, alcoholism, mental deficiency and epilepsy. . . . Thus, in general, the laws of hospitalization define mental illness not in terms of current psychiatric theoretical models but in terms of social disability which describe loss of capacity for minimal social reality adaptation [pp. 411-412].

> The enlarging scope of mental illness [thus] embraces the maladjusted, the senile, mentally defective, epileptic, drug addict, alcoholic and the destitute aged and the line between the psychotic and the anti-social is becoming less and less distinct [p. 412].

In 1961, the American Bar Foundation published an analysis of the law concerning the mentally disabled in an effort to clarify the concepts used in them.[17] They recommended revision of relevant statutes to make them more uniform and more specific so as to protect the rights as well as the property of the individuals who are affected.[17] Their report draws attention to the tautological use of the terms "incompetence" and "hospitalization"* and recommends a statutory clarification of the relationship between "discharge" and the "restoration of capacities." They also call attention to the absence of definition in the statutes as to which individuals fit such categories as "lunatic," "insane," "mentally unfit," or "mentally disabled." Their analysis points out that despite the vague and unscientific language of these statutes, individuals who fall under their jurisdiction

---

*Roche[21] comments that although incompetency and hospitalization are separate legal concepts, they are sometimes confused. The former is concerned exclusively with the protection of the assets of an individual who is incapable of managing his own affairs; the latter is to protect the mentally disabled from inflicting injury on others or himself and to provide treatment for him. Ross[24] attributes this confusion of the two legal concepts to old cases and statutes which used the term "insanity" to refer to both concepts. This confusion still persists in a few cases in which hospitalization automatically constitutes a finding of incompetency.

are variously limited in different states in their rights to make wills, to execute contracts and conveyances, to sue or be sued, to engage in business, to be licensed professionally, to appoint agents, to secure a driver's license, to vote, to hold public office or to serve on a jury, to pay taxes, to receive pensions and veteran's benefits, and to negotiate various insurance matters.[21]

Our final concern in this regard has to do with the changing focus of analysis and intervention from the individual to his social groups. As related research finds salient causes of the mental illness of an individual in his family, work, or other social groups (the "schizophrenogenic family"[12] and the "alcohologenic spouse" are examples) rather than in his own unique physiology or idiosyncratic history, and when intervention strategies are geared to changing social relationships rather than individual coping mechanisms, new legal issues may be anticipated. The questions in law here have to do with the measures that may be used to motivate or coerce participants in the social groups of mentally ill persons to engage in treatment themselves. Under existing law, so long as they do not come to an agency with a presenting problem, so long as they form no contract for treatment, and so long as they commit no crime and do not present a clear threat to themselves or to others, they cannot be coerced into treatment. Some common questions have to do with how broadly the ramifications of a "threat to others" may be defined. For instance, can welfare payments be withheld until families of clients submit to group therapy? A major issue for those concerned with the maintenance of individual autonomy is that the coordination of services may itself be coercive by withholding some services from individuals as the price of their participation in other services.

In contrast to those issues involving the protection of the rights of the mentally ill, public concern for diminishing social control is already apparent in the public's resistance to some aspects of the community mental health program. Much of this resistance is based on evidence that many categories of the mentally ill, as they are described in the community mental health centers legislation, are associated with crimes in the community. The drug addict may steal to support his habit, for instance, and the alcoholic who drives a car is a threat to highway safety. The court release of criminals pending psychiatric evaluation and the liberalization of criminal sentencing have already aroused public protest, although this protest is most commonly directed toward the criminal justice system, and political relief rather than legal relief is most commonly sought. The problems of the liberalization of sentencing for crimes, especially in the largest cities, may only be the result of the fact that this trend preceded the development of mental health staffs and facilities adequate to serve the affected individuals and to initiate effective education of the public to work with them. Nevertheless, many community members view themselves as victims of conditions for which they may share responsibility but with which they cannot cope. As reforms to protect the rights of the mentally ill take place, questions of social control emerge, and visa versa.

Many unresolved issues remain in determining the relationship between the individual and the public in light of existing law and emerging concerns with the public welfare. Some observers, including Roche, look forward to the time when "involuntary hospitalization . . . is an exception, when mental disability has been denatured of its superstitious elements of distrust, repellance and danger and when it can be regarded with the same objectivity as physical disability, [and] when legal forms can be reduced to a minimum of basic personal rights and property protection" [p. 418].[21] However, attitudes are not solely responsible for the major dilemmas of the new program. The most salient characteristics of the new legislation is that it calls for, and results in, broadly based changes in individual and group relationships, the most formal statements of which appear in the law.

CONCLUSION

The 1963 Community Mental Health legislation has set in motion a massive restructuring of services related to mental health. It directs that populations be reorganized for more effective service delivery and that professional staffs and service agencies, both public and private, be coordinated, in many instances across institutional lines. Since the law is concerned with rules for the maintenance of satisfying and equitable relationships among individuals, it might have been anticipated that the establishment of new social relationships would result in legal dilemmas. Some of the most common concerns of the new program in this regard have been grouped here into three general categories of jurisdictional problems: those relating to established political jurisdictions, those relating to interprofessional relationships, and those concerned with the relationships between the individual and the public. In its large-scale impact on existing social relationships, the development of community mental health as an intent of government for the public welfare is more than a case study in the development of a profession or in the solution of a social problem. It casts some light as well on social processes and the problems of social change.

REFERENCES

1. ADRIAN, C. R.: "The Community Setting," in Adrian, C. R. (ed.): *Social Science and Community Action*. East Lansing, Michigan: The Institute for Community Development & Services, Continuing Education Services, Michigan State University, 1963.
2. BAHN, A. K., GARDNER, R. A., ALLTOP, L., KNATTERUD, C. I., AND SOLOMON, M.: "Admission and Prevalence Rates for Psychiatric Facilities in Four Register Areas." *American Journal of Public Health* 56:2033-2051, 1966.
3. BROWN, BERTRAM: "The Impact of the New Federal Mental Health Legislation on the State Mental Hospital System," in Bindman, A. J., and Spiegel, A. D. (eds.): *Perspectives in Community Mental Health*. Chicago: Aldine Publishing Co., 1969.
4. CONNERY, R. J.: *The Politics of Mental Health*. New York: Columbia University Press, 1968.
5. Community Mental Health Centers Act of 1963. Title II; Public Law 88-164, Regulations. *Federal Register*, 1964.
6. DUHL, LEONARD: *The Urban Condition*. New York: Basic Books, 1963.
7. *Federal Register*, pp. 5951-56; 54:201-215, 1964.

8. GRAS, N. S. B.: *An Introduction to Economic History.* New York: Harpers, 1926, p. 183.

9. GREER, SCOTT: *The Emerging City.* New York: Free Press, 1962.

10. "Guide to the Essentials of a Modern Medical Practice Act," adopted by the Federation of State Medical Boards and reprinted in *Selected Readings for Legal Problems in Practice of Medicine.* Chicago: University of Chicago Press, 1961.

11. GUTTMACHER, MANFRED S.: *The Role of Psychiatry in Law.* Springfield, Illinois: Charles C. Thomas, 1968, p. 85.

12. HALEY, JAY: "The Family of the Schizophrenic: A Model System," in Bergen, B. J., and Thomas, C. S. (eds.): *Issues and Problems of Social Psychiatry.* Springfield, Illinois: Charles C. Thomas, 1966.

13. JAHODA, MARIE: *Current Concepts of Positive Mental Health.* New York: Basic Books, 1958, p. 22.

14. JAHODA, MARIE: "Mental Health," in Kotinsky, Rugh, and Witmer, Helen L. (eds.): *Community Programs for Mental Health.* Cambridge: Harvard University Press, 1955, p. 298.

15. KRAMER, MORTON: "Epidemiology, Biostatistics and Mental Health Planning," in Monroe, Russell R., Klee, Gerald D., and Brody, Eugene B. (eds.): *Psychiatric Epidemiology and Mental Health Planning,* Chapter I. Washington, D.C.: American Psychiatric Association, 1967.

16. LEIGHTON, ALEXANDER: "Is Social Environment a Cause of Psychiatric Disorder?" in Monroe, Russell R., Klee, Gerald D., and Brody, Eugene B. (eds.): *Psychiatric Epidemiology and Mental Health Planning.* Washington, D.C.: American Psychiatric Association, 1967.

17. LINDEMAN, F. T., AND MCINTYRE, D. M., JR.: *The Mentally Disabled and the Law.* Chicago: The University of Chicago Press, 1961.

18. LINSANSKY, EDITH, AND SROLE, LEO: "Discussion of Papers by Hogarty, Locke, and Gardner," in Monroe, Russell R., Klee, Gerald D., and Brody, Eugene B. (eds.): *Psychiatric Epidemiology and Mental Health Planning,* pp. 283-285. Washington, D.C.: American Psychiatric Association, 1967.

19. NIMH Guidelines for State Plans, 1965. Submitted under the Community Mental Health Centers Act of 1963, DHEW, PHS, NIH. Washington, D.C.: U. S. Government Printing Office, 1965.

20. NEWBROUGH, J. R.: "Community Mental Health: A Movement in Search of a Theory," in Bindeman, A. J., and Spiegel, A. D. (eds.): *Perspectives in Community Mental Health.* Chicago: Aldine Publishing Co., 1969, p. 70.

21. ROCHE, PHILLIP Q.: "Psychiatry, Law and the Community," in Bellak, Leopold (ed.): *Handbook of Community Psychiatry and Community Mental Health.* New York: Grune and Stratton, 1964.

22. SIGERIST, H. E.: "Physician's Profession through the Ages," in Marti-Ibanex, F. (ed.): *Henry E. Sigerist on History of Medicine.* New York: MD Publications, Inc., 1960.

23. Report of the National Advisory Committee on Health Manpower, Vol. II. Washington, D.C.: U. S. Government Printing Office, 1967.

24. ROSS, H. A.: "Commitment of the Mentally Ill: Problems of Law and Policy." *Michigan Law Review* 57:945-1018, 1959.

25. SHINDELL, SIDNEY: "Survey of the Law of Medical Practice. I. The Legal Status of the Physician." *JAMA* 193:601-606, 1965.

26. SHINDELL, SIDNEY: "Survey of the Law of Medical Practice. II. Contractual Aspects of the Physician-Patient Relationship." *JAMA* 193:935-940, 1965.

27. SHINDELL, SIDNEY: "Survey of the Law of Medical Practice. IV. Negligence in the Practice of Medicine." *JAMA* 194:281-287, 1965.

28. SMITH, M. B., AND HOBBS, N.: "The Community and the Community Mental Health Center," in Bindeman, A. J., and Spiegel, A. D. (eds.): *Perspectives in Community Mental Health.* Chicago, Aldine Publishing Co., 1969.

29. STETLER, C. J., AND MORITZ, A. R.: *Doctor and Patient and Law,* ed. 4. St. Louis: A. B. Mosby Co., 1962.

30. COHEN, ROSALIE: "Some Legal Constraints on the Effective Operation of 'The Team' in Medical Settings." Paper read at the annual meeting of the Southern Sociological Society, New Orleans, April, 1969.

CHAPTER 5

Private Rights versus Community Needs: The New Haven Experience*

AUGUST B. HOLLINGSHEAD

In recent years there has been a marked increase in the fear of the invasion of private rights by organized groups of one kind or another, such as political and business groups and governmental agencies. While Congressional hearings and civil rights groups call our attention to this concern, the general public and specific interest groups demand the solution of social problems, particularly in our cities. Viewed broadly, we in the United States have developed a society that requires the accumulation of information about individuals, social groups, and institutions for effective functioning. At the same time, we value our individual freedom and privacy. In other words, while Americans attempt to keep their private lives private, they demand public solutions to personal problems. Thus there is a cleavage between the "rights" of individuals and the "needs" of the community for information for planning purposes. Individuals demand that their private rights be protected from invasion by the very agencies that need such information to help solve the personal problems that plague our society.[10] The situation poses dilemmas for social researchers. This chapter presents some of these dilemmas by discussing selected aspects of a research program in which I have been engaged in recent years.

Increasingly, sociologists are becoming enmeshed in the pressing social issues of our times. We are being called upon to apply our knowledge to various kinds of social problems, including the problem of mental illness. Although mental illness is only one of the problems facing society today, it is one of the most sensitive areas of public concern. It is also one of the most handicapping conditions to afflict individuals and families.

*Revision of a paper presented to the Committee on Psychiatric Sociology of the Society for the Study of Social Problems during its Annual Meeting in San Francisco, August, 1969.

The study of the distribution of treated mental illness in the population of the New Haven community was begun over 20 years ago by Dr. Fredrick C. Redlich, now Dean of the School of Medicine, Yale University, and myself. In the ensuing years, I have been involved in four large-scale studies that attempted to determine interrelations between the social structure and the treatment patients received for their health difficulties. These studies have been completed and several volumes have been published on the findings.[3,6,7,5,1] These were done without undue public resentment. Times, however, have changed! The present study was hardly out of the planning stage when psychiatrists, lawyers, and social workers challenged what we intended to do. Before the research could proceed, we had to face the challengers and satisfy the questioners.

Currently, the New Haven community encompasses the city of New Haven and a number of suburban towns. For all practical purposes, the communal area, as we define it ecologically, and the Standard Metropolitan Statistical Area of New Haven, as the United States Census defines it, are coterminous. The city of New Haven has been losing population for some 20 years while the suburban towns around it have more than doubled in population. Between 1960 and 1970, the city's population declined 9.4 per cent whereas the population of the suburban towns increased by 29 per cent. There is a sharp contrast racially and economically between those who reside in the city and those who reside in the suburban towns. Moreover, between 1960 and 1970 the white population in New Haven declined by 27.7 per cent and the nonwhite population increased by 66.4 per cent. The city today faces many economic, political, racial, and health problems, not the least of which is the concentration of mental illness in the worst slum area, which is populated in large part by blacks and Puerto Ricans.*

Health and welfare agencies serving clients and patients in the metropolitan area are concentrated in the city of New Haven. Generally, public and eleemosynary private agencies established to deliver health and welfare services to the public are members of the Community Council of Greater New Haven, Inc., while health and welfare agencies catering to private clients or patients— the private sector of the helping professions and their ancillary agencies—do not hold membership in the Community Council. The present study is focused on the public sector of the health and welfare complex. The research under discussion was initiated by the Community Council and was carried out under its auspices.

The Community Council has three goals: The first is to function as a clearinghouse for the many activities of individual agencies and communal groups concerned with seeking solutions to the community's many social problems. The second is to improve available services in existing agencies. The third is to plan for more adequate services to members of the community in the future.

The Community Council is enmeshed in the vortex of social, economic,

---

*Statistical data in this paper have been brought up to date as of March 31, 1971, wherever information was available.

political, and population changes taking place in the New Haven community. Its officers are busy "putting out brush fires" that break out almost daily, kindled by problems developing around its responsibilities to function as a clearinghouse and to improve existing services. Thus, little time or energy has been left to meet its third responsibility—that of planning for improved services in the future. For several years the officers of the Council and professional workers in particular agencies have been aware of the overlapping of services, confusion, interrelatedness, and complexity of the programs being carried out by its member agencies. A number of Council officials have wanted to plan for more efficient services, but they have been thwarted by a lack of information about what its member agencies were doing, for whom they were doing it, and with what effect.

Although each agency maintained office files on its patients or clients, it was rare for an agency to have basic information on individuals by the types of service rendered and by family groups in which more than one member might be receiving service. No data were available to link the individuals served to the population of the community, its subareas, or subsegments, as, for example, by age, sex, race, and socioeconomic group. Individual agencies periodically furnish the Community Council with summary statistics on services they rendered during a given time interval, usually the preceding year, supplemented by a statement by its staff of the agency's services and needs. Professional and lay persons in the Council were then asked to make decisions in the interest of the community. These decision-makers often relied on their own subjective judgments of what an agency was doing and what it needed. As a result, decisions were based upon a variable mix of statistics and opinion, with opinion usually the major component. Stated bluntly, the Community Council had little or no information on the sociobiographical characteristics of persons and families being served by individual health and welfare agencies on which to base the allocation of funds and their plans for the administration of services.

Faced with this issue, in January, 1967, the officers of the Community Council requested my services in finding solutions to some of their problems. It soon became clear to me that the first step necessary in the planning process was to gather community-wide information more adequate than the simple statistics available to the Community Council at that time. The key question was: *Who does what for whom* in the public sector of the community's health and welfare agencies? If an answer could be supplied for this question, the users of health and welfare services in this community could be compared with the total population. Thus, we needed and designed a system that would: (1) record the delivery of services of an agency to individuals and households; (2) collate the record of services received by a given individual or member of a household in more than one agency; and (3) determine the utilization of each health and welfare agency by particular population aggregates. In brief, the information system would reveal who was being served, where he was being served, what type of service he received, when and how often he received it, and if he received the same service from more than one agency. If more than one member of a household received a service, the system would record when, how often, and in what agency. The system would provide information over the years to answer such questions as: Does the use of service by individuals and household units shift agency by agency or by groups of agencies as a result of population, economic, or other changes in a specified area of the community? How can changes in the clientele of an agency be anticipated? How can changes in the community's need for services be forecast? What kind of planning should precede anticipated needs?

In designing the proposed information system, we knew we could not expect to use much of the client's or agency personnel's time in completing lengthy schedules of questions. We therefore automated procedures to the greatest extent possible. The key to this automation was a plastic card similar to the charge plates so widely used in industry and commerce. We called this item the Personal Service Card. The Personal Service Card would be interchangeable from agency to agency. It was to be the property of the individual to whom it was issued, and he was expected to present it to an agency when he sought a service. The information on the Personal Service Card would be transferred mechanically to a special form by a commercial imprinter that also identified the agency rendering the service, the date, and the type of service rendered. By a single movement of the imprinter's handle, these data would be transferred to a back-up card that, in turn, would be read by an optical scanner that would electronically punch the coded items on to a standard 80-column IBM card. The IBM card would be verified, then stored for transfer of the coded information to computer tape. Periodically, the tapes would be collated and summarized by the categories of individuals, household units, and agencies.

As originally designed, the Personal Service Card was to carry the name and address of the individual applying for service, his Social Security number (if he had one), and his age, sex, race, and marital status. In addition, we planned to gather information about the household in which the applicant lived: the name of the head of the household, his Social Security number, age, sex, race, marital status, years of school completed, exact occupation, and the number of persons living in the household. This background information would be placed in a computerized data bank. Overall, the system was planned so that we could trace the path of an individual from a referral agency to a treatment agency and to other agencies. We also intended to develop a master file on computer tape that would be a running record of the services every individual in a household unit received from week to week, month to month, and year to year. In April, 1967, the Board of Directors of the Community Council approved our plans.

What gave rise to this favorable action on the part of the Board of Directors? To answer this question meaningfully it is necessary to outline some of the forward-looking actions taken by community leaders in New Haven in the preceding 15 years. From 1953 to 1967, the city of New Haven had been in the forefront of urban renewal among American cities. A local action agency, Community Progress, Inc., financed originally by a Ford Foundation grant, antedated the Federal Economic Opportunity Act by more than two years. In 1966

86

and 1967, leaders in the community were proud that New Haven had been selected by the Department of Commerce as a site for a pretest of the 1970 United States Census. In addition, the city of New Haven, in cooperation with the International Business Machines Corporation, was initiating a program planning and budget system. The Community Council believed the planned information system would, in time, provide a factual base for planning more adequate services for the community's population, and the officers of the Council thought that this combination of circumstances had provided them with a unique opportunity to launch the first comprehensive effort to gather data on the delivery of personal services to individuals and families in a metropolitan community.

The development of a plan is one thing and its translation into action is another. In the fall of 1967, we became aware of a series of danger signals in the community which resulted from a number of different and apparently unrelated incidents:

First, friction was created in some segments of the community by the Federal test census of April, 1967. The Census Bureau required every fourth household to report detailed information on income and other sensitive personal items. The fact that the trial census occurred on April 5 and income tax returns were due on April 15 aroused suspicions that the Federal government might link figures on income given in the census schedule with figures given to the Internal Revenue Service, especially since both the Test Census Schedule and the familiar Form 1040 required the respondent to list his Social Security number. With the computers now used by the Bureau of the Census and the Internal Revenue Service, such a procedure would be possible, but illegal. The knowledge among community leaders and agency executives that our planned information system also intended to collect Social Security numbers from the users of services became a source of tension among a considerable number of professional men in private practice and entrepreneurs in personally owned businesses. The primary source of this tension, we believe, was traceable to distrust of the government and the threat posed by "data banks."

Second, the State of Connecticut announced that it would participate in an interstate study of mental patients, known at that time as the Seven State Study. This study required that each publicly supported psychiatric treatment agency communicate detailed data on its patients to the Commissioner of Mental Health. These data, in turn, would be sent to Rockland State Hospital in New York. Although there was no connection between the Seven State Study and our local project, the anxiety of some psychiatrists and social workers in several agencies concerning the patients' rights to privacy originally aroused by the interstate study was carried over to our information system.

Third, in mid-August, 1967, New Haven experienced a city-wide racial disturbance. After the "model riot in the model city" (as a psychiatrist called it a public meeting), concern was expressed about arousing antagonism among racial and ethnic minorities in the city who were assumed to be the largest users of the services of the community agencies. Thus, more questions were raised about the planned information system.

Fourth, in 1967, the United Fund was not able to meet its goals in its annual drive. The gap between hopes and pledges meant that some agencies were not going to receive the amount of money they had requested from the United Fund. When this became clear, some agency executives began to express doubts about the wisdom of starting a new program, even though it was to be financed for several years by grants from outside agencies.* These executives were concerned that in the future the information system would have to be financed by the United Fund, and they looked upon the United Fund's dollars as their dollars for service, not dollars for administrative functions. These fears were realistic. Each fall the United Fund has experienced difficulties in raising funds to meet the demands of social agencies in the community. There was a wide gap in 1969 and a wider gap in 1970 between voiced "needs" and available funds.

Fifth, and last, during the fall of 1967, Community Progress, Inc., the New Haven action agency mentioned earlier, received widespread publicity in the local media as being investigated by the area's Congressman. Some of his conclusions on the functioning of Community Progress, Inc. (C.P.I.) were as follows:

It is clear that C.P.I. is an overly centralized, paternalistic, big brother institution, manned by "planner-administrators" who believe that they know what is best for everyone. We have had these people in our midst for a long time in New Haven but at long last their ineffectiveness is beginning to show through. They serve themselves rather than the poor whom they are supposed to help. The investigation proves conclusively that they know how to take care of themselves. At the same time, it is quite clear to me that they have accomplished little if anything at all in bettering conditions among the poor in our cities. Salaries are extremely high, especially when one considers the 35-hour work week and liberal fringe benefits. Telephone costs are outrageous. Travel costs are high. Leasing procedures are very questionable, and I intend to look further into this practice.

Research costs have contributed nothing and have wasted $625,000. An $800,000 grant for a juvenile delinquency program went down the drain and accomplished nothing. C.P.I. must develop a better relationship with business and industry if it is to succeed in reducing unemployment. To date it has not done so and may well have alienated business and industry because of some of its philosophical attitudes.

The most serious indictment of C.P.I., however, is its attitude toward local existing agencies. Its attitude that these agencies had done nothing to solve local problems is incorrect. Its attitude that if it could not control the local agency it would have little or nothing to do with it is wrong.

---

*Preliminary design of the information system was supported by a small grant from the New Haven Foundation. The National Institute of Mental Health (Grant No. MH-15076) is furnishing the major part of the funds to support the information system during its early years.

I am convinced that we have many fine local agencies in New Haven which could do a much better job than C.P.I. and with much smaller overhead costs. The involvement of local organizations with their expertise, with their fine relationships with business and industry, labor, City Hall, the financial and charitable institutions and with the populace in general would result in a much more effective job in the antipoverty war. I am certain that if the 18 million dollars C.P.I. has received had been given to these local agencies without the C.P.I. hierarchy and superstructure draining off most of the money, we would have had more effective accomplishments in the anti-poverty war. They hardly could have done worse.[2]

By early 1968, a general mistrust of information-gathering and action agencies was voiced in the community. This distrust has not been mitigated by time.

From the inception of our plans, we realized that the idea of a community-wide information system would have to be carefully outlined, interpreted, and justified to the many segments of the community's population before we could hope to have the plan accepted. To allay any aroused anxieties, we planned to attend meetings of racial, religious, ethnic, and civic organizations and to arrange to give expository talks about the information system and to answer questions. Above all, we would have to explain the proposal thoroughly to the local mass media in the hope of sympathetic treatment. We did not, however, anticipate the resistance we met in late 1967 and on into 1968. (By 1969 and 1970, resistance became focused in the agencies we had selected for a trial run of the information system, but this is a story that cannot be told here.)

When dissent began to focus on our proposed information system, the president of the Community Council, a prominent attorney, made a thorough examination of the legal implications of what we planned to do. He reached the conclusion that what we were planning was legal but that the data we planned to put into the information system would be subject to subpoena in a court of proper jurisdiction. The privilege of confidentiality is defined by state law and, thus, varies from state to state. In Connecticut, sociologists are not privileged. Therefore, any data we might collect (questionnaires, interviews, tape recordings, diaries, etc.) would be subject to subpoena. The president of the Community Council also asked an advisory committee (originally appointed during the planning of the information system and composed of a distinguished New Haven psychiatrist in private practice, an officer of the largest private corporation in the community with a sophisticated knowledge of computerized data systems, and a Yale University professor with wide community contacts and competent in field studies in the behavioral and health sciences) to represent the interests of the Council in the controversy.

The research staff,* the officers of the Community Council, and the advisory committee decided to meet our critics face to face to discuss the issues that had

*August B. Hollingshead, principal investigator; Melvyn R. Diamond, project director; and Joan Jenkins, research assistant.

been voiced in disparate groups and through gossip. We met with spokesmen for several groups that were concerned about the planned information system. These spokesmen were mostly psychiatrists, lawyers, and social workers. The discussions during the meetings ranged widely over community issues and problems. Several lawyers raised the point that an investigator for a state or Federal agency might subpoena the records of the information system on a specific individual and find that he had been a mental patient or on welfare. This might be a barrier to employment. The fact that a person had received services from two or more agencies might subject him to "double stigmatization."[4] A lawyer representing the American Civil Liberties Union argued that the system would be an infringement of civil rights. Several psychiatrists charged that the system would be an invasion of privacy and a detriment to the confidential relationship between patient and physician so necessary for a healthy therapeutic outcome. This was an extreme position, since in a clinic or agency a number of different persons have access daily to patient records. The stigma of mental illness was always a factor in our conversations.* A crucial point was the fear that a future crusade, such as the late Senator Joseph McCarthy led in the early 1950s, could gather material on an individual or family from the master file that might destroy a political or occupational career. This was a real threat, as recent events in the nation have indicated.

Another area of controversy was our stated intention to link our data on individuals who used the agencies in the system with data collected by the United States Census. We planned to compare statistical data on individuals who used the agencies with those who did not, census tract by census tract. In the course of our sometimes heated conversations, the fact became clear that our critics had only the vaguest idea of the way the Bureau of the Census operates and little or no knowledge of the legal safeguards surrounding data in the custody of the Bureau of the Census.† Our critics could cite no incidents in which the Bureau of the Census had violated the law or the spirit of the Decennial Census, but such was the anxiety on this point that a number of persons expressed suspicions about the confidentiality of census data.[8]

"Informed consent" of patients or clients was another issue in our conversations. From the beginning of our study, we had stressed our intention of explaining the system to each patient or client and inviting participation. The patient or client would be *free* to accept or reject our invitation to enter the in-

---

*An early tangible outcome of the discussions we had with representatives of the local Mental Health Association, psychiatrists, lawyers, and social workers was the introduction of a bill in the 1969 Session of the State Legislature that redefined the confidentiality of psychiatric records. This bill was passed and is now on the statute books: An Act Concerning the Confidentiality of Communications and Records of Mental Patients. *General Statutes, State of Connecticut,* Section 52-146 a.

†Section 214, Title 13 in the United States Code provides: "Whoever, being an employee . . . , publishes or communicates, without written authority of the Secretary or another authorized officer or employee of the Department of Commerce or bureau or agency thereof, any information coming into his possession by reason of his employment under the provisions of this title, shall be fined not more than $1,000 or imprisoned not more than two years or both."

formation system. We realized, however, that it is difficult to explain to a sick or disturbed individual, sorely in need of help, how the system works. The patient or client might fear that if he did not go along with the invitation to join the information system he would not receive care in that agency. We had stressed that no one would be refused service because he would not participate in the information system. But even this was unacceptable to some of our critics.

By the spring of 1968, we concluded that we either had to modify our original design or drop the idea of a community-wide data-gathering system designed to determine who uses public health and welfare agencies. As we were not prepared to give up our plans at that time, we turned to the task of modifying the information system to meet the objections that had been raised during our conversations with different groups during the course of the winter.

Our intention to use Social Security numbers had been the focus of the most anxiety and hostility, whereas in our judgment, the use of Social Security numbers was the most efficient device for follow-up of individuals from agency to agency or address to address and for linking our data with those of the Census Bureau.* Another point of great concern to our critics was the inclusion of names and addresses of individuals in a central file in the research office. After considerable discussion within the research staff, we decided *not* to collect Social Security numbers or to use names and addresses, but we did decide to collect the remaining data as we had originally planned.

The data gathered in the revised information system are divided into three segments: (1) information on the Personal Service Card; (2) the date and the agency performing a service for a client; and (3) the nature of the service performed. The items on the Personal Service Card are: the serial number of the client (six figures), the age, race, sex, and marital status of the client, the race, sex, age, marital status, exact occupation, and years of school completed of the head of the client's household, and the number of persons living in the client's household. These items are coded numerically for transfer to an IBM card. The date on which a given agency performs a service and the agency's code number are recorded on the second segment of the IBM card. The nature of the service performed by the agency for the particular client is recorded on the last segment of the IBM card. Each time a service is performed for a client, a new card is made to record the action.

The redesigned system focuses attention upon sociobiographical data associated with unnamed individuals in household units in specified geographical areas of the community. The Standard Metropolitan Statistical Area is divided into census tracts. Individual and household units are coded by census tracts in the suburban towns, each containing some 500 household units, and by quarter-tracts in the city, each containing from 200 to 600 household units. This change met the major objections of concerned citizens and agency

*The 1967 test census had included Social Security numbers, and we were told that the 1970 Decennial Census would ask for them. The Bureau of the Census later decided not to ask for Social Security numbers in 1970.

personnel. Therefore, the decision was reached to move forward with this information system.

Methodologically, the changes made in the redesigned system do not weaken the possibilities for analysis at the community level. Although comparisons between the users and nonusers of agency services are more difficult, they are not impossible. This phase of the research plan involved linking data from our information system with data gathered in the test census of April 1967 and the Decennial Census of 1970. These plans were worked out in close consultation with officers of the Census Bureau. I stress very strongly that the projected comparisons between users and nonusers of services in the population would be made by the Bureau of the Census, not by the research staff of the Community Council. Thus, individual can be identified as being in either category by persons in the Research Office of the Community Council or in the New Haven community.

In July, 1968, the Community Council approved our new plan. The researchers and the executive secretary of the Community Council assured the Board of Directors of the Community Council that participation in the information system would be voluntary for each agency and each client. Thus, we proceeded to assemble the necessary supplies and machines and by late October, 1968, we were ready to begin the data gathering phase of our activities.

We first planned to test the feasibility of the information system in a limited number of agencies that performed different types of services. With this field trial in mind, we selected thirteen agencies: the New Haven City Welfare Department; the smaller of the community's two general hospitals; four mental health agencies; two family agencies; a dental clinic; a rehabilitation center; a homemaker's service; a neighborhood action agency; and a visiting nurse association. During the summer and fall of 1968, the project was outlined to the executive director of each agency, which was then invited to participate in the information system. Negotiations went on for several months. The directors needed time to discuss the invitation with their governing board and staff, and their decisions were reached slowly. One difficulty was that some directors were insecure in their relations with their governing board and/or their staff. Also, the meetings of the board of directors of most of the agencies were infrequent, and often the agenda for the next meeting was full, or our project was given a low position on the agenda so that a decision was often postponed for another month or two.

After a board gave its approval, the research staff had to explain the project to the agency's staff and train those who would be responsible for client intake and records. We soon learned that we had to adjust to the work patterns of each agency. Because the intake personnel in each agency were not prepared to explain the system to clients who were already receiving service, we had to alter our plans by limiting the project to newly admitted clients. This decision enabled us to initiate data collection in twelve of the thirteen agencies. With this new plan, we expected to be able eventually to enroll all clients who were willing to participate in the information system. We began to gather data in one agency on November 1, 1968, and activated the system in the eleven other agencies during the first nine months of 1969.

One of the questions of interest to the researchers, staff personnel, and concerned citizens was the proportion of clients willing to participate in the information system. Having asked each agency to record each individual's responses to the invitation to enter the system and to forward the information to the Research Office, we believe that we have enough information at this date to answer this question. The responses of individuals vary from agency to agency. The highest percentage of acceptance was in the dental clinic: 99.5 per cent of the patients were willing to participate in the project. The lowest percentage of acceptance occurred in one of the family agencies where the acceptance rate was 72.9 per cent. Overall, the acceptance rate in the 12 agencies participating in the feasibility trial was 92.7 per cent. By December 31, 1971, 7134 persons had entered the information system from the 12 participating agencies. Currently, data collection is going forward, and the data collected before January 1, 1971, are being analyzed. In due course, we expect to report our experiences and findings in a monograph.

Reactions to the idea of the information system can be characterized by groups. Generally speaking, the officers of the Community Council represented the interests of the larger society, as they conceived them, in assuming the responsibilities of coordinating the delivery of welfare services and in their desire to improve services. The psychiatrists generally feared that the information system would breach the confidential relationship between physician and patient. The lawyers were concerned with the client's right to privacy and the potential threat to an individual or family from governmental agencies. The social workers and agency executives were particularly sensitive about supplying data on their activities and their relations to other agencies to the Community Council and the United Fund. Lawyers, psychiatrists, and social workers were all sensitive to the issue of informed consent.

Representing the point of view of the researcher with a knowledge of the community and the experience to apply data gathering and processing techniques to a specific problem, I hoped to be able to link our data to the comprehensive data gathered by the Bureau of the Census. I believed that the study might well provide new insights into interrelations between social conditions in the community and the use of social agencies by its population. The opportunity to apply sociological knowledge to the solution of social problems was personally important to me. Having worked in this community for twenty years, I was personally and professionally identified with the New Haven area. Moreover, Yale University was concerned with the contribution its faculty could make toward improving the quality of life of the disadvantaged segment of the community's population.

Our experiences since early 1967 with the representatives of these differing points of view indicate that partisan interests need to be measured against the

93

general interests of the community. The individual's right to privacy must be respected, but this right is offset by a complex society's requirement for information to plan better services for those in need. In view of the increasingly high costs of health and welfare services in urban areas and the increasingly strident demands of minority groups for more services, the need for a social accounting system is particularly critical. The obligation to protect the privacy of those receiving services of any kind—whether aid to dependent children or treatment for mental disturbance—should be balanced by the need of duly constituted community authorities to know the sociobiographical characteristics of those who are served.

The issues raised in this discussion will continue to be of intense interest to lawyers, health professionals, social workers, social scientists, and concerned citizens. I believe our attempt to solve the problems posed by urban crises is likely to increase the need for information about individuals and their ways of life. This is likely to result in open conflict between partisans for and against the development and use of computerized data files. In the final analysis, access to data obtained by an information system such as the one I have discussed here will be a matter for determination by the courts.[9] It is the judiciary who must weigh and balance the need of the community for sociobiographical data against the right to personal privacy. Such a balance is needed to guide more adequate solutions to our social and psychiatric problems than are now at hand.

REFERENCES

1. DUFF, R.S., and HOLLINGSHEAD, A.B.: *Sickness and Society.* New York: Harper & Row, 1968.
2. GIAIMO, R.: "Report Criticizing C.P.I." *The New Haven Register,* New Haven, Connecticut, January 4, 1968.
3. HOLLINGSHEAD, A.B., AND REDLICH, F.C.: *Social Class and Mental Illness.* New York: John Wiley and Sons, 1958.
4. MORRIS, N.: "Psychiatry and the Dangerous Criminal." *Southern California Law Review* 41:514-547 (especially pp. 524-525), 1968.
5. MYERS, J.K., AND BEAN, L.L.: *A Decade Later: A Follow-Up of Social Class and Mental Illness.* New York: John Wiley and Sons, 1968.
6. MYERS, J.K., AND ROBERTS, B.H.: *Family and Class Dynamics in Mental Illness.* New York: John Wiley and Sons, 1959.
7. ROGLER, L.H., AND HOLLINGSHEAD, A.B.: *Trapped: Families and Schizophrenia.* New York: John Wiley and Sons, 1965.
8. TAEUBER, CONRAD: "Invasion of Privacy" [a comprehensive discussion of the issue of confidentiality in relation to the Bureau of the Census]. *Eugenics Quarterly* XIV:243-246, 1967.
9. WESTIN, A.F.: *Privacy and Freedom.* New York: Athanaeum (pp. 7, 27, 48, 49, 61-62, 356, and 386), 1967.
10. WHEELER, S. (ed.): *On Record: Files and Dossiers in American Life.* New York: Russell Sage Foundation, 1969.

CHAPTER 6

Strategies of Preventive Psychiatry and Social Reality: The Case of Alcoholism

PAUL M. ROMAN AND HARRISON M. TRICE

A principal goal included in the community mental health mandate is to eradicate or reduce the rates of undesirable behaviors defined as psychiatric disorders or as stemming from psychiatric disorders. The spectrum of existing and projected efforts toward this end is included under the rubric of "preventive psychiatry." In this chapter, we critically evaluate various preventive strategies and attempt to delineate the roots of the "prevention movement." Alcoholism and alcohol abuse, which tend to be classified on the borderline between deviant behavior and psychiatric disorder, are the focus of the present consideration as an area of intervention marked by a considerable range of preventive strategies. Much of our analysis of this area can be generalized to other preventive efforts where the targets are other forms of aberrant behavior.

Preventive activities may be defined as attempts to reduce the incidence of a disorder or type of deviant behavior and to minimize the impact of such behavioral patterns on the afflicted individuals and on the community at large.[10] Within preventive psychiatry, three types of prevention have been delineated: Primary prevention comprises those strategies designed to "lower the rate of onset of emotional disorder in the community."[59] Secondary prevention comprises those strategies oriented to locating instances of disorder early enough to reduce the incidence of "full-blown" disorder.[5] Tertiary prevention comprises those strategies oriented to "reducing the rate of defective functioning caused by mental disorder."[19] The present concern is solely with primary and secondary prevention, since tertiary prevention, i.e., studies of the outcome of therapy or rehabilitation efforts, has been given considerable attention elsewhere.[50]

Problems related to excessive use of alcohol have long been a concern of government, public health, religious, and medical professionals in American society.[2] The history of this country has been marked by sporadic efforts, sometimes of great social intensity, to reduce the disruptive effects of alcohol use through the manipulation of structures of social control. There have been periods in history when this concern was minimal.[49] However, at the present time, the prevailing image and definition of chronically excessive alcohol use is as a severe social problem.[40,11,17] One of the unique features of the current definition is that it attaches disease definitions to problem drinking of various types. These definitions are sanctioned by the American Medical Association, the World Health Organization, and nearly all other Western medical organizations and have brought alcohol problems under the aegis of medicine and psychiatry, although the definition of deviant drinking as a disease, as a psychiatric disorder, or as reflective of psychiatric disorder has not been universally accepted in either professional or lay circles.[64,35,9,57] Nonetheless, the disease model of alcoholism appears to have permeated the psychiatric profession and parapsychiatric occupations to such an extent that most preventive programs have been planned or executed within a medical or public health frame of reference. The history of public health had indicated that the prevention of disease is possible, the classic examples being Snow's work on cholera and Goldberger's studies of pellagra. Thus, by analogy, it is widely assumed that conditions labeled as diseases are preventable. This is the basic paradigm underlying the preventive efforts that are the focus of this chapter.

At the present time, the prevention of alcohol-related problems and disorders is a high priority activity of the Federally-funded National Institute of Alcohol Abuse and Alcoholism. Through its Division of Prevention, this agency is funding a range of activities designed for preventive outcomes, some of which are designed at the national level while others stem from local initiatives.

The twelve preventive strategies delineated here overlap. Frequently an actual preventive program uses several strategies in concert. For the sake of evaluation, however, they are separated here. The first five strategies are basically oriented toward individuals, with an emphasis on behavior change, protection, or treatment in specific populations; the remaining seven are focused on changes in the social structure. We outline the basic orientation of each strategy, its general use in prevention, and its specific use in alcoholism prevention. After considering these strategies and their deficiencies, we develop an account for the wide acceptance and support given to the prevention movement in contemporary American society.

INDIVIDUALLY ORIENTED PREVENTION

Differential Risks

A prominent preventive strategy that stems directly from public health experiences is the location of a subpopulation within a general population in which there is a higher risk for the individual of the development of a particular disorder or pattern of deviant behavior than in other subpopulations. Such a

96

subpopulation may be identified by genetic background, biochemical characteristics, membership in a cultural group found to have high rates of the disorder, or the location of individuals who have experienced specific stress risks believed or known to lead to the disorder. The major tactics in this strategy are that the subpopulation be (1) closely watched for signs of the development of the disorder, (2) kept in relative isolation from the stressors known to create risks for the disorder, and/or (3) treated in some way that reduces susceptibility to a particular disorder. Examples of this strategy in public health are tests for phenylketonuria to identify risk of mental retardation and the addition of niacin to diets of poor Southerners to prevent pellagra. This strategy has been used in preventive psychiatry as "crisis intervention" at known points of risk; examples are the close surveillance of mothers immediately following childbirth and intervention directed toward the bereaved.[59, 29] In the prevention of alcohol abuse, this strategy has been advocated,[39, 6] but no specific use of it is known.

Social Inoculation

With this strategy, the location of special risk populations is not necessary, since the major tactic is to make an entire population "immune" to a particular disorder through a uniform intervention designed to make the entire population nonreactive to stressors which may lead to the undesired condition. Within public health, examples of this strategy include inoculation and vaccination for the prevention of such major diseases as diptheria, smallpox, and poliomyelitis. More generally, early religious training and other types of specific education are frequently attempts at social inoculation. Programs that attempt to fortify young children for coping with stress are further examples of this strategy.[25, 59] In the prevention of alcohol abuse, state legislation regarding alcohol education in elementary and secondary schools[60] is an example of this strategy, although such program designs vary widely in scope and quality. This education has traditionally been "against alcohol," teaching that all alcohol use is harmful, a threat to health and society, etc.[53]

Plaut[39] has advocated a form of this strategy in what he calls "non-specific primary prevention." He argues that "since alcoholism can be viewed as a maladaptive means of dealing with personal problems or tensions, its rate would be reduced if, generally speaking, the psychological functioning of persons would be improved" [p. 66]. He cites successful examples of such prevention in preparing Peace Corps trainees for service abroad and in preparing patients for surgery, but does not specify the tactics for "improving psychological functioning." A similar argument has been advanced by Chafetz and Demone,[12] but here also there is no specification of means.

Education

With assumptions similar to the social inoculation model, the education model of prevention is broader in scope and is much more widely used. While social inoculation might attempt to project negative role models associated with undesirable behavior patterns, educational efforts emphasize the means for early identification of the disorder and drawing the line between acceptable and unacceptable types of behavior.[36,40] Education is designed to create a sense of responsibility rather than fear. "Education for positive mental health,"[13] "education for child-rearing,"[8,59] and sex education are examples of this approach.

In the prevention of alcoholism, education attempts to change attitudes and behavior regarding the appropriate or inappropriate uses of alcohol and to encourage toleration of abstinence and intolerance of drunkenness. This type of education has also been used in training personnel in work organizations to produce more realistic attitudes toward alcohol abuse and to attune supervisors to behavioral cues, such as job performance, that may identify deviant drinkers.[56] Thus, educational efforts may be oriented to preventing subsequent alcohol abuse among the trainees and to making them agents in an early identification program of secondary prevention. In 1973, the National Institute of Alcohol Abuse and Alcoholism created the National Center for Alcohol Education, giving it the mission of developing innovative strategies in the use of education as a preventive strategy.

Early Identification

This is the basic strategy of secondary prevention, which oftentimes subsumes the differential risk and education strategies. Rather than being oriented towards reducing the incidence of the outbreak of a disorder, the orientation is toward locating persons in the early stages of the disorder and intervening to alter the developing process. This strategy stems directly from the medical definition of aberrant behavior. Since one of the basic characteristics of disease is that it will get worse if not treated,[7] early identification is a logical step. Early identification generally involves locating a subpopulation in the early stages of a disorder by using physiological, psychological, or behavioral indices. Following identification, intervention is attempted, which, in accord with the strategy's assumptions, usually involves treatment to curb the disorder's progression. This strategy has been applied to many types of psychiatric disorders, to deviant behavior such as juvenile delinquency, and to alcohol abuse.

Direct Constructive Confrontation

This secondary prevention strategy operates on the assumption that if the occurrence of certain behaviors can be reduced or eliminated, the disorder will cease to be a problem. Thus, the focus is upon altering the central symptoms. Such efforts can take many forms, but they should not be confused with behavior therapy techniques used among persons with full-blown symptoms. Confrontation is directed toward early-stage cases. The strategy attempts to reduce the development of severe cases through the early identification of a surfacing problem and the early manipulation of exchange relationships in which the individual is involved. Those who possess greater social power than the problem individual may alter his behavior through threatening the removal of certain rewards. The usefulness of this strategy is affected by the clarity of the rewards and the roles involved; thus it can have more impact on the job than in the family.

The most clearcut example of this strategy in alcoholism prevention is in work organizations in "troubled employee" or employee alcoholism programs.[41, 57] Within the work role relationship, the employer demands a certain job performance in exchange for a specific remuneration to the employee. If the employee fails to perform adequately, the employer has the right to intervene. If the employee fails to alter his behavior or fails to seek help for his problem after a reasonable number of warnings, disciplinary action may be taken. The threat of such discipline is often adequate to motivate efforts towards behavior change, depending on how the individual values his job and job security. Since job performance is usually affected early in the progression toward alcohol addiction, job-based intervention has high potential effectiveness. Essential to the success of such efforts are the ability of supervisors to identify impaired job performance and to take appropriate action and the availability of means for referring cases for help supplemental to direct confrontation. A wide range of demonstration projects to diffuse the concepts of work-based alcoholism prevention programs are currently being supported by the Occupational Programs Branch of the National Institute of Alcohol Abuse and Alcoholism.

SOCIALLY ORIENTED PREVENTION

Reduction of Risks

This strategy is one of those aimed at changing the social circumstances surrounding individuals who may develop the disorder. Instead of attempting to provide individuals with increased resources to cope with etiological agents, this strategy is designed to reduce the incidence of stressors in the environment so that overall risk is reduced. In the history of public health, strategies to reduce environmental stress include the creation of closed sewage systems, the eradication of animals or insects which carry disease agents, and the provision of improved housing.

In alcoholism prevention, the lead of community psychiatry has been followed, and alcoholism specialists have advocated the strategy of "improving the community";[33] the means for accomplishing this laudable goal are not specified.

Replicating Immune Social Conditions

This strategy also follows the public health model and involves the location of populations or subpopulations that are relatively "immune" to certain disorders.[13] When such low incidence populations are located, research develops explanations for the low incidence which then provide the basis for preventive programs in other populations.

In alcoholism prevention, such attention has been focused upon the low rates of alcoholism in Jewish[46] and Italian[30] cultures and subcultures. Research has indicated that alcohol typically has a ritual and religious connotation in Jewish populations causing less tolerance for its abuse. Lolli and his associates[30] conclude that in Italian populations, alcohol is used in a family setting primarily as a foodstuff (in sharp contrast to the cocktail hour usage). This has created a set of attitudes that also sharply reduces tolerance for abuse. Researchers conclude that a common factor in both subcultures in accounting for low rates of alcohol abuse is the introduction of alcohol to children at an early age.[11] These observations have led to the advocacy that all children be introduced to alcohol at an early age[11] and that alcohol be used primarily with meals so that it is defined as a foodstuff and associated with the valued setting of the family.[40] No effort has been made to implement these preventive strategies on a major scale, but they have generated considerable debate.[21]

Normative Change

Closely related to replicating immune circumstances and to the education model is the advocacy of change in societal norms as a way of reducing alcohol addiction. Observers argue that excessive drinking is tolerated within American society, that abstinence is frequently the source of negative social sanctions and embarrassment, that alcohol is widely defined as a useful tranquilizer for "relaxation" and relief from personal problems,[40] and that official age norms for the use of alcohol make its use by teenagers a means for a role passage from adolescence to adulthood, i.e., the use of alcohol as symbolic of adulthood.[32] Likewise, we have suggested that emerging forms of approved drinking, such as that presently common on airlines, be discouraged from further development lest they become normative and thus difficult to reverse.

The straightforward argument of the advocates of normative change is that these things *should* not occur as they do; i.e., drunkenness should not be tolerated, abstinence should be tolerated and perhaps encouraged, alcohol should not be used as a means of personal relief, and social situations where alcohol use is strongly encouraged should be avoided. The means for bringing about such a widespread normative change are not, however, clearly specified. Apparently they might come from pervasive social change, specific campaigns, through the assumption of greater responsibility on the part of alcoholic beverage distributors and the mass media, and the cocktail party hosts who discourage inappropriate uses of alcohol.[40]

Prohibition

The premise of this preventive strategy is that the legal prohibition of potentially dangerous substances along with strict controls and punishments of their use will prevent addiction. It is assumed that a scheme of prohibition can be devised that will successfully eliminate the manufacture and use of these substances, even though a market demand exists for them. The American experience in the first quarter of this century with the prohibition of alcohol[45] and the current attempts at prohibiting the sale and use of opiates, psychedelic drugs, and marijuana exemplify this approach. In contrast to other preventive schemes we have considered, this one is obviously limited to disorders involving substance abuse.

Severe Sanctions

This preventive strategy is similar to prohibition but does not include the assumption that control of the manufacture and sale of the deviance producing substances will be effective. Therefore the use or inappropriate use of these substances is met with severe sanctions that presumably lead to the deviant's realization that the cost of a particular behavior pattern is too high for its continuation. This realization may come through personal experience or by witnessing examples of sharp societal punishment of deviant behavior. Legal sanctions accompanying conviction for "crimes without victims," e.g., homosexuality or drug use, are illustrative of this approach.[44]

Examples of this preventive approach in the area of alcoholism are criminal punishments for public drunkenness and immediate suspension of a motor vehicle operator's license of persons who drink and drive. Several European countries have gone so far as to immediately imprison the drinking driver.

Severe sanctions in regard to alcohol use in some relatively isolated subcultures are instances of successful uses of this strategy. For example, Barnett[3] accounts for low rates of alcoholism among the Cantonese Chinese by the social ostracism of heavy drinkers in this group.

Functional Substitutes

An alternative to the strategy of prohibition is the use of substitutes that serve some of the same functions as the precursors of undesirable disorders but do not contain the harmful elements. The most clearcut example of functional substitutes is found in methadone maintenance,[16] which constitutes an attempt at the tertiary prevention of opiate addiction. Here the functional substitute is designed to eliminate the craving for and the rewards of the addictive substance, essentially creating a substitute addiction.

In terms of alcohol abuse, it has been advocated that research be undertaken to locate the addictive elements in alcoholic beverages, which could then be removed apparently to make any form of alcohol use "safe."[40] It has also been suggested that the alcoholic content of various legal beverages be reduced as a means of reducing addictive potential,[40] or that the use of beer and wine be encouraged as alternatives to "hard" liquor. In regard to the use of alcohol on airlines, we have suggested that entertainment of passengers through music or movies be extended to more flights and that a more desirable selection of nonalcoholic beverages be offered. Lemert[27] has approached the issue of functional substitutes for alcohol from a sociological frame of reference. He argues that alcohol use in American society is serving numerous functions, some of which are more obvious than others. Lemert believes that research must delineate these functions and their interconnections before effective substitutes for alcohol can be located.

Revision of Societal Definitions

This relatively unique preventive strategy stems from action by the group labeled deviant rather than by mandated societal agencies. The strategy calls for a reduction in the incidence of certain abnormal behaviors by changing the societal definition of categories of behavior from abnormal to normal. Illustrative are the efforts by organized homosexual groups to create normative acceptance of their patterns of sexual behavior.[44, 23, 65] Efforts to legalize marijuana are another example.

The widespread campaign to redefine alcohol abuse as a disease rather than as a form of immoral behavior was initially an attempt of this type of preventive strategy.[24] We do not know whether this attempt at destigmatization has made alcohol abuse more respectable and therefore less threatening to potential problem drinkers or whether it has reduced its incidence, but it does seem clear that this redefinition paved the way for societal acceptance of efforts to deal with the problem in a humane fashion. This may in turn pave the way for societal investment in preventive activities.

DATA-BASED EVALUATION

Although several of these preventive approaches have been implemented in varying degrees, relatively little evaluation data are available for assessing their effectiveness. The education strategy has been most widely used. One widely cited effort geared at preventive results through mental health education[14] revealed a small increase in negative attitudes toward the mentally ill following the education program. Evaluation of the well known Cambridge-Somerville project, a carefully organized guidance-counseling project for youth judged to be at risk for developing delinquent behavior, showed minimal effects. A range of studies of the effectiveness of drug education have reported minimal reduction of drug abuse. In some instances it is believed that educational programs have served to inform youth about drug abuse alternatives rather than leading them to drug avoidance.

Turning to evaluations of alcoholism prevention, Williams and his associates[61] evaluated an alcohol education program directed at male high school students and found reduction of deviant drinking practices a month after the end of the program, but a general return to previous behavior patterns a year later. Trice and Belasco[56] reported increases in negative attitudes toward alcoholics among some supervisors following an extensive job-based training program. Negative evaluations of the "noble experiment" of Prohibition abound, emphasizing its adverse side effects. There are no available data to support the preventive value of age constraints on drinking. On the other hand, data have been accumulating for some time on the secondary preventive value of programs based in work organizations which employ a combination of early identification and constructive confrontation, beginning with the evaluative study of Franco[18] in a large metropolitan utility company. A recent descriptive study of similar programs in 11 large companies supports the effectiveness of this strategy.[22] Drinking-driver programs have been reported to reduce traffic accidents and fatalities, but their impact on the incidence of problem drinking is unknown.

ASSUMPTIONS OF PREVENTIVE STRATEGIES

Definition of Alcoholism

At base in the problem of developing effective prevention strategies are the questionable assumptions that underlie them. We now turn to a review of these assumptions. While we focus on alcoholism prevention, many of these problems can be generalized to other foci of preventive psychiatry. One assumption that underlies all these preventive strategies is that undesirable behavior can be defined and delineated. But perusal of the numerous "official" definitions of alcoholism and deviant drinking[64] reveals that the definition of the so called "disease" condition is highly dependent upon normative traditions and situational tolerances, such as the nature of ongoing activities in particular social systems. Thus alcohol abuse in one setting may be acceptable use in another. A crucial point is that most deviant drinkers have not developed physiological addiction, and intake of alcohol is still under their control. Until the individual is intensely addicted both physiologically and psychologically, the use of the disease concept may be inappropriate in prematurely labeling the individual and absolving him of responsibility for his drinking problem. There is considerable ambiguity and variation in definitions of alcoholism employed by psychiatrists and other professionals. Thus, the use of the public health model of prevention may be inappropriate since the target disease state cannot be identified by agreed upon physiological criteria. This problem would be partially solved by acceptance of physiological addiction to alcohol as the criterion for the target behavior, but this criterion would miss the vast majority of problem drinkers. Expansion of the definition of alcoholism through the use of more prevalent clinical criteria seems to create the reverse problem of including a vast number of persons whose behavior is not disordered. One example of expansion is Chafetz's definition of the alcoholic population to include those who by their own or someone else's judgement have been intoxicated four times in one year and those who have acted

103

under the influence of alcohol in ways they would not have acted otherwise.[11] Another suggested definition of alcoholism is via the reactions of others to the drinker's role performance;[9, 57] i.e., intervention is called for when others cease to tolerate the individual's behavior. While such a definition seems more feasible and eliminates the problem of setting criteria, it contradicts the basic disease model assumptions. In sum, while the disease definition may set the stage for preventive intervention, it raises sharp problems in the designation of a target population. Those of us who employ the behavioral definition attempt reconciliation by minimizing the use of the term alcoholism and by referring to alcohol abuse as a health problem.[57]

Known Etiology

A second major assumption of all the preventive strategies, except early identification, prohibition, severe sanctions, and revision of societal definitions, is that the etiology of problem drinking or alcoholism is known. However, no clearcut empirical evidence has specified genetic, biochemical, psychological, or sociological attributes as the cause of alcohol problems. While risk factors have been hypothesized,[42] they do not provide for isolation of specific subpopulations, thus impeding preventive strategies. Likewise, programs oriented toward educating persons in the appropriate uses of alcohol are hampered by lack of knowledge about patterns of alcohol use that lead to drinking problems. The history of public health clearly indicates that the discovery of etiology preceded the effective prevention of deficiency conditions such as pellagra and of infectious diseases. In certain instances, effective treatments were discovered previous to the discovery of etiology, e.g., some psychotropic drugs, the mechanisms of which are largely unknown. However, prevention without knowledge of etiology involves risks, which can also be illustrated by the use of psychotropic drugs, e.g., the incidence of undesirable long-term side effects and unanticipated allergic reactions.

Means of Social Change

A third important assumption underlying most preventive strategies is that normative structures can be manipulated and changed, and, furthermore, that such change can proceed with minimal disruption to existing social structures. Without detailing arguments about social equilibrium, it seems obvious that normative structures have degrees of interdependence such that their removal and replacement can generate large scale disruptions in other parts of the structure.[47, 37]

Most preventive strategies are designed without a knowledge of how normative structures are changed. It appears summarily naive to assume that a particular pattern of behavior can simply be "grafted" into a culture by education, prohibition, or functional substitution. It is also important to consider what desirable latent functions certain undesirable behavior patterns, such as certain types of drinking, may be serving. For example, a clearcut mode of passage from adolescence to adulthood appears to be crucial for youth to internalize adult identities and to undertake socially responsible adult behavior.[63] One of the neglected findings of Maddox and McCall's research on teenage drinking[32] was that adolescent drinking appeared to create symbolic rites of passage into adulthood that are typically lacking in other segments of a complex industrial society. Another obviously desirable function of alcohol is the "social lubrication" of gatherings of relative strangers, leading in many instances to valuable relationships. The removal of these functions might have disruptive consequences for the system as a whole.

Behavior Change

A fourth assumption directly underlying the social inoculation and education strategies is that effective means of individual behavior change are known. The meager evaluation data available indicate that actual behavior change is most difficult to bring about through education.[61, 56, 1] In other words, although education and training programs proceed at a large scale at nearly every level of society, rigorous evaluation of the actual impact of such attempts is rarely undertaken, and when it has been carried out, has yielded disappointing results. Preventive programs are conducted with little knowledge of effective tactics for behavior change, and program advocates appear to assume that rigorous evaluation is impossibly disruptive or that trial equals success.

Lemert[28] and Roman and Trice[43] have described the insidious process of "normalization" in social groups as a covert block to preventive schemes that attempt to make persons more sensitive to their fellows' deviance. An example is the tendency for groups to concentrate on goal attainment, resulting in a broadening of tolerance once deviance occurs. That is, in order for the group to continue functioning without the disruption of a labeling process and the removal of a group member, deviant acts are "normalized" and made acceptable. This process may continue until the deviance itself prevents the group from continuing to attain its goals. Other forces leading to normalization are the use of deviant group members as scapegoats, the fact that a deviant may occupy the lowest status in the group and thus elevate others' statuses, the fear of "boomerang labeling" should attempts at early identification lead to retaliation, and concern over being imputed as a causal factor in generating a fellow's undesirable behavior. This formulation clearly points to a pragmatic element in social life that may render laymen's intervention relatively ineffective.

Right to Intervene

A fifth assumption that underlies all the strategies is the right of certain individuals or groups to intervene. Assuming that a population at risk could be identified, what assurance is there that a program of early identification and treatment or ongoing surveillance would be met with cooperation? Without doubt, Americans intensely value their right to privacy and enjoy Constitutional protection of this right. To a considerable extent, the legitimacy of mandates has sidestepped this difficulty when the target disorders are defined as medical problems.

What degree of cooperation could be expected in proposed programs of "social overhaul" which, for example, would require families to use alcohol only with meals or agree to introduce alcohol to their children at an early age? The thorny issue of the "right to treat" has led to considerable controversy in both psychiatry and law in recent years.[51, 52]

Side Effects

A sixth assumption underlying all the strategies is that undesirable side effects stemming from the involvement of the population in preventive programs will be minimal. As Lemert[27] has pointed out, there is no assurance in a society undergoing rapid change that values and attitudes indoctrinated in childhood will be subsequently serviceable in adulthood. Recent sociological research and theory indicates that a major undesirable consequence of preventive efforts may be the premature labeling of a person as "sick," as when, for example, his use of alcohol is still under his personal control.[41] Premature labeling may provide the individual with an excuse for subsequent deviance and may also result in a change in self-concept from "normal" to "deviant," in which case a self-fulfilling prophecy may ensue.[26] While labeling effects have been exaggerated,[20] evaluative research may produce insights into the mix of intended and unintended impacts of implemented preventive strategies.

Effective Treatment

A final assumption underlying most of these strategies is that some effective form of treatment is available for those who are identified in the early stages of alcohol addiction. Although research indicates that treatment during the early stages has a higher degree of effectiveness than that which begins subsequent to physiological addiction,[54] no clearcut form of widely effective treatment has yet been delineated. While systematic selection for different treatment modalities is a potential use of treatment evaluation data,[58] little progress along this line has been made. Thus many individuals revealed in a program of early identification may simply be put through a premature labeling process and subjected to ineffective treatment, the overall consequence of which may be relatively long term careers in deviant drinking. Furthermore, as McGavran[33] has argued, in the history of public health, successful prevention has not been associated with early identification, but rather with knowledge of etiology.

Three preventive strategies are relatively independent of the unsubstantiated assumptions outlined above. These are constructive confrontation based in exchange relationships, attempts to halt or discourage disordered behavior through the administration or threat of severe sanctions, and elimination of the problem through societal redefinition. The strategies of constructive confrontation and severe sanctions are somewhat similar, except that constructive confrontation attempts to manipulate existing rewards and punishments through the threat of job loss, while severe sanctions involve the introduction of new punishments. In the use of the latter, it is assumed that the individual can be shown the relative costs of negative sanctions, while constructive confrontation is essentially a private demonstration of potential costs. Finally, and perhaps most important, severe sanctions involve negative imagery and their administration may involve abrupt labeling and severe role disruption; by contrast, constructive confrontation is positively oriented to maintaining role performance.

The exchange relationship between employer and employee is much clearer than most role relationships. Of great importance is the recognition by both parties of the employer's legitimate *right* to intervene. Furthermore, in the constructive confrontation in a work situation, the deviant is still within the context of stable relationships and social control so that the risk of rejection with a consequent drift into deviant drinking subcultures is somewhat reduced.[55] Finally, this approach involves offering help in dealing with the disorder rather than relying solely on the threat of discipline or job loss. Constructive confrontation is, however, limited to employed adults, who are the majority of early-stage deviant drinkers, but it does not reach a minority of the target population, the housewife with a drinking problem. Nor should we imply that this strategy is free from operational difficulties. Work supervisors are usually reluctant to engage in early identification because of the pressures for normalization found in work groups.[43, 57] Furthermore, while the *right* of employer intervention is clear, the *grounds* for intervention, e.g., impaired job performance, are ambiguous in many occupations, particularly middle- and upper-status white collar jobs.

The strategy of changing societal definitions seems to hold considerable merit. The definition of a range of patterns of deviant alcohol use as disease conditions is not only ambiguous but often inappropriate. Broadening definitions of many disorders produces the rising rate estimates that appear in the publications of various agencies concerned with alcoholism and points to a phenomenon novel to industrial societies, namely the "social problem industry." So called social problems receive a large proportion of national resources and, as is the usual case with expenditures of large sums of money, vested interests develop in regard to the continued existence and expansion of these problems. The expansionist trend in medicine and psychiatry has been aided by epidemiological studies of untreated populations which have labeled the vast majority of the non-help-seeking population to be "psychiatrically impaired" to some degree.[48] The present "crises" in American society in regard to alcohol abuse may be in some part an artifact of these ongoing redefinitions which expand the problem and attract allocation of more resources for its solution. Therefore, definitional changes stemming from recognition of the fact that many patterns of alcohol abuse can be controlled by laymen through "constructive persuasion" may lead to substantial reductions in the statistics on the incidence of the disease of alcoholism.

SUPPORTS FOR THE PREVENTION MOVEMENT

Given the wide range of unsubstantiated assumptions that cast doubt on the effectiveness of most preventive strategies, why have activities directed toward prevention attracted such wide attention and resource investment? There are several interacting factors that account for this phenomenon.

First, within the humanitarian value orientation traditional in American society,[62] disease conditions are regarded as undesirable and worthy of attention. Thus the broad definition of psychiatric disorder to cover various types of alcohol abuse and myriad other types of deviance[15] lends positive social sanctions to efforts preventing these conditions. As pointed out, the use of the disease model coupled with the history of preventive success in public health creates the assumption that the prevention of other, new disease conditions is also possible.

A second and related factor is the pragmatic "action" orientation so highly valued in American society.[62,34] The activist orientation, in contrast to the fatalistic view that it is impossible to alter undesirable conditions, calls for taking action to solve social problems rather than allowing their continued existence. Moreover, immediate preventive efforts are more compatible with American values than long-term, tedious processes of scientific theorizing and research. Doing something *now*, regardless of realistic impact, is largely acceptable within this cultural framework. The allocation of resources to "shot in the dark" preventive efforts is also greatly bolstered by their identification with the highly prestigious medical profession.

A third factor that has influenced the allocation of resources and attention to the prevention movement is the attempt by the medical profession to broaden its societal mandate and thereby its power, authority, and prestige. Undertaking the new role of prevention, in addition to the traditional roles of identification and treatment, creates a large new area for the expansion of the authority of the medical profession. The nature of this role is parallel to Becker's concept of the "moral entrepreneur," i.e., "crusader" who undertakes to prohibit certain behaviors in society.[4] Becker contends that the medical professionals' aid may be eventually enlisted by the crusader. However, in contemporary preventive psychiatry, physicians, with their allied occupations and professors, may themselves be assuming the "crusader" role.

A fourth factor is the passage of the 1963 Community Mental Health Center Act. This Act set the stage for the burgeoning of community psychiatry, including in its mandate the need for prevention activities at the community level.[10] With specific budgetary allocations for preventive activities, preventive programs move ahead in response to this societal mandate. We thus have a revolution that is relatively devoid of conceptualization and that has been referred to as a case of "the Emperor's new clothes."[38] This revolution grows from resource allocation by formal legislative authority rather than from discoveries and inventions by the scientific community.

As part of the formal mandate of the community mental health movement, prevention has received the least attention and probably represents the least accomplishment. At the same time, it is a concept that generates great enthusiasm and hope, with critiques of its feasibility bound to be unpopular.

CONCLUSION

To conclude, it appears that current attempts to prevent alcohol abuse are based largely on unwarranted assumptions, which may themselves be preventing prevention. The problems outlined extend to preventive efforts with other targets. The legislative mandate for prevention, the tendencies toward expansion of areas of professional authority, and a rapidly growing system of organizations that have vested interests in the expansion of definitions of problems, have led to advocacy of preventive strategies that are largely unguided by systematic principles or supportive data. Perhaps etiological models will develop from preventive experiences that will, in turn, lead to effective prevention. On the other hand, Bordua[7] may have described the situation more accurately: "The specific empirical research done in any period will heavily reflect social interest in specific forms of deviance as evidenced by the availability of public and private research funds, and may not either reflect or foreshadow significant intellectual developments" [p. 149].

REFERENCES

1. ARGYRIS, C.: "Some Unintended Consequences of Rigorous Research." *Psychological Bulletin* 70: 185-197, 1968.
2. BACON, S.D.: "Alcohol and Complex Society," in David J. Pittman and Charles R. Snyder (eds.): *Society, Culture and Drinking Patterns*, pp. 78-94. New York: Wiley and Sons, 1962.
3. BARNETT, M.: "Alcoholism in the Cantonese of New York City," in O. Diethelm (ed.): *Etiology of Chronic Alcoholism*, pp. 179-225. Springfield, Ill.: Charles C. Thomas, 1955.
4. BECKER, H.S.: *Outsiders.* New York: Free Press, 1963.
5. BERLIN, I.N.: "Secondary Prevention," in Alfred M. Freedman and Harold I. Kaplan (eds.): *Comprehensive Textbook of Psychiatry*, pp. 1541-1548. Baltimore: Williams and Wilkins, 1967.
6. BLANE, H.T.: *The Personality of the Alcoholic.* New York: Harper and Row, 1968.
7. BORDUA, D.J.: "Recent Trends: Deviant Behavior and Social Control." *Annals of the American Academy of Political and Social Science* 369: 149-163, 1967.
8. BRIM, O.G.: *Education for Child-Rearing.* New York: Russell Sage Foundation, 1960.
9. CAHALAN, D.: *Problem Drinkers.* San Francisco: Jossey-Bass, 1970.
10. CAPLAN, G.: *Principles of Preventive Psychiatry.* New York: Basic Books, 1964.
11. CHAFETZ, M.E.: "Alcoholism Prevention and Reality." *Quarterly Journal of Studies on Alcohol* 28: 345-348, 1967.
12. CHAFETZ, M.E., AND DEMONE, H.: *Alcoholism and Society.* New York: Oxford University Press, 1962.
13. CUMMING, E.: "Pathways to Prevention," in *Key Issues in the Prevention of Alcoholism*, pp.

11-25. Harrisburg, Pa.: State Department of Health, 1963.

14. CUMMING, J., AND CUMMING, E.: *Closed Ranks.* Cambridge: Harvard University Press, 1957.

15. DUNHAM, H.W.: "Community Psychiatry: The Newest Therapeutic Bandwagon." *Archives of General Psychiatry* 12: 303-313, 1965.

16. EINSTEIN, S.: *Methadone Maintenance.* New York: Marcel Dekker, 1971.

17. FORT, J.: *Alcohol.* New York: McGraw-Hill, 1973.

18. FRANCO, S.C.: "Problem Drinking in Industry: Review of a Company Program." *Industrial Medicine and Surgery* 26: 221-228, 1957.

19. FREEDMAN, A.M.: "Tertiary Prevention," in Alfred M. Freedman and Harold I. Kaplan (eds.): *Comprehensive Textbook of Psychiatry,* pp. 1548-1552. Baltimore: Williams and Wilkins, 1967.

20. GOVE, W.: "Societal Reaction to Mental Disorders." *American Sociological Review* 36: 318-340, 1970.

21. HILTNER, S.: "Alcoholism Prevention and Reality: Comment on the Article by M.E. Chafetz." *Quarterly Journal of Studies on Alcohol* 28: 348-349, 1967.

22. HORN, D., AND RILEY, F.: *Attitudes Toward Alcohol in 11 Companies.* Palo Alto: Stanford Research Institute (mimeo), 1973.

23. HUMPHREYS, L.: *Out of the Closets.* Englewood Cliffs, N. J.: Prentice-Hall, 1973.

24. JELLINEK, E.M.: *The Disease Concept of Alcoholism.* New Haven: College and University Press, 1960.

25. KELLAM, S.G., AND SCHIFF, S.K.: "Adaptation and Mental Illness of First Grade Classrooms of an Urban Community," in M. Greenblatt, P. Emery and B.C. Glueck, Jr. (eds.): *Poverty and Mental Health,* pp. 79-91. Washington, D.C.: American Psychiatric Association, 1967.

26. LEMERT, E.M.: *Social Pathology.* New York: McGraw-Hill, 1951.

27. LEMERT, E.M.: "Alcohol, Values and Social Control," in David J. Pittman and Charles R. Snyder (eds.): *Society, Culture and Drinking Patterns,* pp. 553-571. New York: Wiley and Sons, 1962.

28. LEMERT, E.M.: *Human Deviance, Social Problems and Social Control.* Englewood Cliffs, N.J.: Prentice-Hall, 1967.

29. LINDEMANN, E.: "Recent Studies on Preventive Intervention in Social and Emotional Crises," in Ralph H. Ojemann (ed.): *Recent Research Looking Toward Preventive Intervention,* pp. 12-41. Iowa City: State University of Iowa, 1961.

30. LOLLI, G., SERIANNI, E., GOLDER, G.M., AND LUZZATTO-FEGIZ, P.: *Alcohol in Italian Culture.* New Brunswick, N.J.: Rutgers Center of Alcohol Studies, 1958.

31. LONDON, P.: *Behavior Control.* New York: Harper and Row, 1969.

32. MADDOX, G.L., AND McCALL, B.C.: *Drinking Among Teenagers.* New Brunswick, N.J.: Rutgers Center of Alcohol Studies, 1964.

33. McGAVRAN, E.: "Facing Reality in Public Health," in *Key Issues in the Prevention of Alcoholism,* pp. 55-61. Harrisburg, Pa.: State Department of Health, 1963.

34. MERTON, R.K.: "Social Problems and Sociological Theory," in Robert K. Merton and Robert A. Nisbet (eds.): *Contemporary Social Problems,* pp. 715-716. New York: Harcourt, Brace and World, 1966.

35. MULFORD, H.A., AND MILLER, D.E.: "Measuring Public Acceptance of the Alcoholic as a Sick Person." *Quarterly Journal of Studies on Alcohol* 25: 314-321, 1964.

36. NATIONAL CENTER FOR THE PREVENTION AND CONTROL OF ALCOHOLISM: *Alcohol and Alcoholism.* Washington, D.C.: Government Printing Office, 1966.

37. PAUL, B.D.: *Health, Culture and Community.* New York: Russell Sage Foundation, 1955.

38. PIEDMONT, E., AND DOWNEY, K.: "Revolutions in Psychiatry: The Emperor's New Clothes." Presented to the Society for the Study of Social Problems, San Francisco, August 30, 1967.

39. PLAUT, T.F.A.: "Translating Concepts into Action," in *Key Issues in the Prevention of Alcoholism,* pp. 62-72. Harrisburg, Pa.: State Department of Health, 1963.

40. PLAUT, T.F.A.: *Alcohol Problems: A Report to the Nation.* New York: Oxford University Press, 1967.

41. ROMAN, P.M., AND TRICE, H.M.: "The Sick Role, Labeling Theory and the Deviant Drinker." *International Journal of Social Psychiatry* 13: 245-251, 1968.

42. ROMAN, P.M., AND TRICE, H.M.: "The Development of Deviant Drinking." *Archives of Environmental Health* 11: 242-257, 1970.

110

43. ROMAN, P.M., AND TRICE, H.M.: "Normalization." Paper presented to the American Sociological Association, Denver, 1971.
44. SCHUR, E.M.: *Crimes Without Victims*. Englewood Cliffs, N.J.: Prentice-Hall, 1965.
45. SINCLAIR, A.: *Prohibition: The Era of Excess*. Boston: Little, Brown and Co., 1962.
46. SNYDER, C.R.: *Alcohol and the Jews*. New Brunswick, N.J.: Rutgers Center of Alcohol Studies, 1958.
47. SPICER, E.M.: *Human Problems in Technological Change*. New York: Russell Sage Foundation, 1954.
48. SROLE, L., LANGNER, T.S., MICHAEL, S.T., OPLER, M.K., AND RENNIE, T.A.C.: *Mental Health in the Metropolis*. New York: McGraw-Hill, 1961.
49. STRAUS, R.: "Alcohol," in Robert K. Merton and Robert A. Nisbet (eds.): *Contemporary Social Problems*, pp. 236-280. New York: Harcourt, Brace and World, 1966.
50. SUSSMAN, M.B.: *Sociology and Rehabilitation*. Washington, D.C.: American Sociological Association, 1966.
51. SZASZ, T.S.: *Law, Liberty and Psychiatry*. New York: Macmillan, 1963.
52. SZASZ, T.S.: *Psychiatric Justice*. New York: Macmillan, 1965.
53. TODD, FRANCES: *Teaching About Alcoholism*. New York: McGraw-Hill, 1964.
54. TRICE, H.M.: "Reaction of Supervisors to Emotionally Disturbed Employees." *Journal of Occupational Medicine* 7: 177-188, 1965.
55. TRICE, H.M.: *Alcoholism in America*. New York: McGraw-Hill, 1966.
56. TRICE, H.M., AND BELASCO, J.A.: "Supervisory Training about Alcoholics and Other Problem Employees: A Controlled Evaluation." *Quarterly Journal of Studies on Alcohol* 29: 382-398, 1968.
57. TRICE, H.M., AND ROMAN P.M.,: *Spirits and Demons at Work: Alcohol and Other Drugs on the Job*. Ithaca, New York: Cornell University, 1972.
58. TRICE, H.M., ROMAN, P.M., AND BELASCO, J.A.: "Selection for Treatment." *International Journal of the Addictions* 4: 303-317, 1969.
59. VISOTSKY, H.: "Primary Prevention," in Alfred M. Freedman and Harold I. Kaplan (eds.): *Comprehensive Textbook of Psychiatry*, pp. 1537-1541. Baltimore: Williams and Wilkins, 1967.
60. WILKINSON, R.: *The Prevention of Drinking Problems*. New York: Oxford, 1970.
61. WILLIAMS, A.F., DICICCO, L.M., AND UNTERBERGER, H.: "Philosophy and Evaluation of an Alcohol Education Program." *Quarterly Journal of Studies on Alcohol* 29: 685-702, 1968.
62. WILLIAMS, R.M., JR.: *American Society*. New York: Knopf, 1960.
63. YOUNG, F.W.: *Initiation Ceremonies*. Indianapolis: Bobbs-Merrill, 1964.
64. KELLER, MARK: "The Definition of Alcoholism and Estimation of Its Prevalence," in Pittman, David, and Snyder, Charles (eds.): *Society, Culture and Drinking Patterns*. New York: John Wiley & Sons, 1962.
65. HOFFMAN, MARTIN: *The Gay World*. New York: Basic Books, 1968.

Part II

COMMUNITY MENTAL HEALTH IN ACTION

INTRODUCTION

Having explored a series of general issues and problems in carrying out community mental health programs, it is appropriate to describe and evaluate specific programs in action from several sociological perspectives. The five chapters in this section cover a wide range. Chapter 7 describes the panorama of programs in community mental health practice and the myriad problems encountered in evaluating them. Chapters 8 and 9 describe interorganizational and interprofessional problems raised with the addition of community mental health activities to ongoing treatment institutions. Chapter 10 describes a unique and partly unexpected positive impact rendered by a community development program that was essentially a spin-off from a large scale social psychiatric research project. This chapter, with the dramatic nature of some of the results reported, tends to temper the critical tone of some of the foregoing chapters. A similar positive tone is set by a summary of evaluations of home treatment in Chapter 11.

Although these are our dominant themes, others emerge in the process of analysis. After delineating the plethora of therapeutic actions included under the umbrella of community mental health and community psychiatry, Trice and Roman in Chapter 7 discuss the basic problems of evaluative research in community psychiatry. Simply put, evaluative research in community mental health calls for the interaction between two alien groups: action oriented practitioners and intellectually oriented researchers. We locate the sources of this nearly fatal flaw in the nature of evaluative research in the makeup of the community mental health movement and in the role of the evaluative researcher himself. Because much resistance to evaluative research derives from its tendency to use the goal attainment model and the experimental designs associated with it, we examine other models, such as systems analysis and ceremonial approaches, and offer a somewhat radical departure from all of these, urging evaluative researchers to use the indigenous evaluative efforts of practitioners themselves as their starting point. Despite the biases of practitioners, such a starting point gives the evaluative researcher a basis for harmonizing his activities with those evaluative processes indigenous to the action program and places the evaluator in a position to refine the strategies native to and understood by practitioners. We put forth suggestions for adapting evaluative research to community mental health programs and describe less irritating versions of experimental designs, suggesting, for example, that two types of distinct treatment programs can be legitimately compared as an alternative to seeking illusive and potentially controversial "control groups," a strategy explored by Angrist and Dinitz in Chapter 11. We urge practitioners to explore the system integration model for evaluative research since it seems more realistic for community mental health programs than the traditional goal attainment model.

In Chapter 8, Ellison, Rieker, and Marx thoroughly examine "the most significant and unique profession-relevant change introduced by a community mental health center," namely, a blurring of the boundaries between professionals and nonprofessionals. They describe in detail the organizational setting, service structure, and internal functioning of one center as it sharply contrasted with the traditional psychiatric organization into which it was introduced. Such centers are probably not representative since diversity is the hallmark of community mental health, but the authors' comparison of psychiatrists in various units of the community mental health center they observed with the more traditional psychiatrists in the sponsoring psychiatric hospital sets the stage for a larger study. Particularly in regard to the education and consultation unit, the psychiatrists' roles, tasks, and responsibilities contrast sharply with those of more traditional psychiatrists.

In Chapter 9, Beran and Dinitz generate the hypothesis that "the community mental health system is pressuring its personnel to think and act in a manner to which they are unaccustomed and for which they are unprepared." That is, many nurses, psychologists, and social workers find it difficult to take over roles and responsibilities traditionally ascribed to the doctor in their new role of "case manager" for patients. In addition, patients themselves become upset over the substitution of other staff members for the doctor. Their observations of the social processes accompanying the introduction of a community mental health center into traditional psychiatric services suggests that professionals themselves do not readily yield their roles to paraprofessionals and nonprofessionals. The "mystique of medicine" remains firmly established in the minds of many (probably most) Americans. For Beran and Dinitz, this difference in role definition between traditional and community psychiatry is only one of many sharp contrasts "evident on every ideological and procedural dimension examined." The authors were able to examine the extent of these differences when a "natural experiment" presented itself that permitted the authors to observe the reactions of the nonmedical case managers and other treatment team members when the teams were left without a medical representative.

These two ethnographic chapters suggest that longitudinal studies of organizational and occupational adaptation to community psychiatry is a fruitful approach. Obviously the introduction of community mental health centers has triggered dynamic forces. What processes of accommodation emerge? What changes in the role behavior of traditionalists take place as a consequence of interaction with ideologies and strategies often viewed as radical departures from past practices? Where the community mental health center is not grafted onto an existing organization, how do more traditional treatment facilities in the community react? These are pressing questions for further consideration.

While relatively infrequent at present, innovations in community mental health occasionally surface which tend to be characterized by the conflicts described in Chapters 8 and 9. A report by Holden[1] opens with the strong statement that "any doctor who tangles with the politics of established medicine is likely sooner or later to get his wings clipped." She describes an attempted community mental health innovation in northern New York where a publicly financed psychiatrist regularly placed patients in the medical wards of local general hospitals rather than constructing local psychiatric inpatient facilities or placing patients in a state institution. Furthermore, he deliberately assigned psychiatric patients to rooms shared with general medical patients. His procedure was based on the belief that "the entire community is responsible for the mental health of its members" [p. 639]. Although a four-year evaluation indicated a sharp reduction in the average hospital stay of patients placed in general hospitals (from 41 to 8 days), conflicts within the community, based in part in the local medical establishment, led to the county legislature's total withdrawal of support of the county mental health program and their rejection of a $100,000 Federal grant received by the psychiatrist for support of services. While this incident demonstrates intraprofessional conflicts, it also points up the need for the political skills emphasized in Chapter 2 by Dunham. These skills were seemingly lacking in the deposed psychiatrist who had openly challenged the competency of several local physicians, including labeling one a "quack," and who in general possessed an "outspoken personality."

In Chapter 10, Leighton and Stone provide a dramatic example of how natural changes in one sector of community life are associated with sizeable reductions in rates of psychiatric impairment. The challenge for community psychiatry in their study is simply that the 10-year improvement happened with practically no intervention by psychiatric or medical personnel. The only influence of this type was a program for improvement devised by the original field researcher who interested school officials in giving the community special attention. Natural community processes took over following an adult education program. Predictably these centered around improvement in work skills and work opportunities; these changes triggered startling changes in community cohesiveness, pride, and cooperation that, in turn, preceded a reduction in psychiatric problems. Apparently the natural processes for improvement are often present in latent form in community life: "These findings clearly suggest the potential significance of community development programs for improving mental health," conclude Leighton and Stone. At the same time, they cannot carry their conclusions much beyond this. By implication, they raise the same questions raised by Dunham in Chapter 2: Does the community psychiatrist possess the skills to manipulate community forces in order to produce desirable results? To what extent are community psychiatrists guided by an overly rational systems model of community behavior? Leighton and Stone do, however, provide a potential answer for a nagging problem—that of how to measure mental health or illness. To this end they describe in detail the development of The Health Opinion Survey for Assessing Mental Health Levels (HOS). This instrument has gone through numerous tests of reliability and validity and has been subject to numerous field applications. The authors believe it is a way to gauge the impacts of various intervention strategies with before and after measurements. Would others agree?

Other questions raised are: How generalizable is the study? Do the processes

116

tapped here tend to be latent in most disintegrated communities? How can the relationship between reduction in psychiatric impairment and change in community behavior be interpreted? To what extent is "research effect" an explanation of the results presented by Leighton and Stone? What social/psychological mechanisms translate changes at the community level into reduced psychiatric problems? Finally, are there negative instances by means of which such processes can be further understood?

In Chapter 11, Angrist and Dinitz discuss home care as an alternative to hospitalization, a strategy that is central to the whole thrust of the community mental health movement. After pointing out the surprisingly wide choice of facilities, these authors focus on why the home-community care movement has "all the characteristics of a religious crusade," and point to recent pressures to humanize treatment, World War II treatment success, and hospital costs. Perhaps most valuable is the authors' review of the literature about the effectiveness of such efforts, giving their chapter a more positive tone than some others. The literature on home care is of relative long-standing and often marked by sophisticated research methods. Studies show that severely impaired patients are much more subject to rehospitalization, and that community based home treatment programs in general yield effective results provided that care is continuous. Without such continuity, the value of such programs tends to wash out after approximately five years. The necessity of continuity of care for home based patients is reiterated in a recent NIMH sponsored review of treatment evaluation.[2] Angrist and Dinitz also examine some basic issues in evaluating home care effectiveness. They conclude that home care can foster certain limited goals, that its realistic possibilities do not include high level patient functioning, and that it involves certain social costs to both families and patients.

Some painful and provocative questions for the future emerge from these chapters. Where does "therapy" stop in human experience? How much can the community mental health movement proliferate without jeopardizing its resources? How can evaluation research distinguish valuable program dimensions from the overall melange? How can such dimensions be preserved without loss of entire programs? How can evaluative research be coordinated to avoid damage to action programs? Finally, all of the authors of these chapters ask by implication the basic questions faced by any radical new innovation—questions especially pertinent in the emerging "decade of accountability": What if your programs had never come into being? What would be different? And if differences can be shown, what is their social value?

REFERENCES

1. HOLDEN, C.: "Mental Health: Establishment Balks at Innovative Psychiatrist." *Science* 181: 638-640, 1973.
2. MOSHER, L., AND GUNDERSON, J.: "Special Report: Schizophrenia, 1972." *Schizophrenia Bulletin* 7:26-50, 1973.

CHAPTER 7

Dilemmas of Evaluation in Community Mental Health Organizations

HARRISON M. TRICE and PAUL M. ROMAN

The numerous claims and counter-claims regarding the value and effectiveness of community mental health strategies point to the need for systematic, data-based evaluation, particularly at this critical time when Federal, state, and local officials face the question of continued funding for community mental health programs. Furthermore, as competition for scarce funds increases, due to the ever widening range of programs to combat "social problems," accountability for the use of funds in existing programs has become a priority concern. With centralized funding at the Federal level, evaluative data have been used heavily to consider the results of demonstration projects in terms of effecting policy change. With competition for the scarce revenue sharing funds at the local level, evaluative data may become the center of political controversy among agencies and programs. At the same time, the technology of evaluation has developed rapidly as funds for evaluation have been made available, increasing the potential for constructive feedback.

In this chapter, we focus on several basic dilemmas facing evaluation research in community mental health. The first of these is the problem of defining what it is that is to be evaluated. The variety of programs under the umbrella of community mental health has grown rapidly since the 1963 legislative mandate, leading to the fact that the concept of a community mental health program means different things to different people. Thus our first task is to delineate "the action" of community mental health centers. Is there *a* program, and if not, how can effective evaluation be undertaken?

Our second goal is to place evaluation research in a perspective broader than simply the mechanics of assessment. What is the relationship between the evaluator and the systems he evaluates? We are specifically concerned with the

119

barriers to the feedback of evaluation results into the ongoing systems of action. This means that organizational dynamics is a key problem of evaluation research. This pivotal concern has received very little attention, despite the obvious fact that an evaluation study may be merely destructive to programs or a useless ritual if results cannot be fed back constructively into program design.

Finally, we scrutinize the various models that underlie different approaches to evaluation, considering how they might be best adapted to some of the unique circumstances of community mental health programs. Drawing upon recent innovations in evaluative research, we offer specific suggestions for improving assessment with the hope of minimizing the potential conflict between the evaluator and his target system and maximizing the possibility that evaluation results will find constructive use.

WHAT IS A COMMUNITY MENTAL HEALTH PROGRAM?

Even a casual review of community mental health programs reveals a panorama of efforts often aimed toward broad goals and involving a perplexing range of techniques and strategies. For the experimentally oriented evaluator, this diversity clearly impedes direct application of his approach except in small sectors of the program. It seems reasonable to assume that this incongruity also adds to the difficulties in harmonious interaction between evaluators and their target systems. Regardless of how rigid or flexible an evaluator is in the design of his study, he cannot escape the necessity of getting a full description of the program's intended agents of change, the type of organizational structure, and the change expected to be produced in specified clients.

The deceptively simple question that must precede successful evaluation is "What is it that is being put to the test?"[57] "It" can range from a projected plan for outpatient treatment of behavior disorders via the "brief therapies" to an entrenched program of aversion therapy for alcoholics in operation for years. Specific efforts take place in a given organizational setting, within a relatively unique environment, with personnel that come and go, and with a target population which may be as broad as an entire census tract.

Hyman and Wright[57] emphasize that "some thread of identity and some common purpose runs throughout, if only because there are central directives emanating from one social agency. Therein lies the justification for the term, a program" [p. 748]. They warn that an evaluator "may attempt a single evaluation of independent programs by different agencies with different goals because his powers of abstraction lead him to see them all as representatives of some common category. . . . [T]he notion of 'program' is extremely deceptive" [p. 749]. The National Institute of Mental Health has instituted a centralized organization in Washington for the administration of community mental health centers,[1] but as Levenson[70] points out, "in order to meet the needs of their respective catchment areas, the centers must differ in regard to program emphases, staffing arrangements, and organizational patterns. . . . When two groups of agencies jointly develop centers in two communities, the two products will be very different even though the lists of participants may be nearly identical" [p. 75]. Obviously for evaluation purposes, a "program" must be carefully designated as a unique local program, not as the misleading abstraction of *the* national program.

Levenson[70] describes various types of centers: those in a general or a state hospital, the multiple agency center, and the independent center. Similarly, different patterns of funding and resource allocation make for program uniqueness. Two programs may look alike in terms of goals and even therapeutic philosophy, but the "muscle" in one may be minute compared with the other. One multiple agency program may be fragmented by each subordinate agency's independence, while in another program subordinate agencies join forces and reduce interagency competition through coordination. The evaluator must also know the extent of resource allocation in relation to program goals, since the behaviors expected to change under the program's impact may be persistent and stubborn, with change achieved only at great cost.[78] Abrupt change in resource allocation may occur in an agency, which, incidentally, provides a situation especially favorable for evaluation.[23] Such changes provide a real chance for comparing two distinctive patterns of programmatic activity.

Recent years have seen not only a "widening definition of mental illness,"[37] but also an increasing diversity in modes of therapy.[47, 29] According to Dinitz and Beran,[34] the community mental health movement "has conceptualized any and all individual and group behaviors and activities as potentially therapeutic in nature. Thus has come the development of art therapy, music therapy, writing therapy, and countless forms of group therapy, and the refinement of occupational therapy and other activity therapies" [p. 102]. Writing poetry, for example, is now regarded as having definite therapeutic potential.[67] Sensitivity training is widely practiced. Desensitizing forms of conditioning therapy appear to be gaining increased popularity among therapists, particularly for disorders such as alcohol abuse. Electroshock is still practiced, particularly for depressive disorders. Recreation therapy remains an old standby.

Thus, centers may differ drastically in types of therapeutic efforts, making it imperative that evaluators limit and define specific, discrete strategies in a program. A brief summary of some distinct change strategies is appropriate here, since evaluation research is totally dependent on accurate description of program components.

Modes of Therapy

Milieu Therapy: This regimen typically comprises frequent patient group meetings in which members discuss the problems they have with other patients and with the staff. Scheidlinger[102] reports that within treatment centers, these groups are sometimes components of a "therapeutic community" and consist of "about 20-30 patients as well as about 6-8 staff members, and may meet from two to five days a week for 1-1/2 hours. In addition, all patient activities are

121

viewed as potentially therapeutic, . . . as a way to promote patient growth" [p. 128]. Many variations of this example can be found.[64]

Family Treatment: Kraft[64] describes a program in which "virtually all relatives are in some kind of group therapy program," and Sager and his associates[100] describe a specific Family Treatment and Study Unit, giving examples of group therapy and specific interventions, such as homework assignments and seeking out male companions for an adolescent in an all-female household. These efforts took place in a clinic setting. Some psychiatric teams have attempted family therapy within the clients' home. A home care strategy in which patients being treated with drugs are visited regularly by public health nurses and seen occasionally by a social worker, a staff psychologist, and a psychiatrist is a family oriented treatment approach described by Pasamanick and associates.[89]

Transitional Communities: These facilities operate as a way station between hospitalization and a full return to community life. Patients practice cooperative living with others. As in therapeutic communities, interactions and relationships among patients and with staff may be manipulated for therapeutic purposes. The halfway house is a prominent example of a transitional community. Typically located in the community, it is not a hospital but a collectivity of patients who are believed not yet ready to return home or to work. Patients live in a supportive environment from which they can explore ways and means of returning to full community participation and independence and avoiding hospitalization. Cahn[20] provides an excellent description of a halfway house for alcoholics. Sheltered workshops, community hostels, and expatient care are also part of this broad therapeutic category.

Partial Hospitalization: In this widely used strategy, patients may spend their days at home or at work and return at night to the hospital for treatment, or the reverse: they may spend their days in a limited, therapeutic hospital environment and return home or to relatives at night. This arrangement may be an alternative to hospitalization or a transition between hospitalization and a complete return to community life. Day care centers are included in this category and provide individual and group psychotherapy, social service consultation, vocational consultation and testing, and occupational therapy during the day.[8]

Brief Psychotherapies: Community mental health center treatment personnel who are oriented towards psychotherapy "attempt to preserve as much of the essence of dynamic psychotherapy as the pressures of time allow and the requirements of the patient demand" [p. 120].[4] The purpose of brief psychotherapy is to relieve present symptoms as quickly as possible, usually within a limit of six sessions.[8,4] Some evidence suggests these may be as effective as much longer comprehensive efforts.[4] Such a strategy, focused on minimizing role disruption, explicitly reflects the ideology of community mental health programs. Therapists rapidly establish a working relationship and use personality indexes to get a quick profile of the individual's strengths. Selection for such therapies centers around the nature of the illness and the inner resources and adaptability of the patient. Barten[4] cautions, however, that "brief therapies have all too often been token treatments. . . . [O]ur sickest patients get the leftovers from the treatment buffet, if they get anything at all" [p. 106]. The fact that community mental health programs seem to attract patients who respond to brief therapies reflects Dunham's[37] foreshadowing observation that the "widening definition [of mental illness] provides an opportunity to overcome frustration that engulfs psychiatrists with respect to their inability to make much therapeutic headway with traditional mental cases" [p. 566].

Walk-In and Trouble-Shooting Clinics: Rome[96] cites evidence that people in the lower social strata are "unlikely to be reached by a clinic because they do not tend to use such facilities. . . . Walk-in clinics have been suggested as a means of overcoming this deficiency" [p. 44]. Zwerling and Rosenbaum describe a walk-in clinic that is part of an outpatient mental hygiene clinic; an attempt is made to have a psychiatrist see "every patient at the time he seeks out-patient help without an intervening work-up. . . . The central purpose is to provide [their] residents with supervised experience in the conduct of brief psychotherapies" [p. 79]. Bellak[8] believes that emotional crises are apt to occur outside of working hours, during the evening, night, and early morning, and he helped organize a clinic for people who need such immediate help. Such services were publicized so that people who had no other services available to them would be encouraged to bring their "problems with living" to the clinic. Kahn[58] indicates that such an informal strategy grew out of a need to "cater to the increasing number of people who were calling the office" [p. 146].

Behavior Therapy and Operant Conditioning: While some of these techniques can legitimately be put in the brief therapies category, they are radically different, based on learning theory and principles of operant conditioning. Aversion to engaging in abnormal behavior can be produced by introducing negative stimuli in conjunction with the undesirable behavior so that the deviant behavior is at least temporarily extinguished. The aversion may be increased by "massed practices" during which a group or an individual with a small number of observers experiences the aversion.[137] Widely applied to the phobias and to hysteria, the strategy ignores the historical factors in the development of the behavior and concentrates on desensitizing the patient to his immediate here-and-now behavioral impairment. Yates offers numerous examples of successful application, including writer's cramp, i.e., hysterical paralysis of the writing arm. Careful observation of these cases suggested that two triggering stimuli precipitated the paralysis: the touch stimulation from the pen itself and a similar tactual stimulation from the hand touching the paper, resulting in excessive pressure on the pen by the thumb and a gross hand tremor [p. 176]. Each symptom was separated out for treatment. The patient was required to insert a stylus into progressively smaller holes and also to perform a tracing task with the stylus. If the stylus touched the metal sides of the hole or the track, the patient received a shock. When heavy pen pressure occurred, the patient received an additional shock. Yates reported that in most cases the writer's cramp was relieved. Phillips

123

and Weiner[91] report that there has been a growing acceptance of operant conditioning during the past decade.

Group Therapy: In group therapy, the therapist may use group features such as norms, leadership, and status to effect change in a specific individual. He may permit natural group forces to emerge with a minimum of intervention. In a well known group procedure, patients voluntarily form groups designed to reduce some commonly experienced behavioral problem, as in, for example, Alcoholics Anonymous. Group therapy is ubiquitous and encompasses a myriad of types and forms. One of its assets is the fact that a group setting may reduce the individual's sense of stigmatization that might be associated with other treatment modalities. This strategy lends itself to outpatient care and can greatly reduce treatment costs by handling a number of patients simultaneously.

This brief and selective review should provide a flavor of the diversity of treatment modalities possible in any single community mental health program. In addition, there are activities based in the community mental health centers that are directed toward community change with the goal of improving mental health and reducing mental illness. A brief review of some of these should further reveal the many-faceted action profile of any given program.

Community Activities

Consultation With Pivotal Community Institutions: As a means of extending psychiatric concepts into the community, Sabshin[99] reports that the center may try to "provide consultative services to a broad network of agencies within the area. . . . Contact has been established with legal agencies, religious groups, school officials, social agencies, physicians, neighborhood clubs, recreational groups, and major political groups within the geographic boundaries" [p. 26]. Consultation is offered to a wide assortment of functionaries concerning a vast array of problems, i.e., delinquency, school failure, school dropouts, mental retardation, child care, and illegitimacy. Daniels[33] speaks of consultations with "firing line professionals" who are not primarily mental health workers: general practitioners, public health and visiting nurses, teachers, lawyers, policemen, and clergymen. Since these persons frequently have initial contact with emotionally troubled people, they have become a target group for community psychiatry.

In addition, community institutions such as colleges, industries, and military units may secure suggestions and guidance from the center in planning psychiatric services, while a family court, a social welfare agency, and a general hospital may be provided regular consultation for staff having considerable contact with persons having emotional difficulties. Thus the essence of consultations, according to Caplan,[25] is "an interaction between two professional persons, one who is a [psychiatric] specialist, and a consultee who asks for help in regard to a troubled client with whom he is working. The consultant may actually treat the client, but the consultee retains professional responsibility" [p. 251].

124

A subsequent step is for the center to launch educational programs for these key community people. The content of these educational programs can range from films and lectures to sensitivity training and role playing with hypothetical problem people.

Prevention: Interpersonal consultation designed to bring about psychological and behavioral change in community leaders with responsibility for diverse nonpatient populations is aimed directly at prevention. Prevention efforts frequently work through community leadership to reach high risk groups in schools, churches, and industry. Emphasis is often on early intervention in youthful populations judged to be at the risk of emotional disorder. Other efforts center around intervention in crisis and transition periods during which persons may be more receptive to help, e.g., leaving home for school, having a first child, and other common points of crises in the life cycle.[25] A more detailed consideration of preventive strategies and problems associated with them is found in Chapter 6.

Treating Communities: Some community mental health activities are based on the interpretation of the principles of community psychiatry and the 1963 legislative mandate that a basic goal is to aim treatment at social collectivities. Therapeutic change efforts are directed to a social structure in an effort to increase the emotional well-being of its members, i.e., this is "treatment at the 'collective level' to eliminate mentally disorganizing social relationships."[37] Sabshin[99] describes a center's plan to "study the way teachers tag first grade students as emotionally disturbed. . . . They are interested in the teachers who do the tagging and the setting in which they make their decisions. . . . Interventions of various types, including attempts at changing the setting, the teachers, the family, and the children, will then be utilized to ascertain deleterious consequences of being . . . labeled as emotionally disturbed" [p. 26]. Far more drastic are the techniques proposed by Dumont[36] in an essay entitled "The City as Patient": ". . . the changes I am talking about, the treatment for this ailing organism, involve a redistribution of the wealth and resources of this country on a scale that has never been imagined" [p. 80]. More pedestrian examples of "community treatment" are efforts to change hiring practices in industrial organizations and attempts to alter their structure in order to improve communications.

Other Relevant Dimensions

Coordination of Services: With this potential range of services, coordination is obviously a central concern. A center typically has a board of directors made up of representatives of different agencies which tends to develop an integrative function for the variety of community mental health efforts, "as a focus of the community's varied efforts."[108] The centers attempt to reorganize therapeutic efforts to focus on keeping the patient in the family and community rather than hospitalizing him. This implies "an increased and workable coordination of diverse social agencies in the community."[37]

125

Underlying these efforts are Federal requirements for the coordination of the center's programs. The community psychiatrist and the center must attempt "to mesh all the resources in a region to maximize service and avoid duplication."[86] Bernard[138] contends that the integrative function in community mental health centers is expressed in guiding concepts and subjective feelings as well as in formal administration. Susser[115] suggests the ever present need for coordination of previously independent activities: "in times of reorganization and rapid changes there is a general tendency to defend old positions in the face of an uncertain future" [p. 235]. The guidelines of the Community Mental Health Centers Act set up the concept of "continuity of care" as a nucleus around which coordinating actions were to be taken for the almost 400 centers existing in 1970. Providing a logical series of services for a large population of troubled persons complicates coordination.

Therapists: The thrust of the community mental health movement has been to include as "therapists" many types of personnel who previously would have been regarded as totally unqualified. Bellak,[8] for example, is shocked by an NIMH program in the mid-1960s that undertook to train middle-aged housewives to perform psychotherapy. But the most emphatic change has been the use of "indigenous mental health workers." One of the persistent themes in the 1963 legislation and its interpretation has been for services to be directed toward the deprived, the poor, the dispossessed, and the uneducated, most of which are presumed to be high risk groups. Smith and Hobbs[108] note, however, that even "when special efforts are made to bring psychotherapy to the disturbed poor it appears they tend not to understand it, to want it, or to benefit from it" [p. 504]. A major factor in such therapeutic failure is that the social distance between middle class professionals and lower class patients can be enormous. A bridge across this gap is needed. Furthermore, many contend that there are many situations where a highly trained therapist is unnecessary. Consequently, some programs have trained lay persons from the community for roles on the therapeutic team. Such trained nonprofessional staffs, attempting to bridge the social and cultural gap are "a significant new development in mental health programs."[102]

We are aware of no systematic evaluation of the effectiveness of this new occupation. Mechanic[81] states, however, that "individual experiences appear to be favorable, and there is theoretical reason to believe that a person who shares the culture and viewpoints of a client may be in a better position to gain rapport and help him than is a therapist with a very different perspective" [p. 106]. Without evaluation data, however, this is only an assumption. The use of indigenous workers may create unanticipated consequences, i.e., demands by lower class, ethnic populations for complete control of the center rather than merely being a "bridge" to it.[1] Community psychiatrists, however, appear to encourage the recruiting and training of mental health aides who strongly identify with their deprived, ethnic communities.[112] Ozarin[86] believes these aids have been valuable

126

in crisis intervention and in collecting information about community needs [p. 72]. Regardless of opinion, the trend toward increased involvement of paraprofessional and nonprofessional workers appears to be established in community mental health.[115]

The status of the social worker as a direct therapist appears to have been greatly enhanced in community mental health systems.[115] Moreover, our field observations indicate that many clinical psychologists have reduced their traditional roles in psychological testing in favor of increased involvement as direct therapists in the community mental health setting. This increased therapeutic involvement by nonpsychiatrists is facilitated by the prominence of techniques such as group therapy.

Settings: Therapeutic action in community mental health may take place in a variety of settings. A basic trend has been to set up activities in close proximity to potential clients, e.g., storefront, walk-in clinics. Treatment activities may also take place in the home, the school, or a hospital. The evaluator(s) must know as much as possible about the specific geography and milieu since these variations can themselves be potent forces in the outcome of change efforts.

Thus, from the viewpoint of the traditional evaluative researcher, the complexities in the community mental health structure that should be considered in attempting its evaluation are manifold: myriad combinations of efforts can come together to form a given program. In many ways, the evaluator encounters what might be called a psychiatric smorgasbord of offerings, established within guidelines which allow almost any function to be carried on in the name of community mental health. The goal is noble: to help just about anyone and everyone with any kind of emotional problem live more effectively and happily. But the task of defining the action is complex, faced by the array of therapies and community interventions by professional, paraprofessional, and lay mental health workers in a wide variety of settings, backed by impressive concepts such as "prevention," all of which represented an investment in Federal funding alone of almost \$300,000,000 by mid-1969.[47] Obviously traditional strategies of evaluation such as goal attainment and experimental designs are useful only in well defined segments (if any can be found). Without doubt, flexibility and adaptibility are called for. Before we detail suggestions for evaluation research in the third part of this chapter, we should consider a broader view of evaluation. If evaluation is to accomplish its goal of constructive feedback into program design, an understanding of the potential pitfalls in the relationship between the evaluator and his target system is in order.

RELATIONSHIPS BETWEEN EVALUATORS AND COMMUNITY MENTAL HEALTH SYSTEMS

Both critics and proponents of evaluation research agree that it faces a swarm of methodological problems. One persistent difficulty is how to distinguish between program results and those outcomes stimulated by the individual practitioner's characteristics. The legitimacy of comparison and control groups is frequently questioned in the interpretation of results. Yet evaluative researchers are resourceful in dealing with these and other problems of contamination. Quasi-experiments, refined followups, and systematic efforts to control for research effects[119] have begun to appear. In short, though never wholly eliminated, many problems of methodology appear to be manageable.

There is another difficulty, however, that can completely defeat almost any evaluation effort. Despite the type or model of evaluation research used and the care exercised to develop and maintain rapport, the program's practitioners and administrators often come to resent and resist the evaluation research and reject the application of its results to their programs. Such resistance may come early or late in the conduct of the research, and it may be covert rather than overt. But such an outcome is all too common. Most evaluation data rarely find their way, as intended, into a reconsideration of policy, technique, or procedures; "most are still filed and forgotten."[124] Without the use of evaluation research results in policy and program alterations aimed at increasing the effectiveness of the organization studied, the effort is, in the main, fruitless.

Thus there is a necessity for an intense consideration of how these two subcultures, community action organizations and research professionals, can relate without crippling conflict. The potential for such conflict looms large. In this section we describe (1) how such conflict can defeat evaluation efforts, (2) sources of conflict within the nature of evaluation research itself, (3) sources of conflict within the makeup of action organizations, and (4) how the evaluator himself can inadvertently create resistance.

Specific field experiences first brought this fundamental problem forcibly to our attention. These experiences were of two kinds: our own long-range evaluation studies[6,121,139] and those of advanced university students during the last three years in a field oriented class entitled "The Evaluation of Social Action Programs." In this course, students worked in twos and threes and attempted to adapt the guidelines of Suchman's *Evaluative Research*[114] to an existing community action program. Both we and the students encountered subtle and various forms of a sharp resistance by action people to evaluation.

We can detail this point from our field work. Despite Herculean efforts to maintain good rapport with the organizations involved, we inevitably wound up as *persona non grata* at best, and, at worst, with some life-long enemies. For example: In six months we had developed a beautiful design with samples of a well defined population randomly placed in several different treatment groups for outcome comparison. These groups were being sustained when a rash of "professional judgments" broke out, destroying the research design. When we reminded the professionals involved that we had a very firm agreement that the randomized placements would be sustained, they reminded us of who knows best for patients when choices had to be made. Thus problems in the relationship between the evaluator and the target system defeated this effort before meaningful data collection could be made, an experience repeated in different forms in most of the other student projects. To our knowledge, none of the other evaluation data that we collected at considerable expense in several organizations over a lengthy time span were ever used within these organizations, despite repeated and conscientious efforts at feedback. However, some reasonably good publications came out of these efforts, proving again the abundance of latent functions.[140]

We find little solace from discovering that others have had similar experiences and also speculate that the problem might be deadly for evaluation. Rossi[97] describes two large, expensive studies in which none of the results were used: "policy remained unaffected." Schulberg and Baker[104] regard potential hostility between evaluation research and clinical efforts as "the most basic question," and feel that the starting point in research should be to decide whether or not such research is so antithetical to the program members that crippling conflict becomes inevitable. The flavor of the conflict that can emerge is dramatized by Freeman and Sherwood[45] who indicate that once an evaluative research design is set up and inaugurated, "the researcher must continue to remain within the environment, like a *snarling watchdog* [emphasis ours] ready to oppose alterations in program and procedure that could render his evaluation efforts useless" [p. 16]. They believe that "conflict between clinician and scientist pervades all fields of medicine but the difficulties that medical researchers have in undertaking experiments with human subjects are minimal in comparison with evaluation efforts in the community" [p. 14].

Weiss and Rein[129] describe a large scale social action program in which the evaluation research group attached to the program initially received a casual reaction to a sound research proposal, namely, that "different change attempts be introduced into different districts of the area" so that a strategy of comparison groups might emerge [p. 99]. When program administrators learned of the proposal, however, they "found the idea charming and unrealistic," and the research suggestion was dismissed. After a series of negotiations during which the practitioners' distrust and fear of negative findings became increasingly overt, the director of the research group left the project, "with bad feelings all around" [p. 101].

The clash is not of recent origin. Writing about the Federal Planning, Programming, Budgeting System (PPBS) initiated in the early 1960s to monitor funded social action programs, Williams and Evans[134] say, "Looking in retrospect at the early PPBS, . . . the conflicts in the system between the analytical staff and the operators of the programs was underestimated. Hence, the politics of evaluation—in essence the clash between methodology, political forces and bureaucracy—looms much larger than was imagined in those early days" [p. 118]. Much the same conclusion came from a 1959 Research Conference on Rehabilitation and the Management of Mental Disorders[59]: "A constant theme . . . referred to the many conflicts between service and research staff" [p. 58].

129

Evaluation Design as a Source of Conflict

Evaluation research is related to basic research but is sharply different from it. In basic research, new knowledge is sought, with relatively little interest in its use.[114] Evaluation studies, in contrast, are designed to test how knowledge is used, with a vital interest in its effective use. Evaluative research is not value free, but judges results in practical terms determined by program goals. For example, an evaluation study of a Head Start program attempted to determine if children in the program increased their intellectual and social-personal development more than comparable children who did not attend.[134] The research focus is on *improvement;* in this instance, improvement in the ability to reason and to show signs of social maturity. Furthermore, evaluative studies must grapple with many variables, often without the conceptual base so prominent in basic research. In other words, the basic researcher is often free to disregard variables that are not a part of the theory or hypothesis he is testing. This does not mean that clearly conceptualized variables have not been used in evaluative efforts, nor does it preclude the possibility that significant theoretical hypotheses can be tested in evaluation studies. But according to Suchman,[114] such opportunities may be rare: "Program testing has almost no generalizability, being applicable solely to the specific programs being evaluated" [p. 77], while basic research is aimed toward valid generalizations about a category of phenomena. "Evaluative research is largely related to a certain time and place; nonevaluative research has as its goal as much 'timelessness and spacelessness' as possible" [p. 78].

At the same time, basic and evaluative research share many common features. Sampling and measurement problems beset both; reliability and validity of data are questions that must be asked about any type of scientific research. Similar problems in data analysis can characterize both types of research. To the extent that evaluative research attempts some degree of experimental design, it shares with basic research the problems of control, i.e., determining whether the presence of a variable creates effects that are not otherwise present. Followup studies in evaluation have their parallel in longitudinal basic research where an attempt is made to determine a temporal series of effects.

Few people question the value of research; it is a hallmark of American progress in areas such as medicine and industrial technology. But evaluation research does not engender such enthusiasm in the target systems. Much of the practitioner's resistance to an evaluative study comes from its explicit, avowed intention to determine if an action program is demonstrably effective, and why or why not. Our exploratory interviews with practitioners and therapists in alcoholism treatment programs suggest that those undergoing evaluation tend to see evaluators as "yes men" or "hatchet men" for funding agencies. At worst, they see evaluation as an effort to "kill us off." In some cases, practitioners fear that evaluators might find the program damaging to some of its recipients. Carol Weiss[124] has summed up the probably reaction as follows:

Program staffs have rarely liked evaluators poking their noses into the operation of programs or measuring outcomes. Whatever soothing explanations are offered about "testing program concepts" or "accountability to taxpayers," the evaluator is a snoop. To the program operator who knows that his program is doing well, evaluation is at best unnecessary and at worst, if it shows few positive effects, a calumny and a threat to the future of the program, his job, and needed help to clients [p. 16].

Practitioners on the firing line tend to believe that outside evaluators have a *strong bias against them from the beginning* and will inevitably come up with negative results. Furthermore, they may believe evaluators will ignore numerous program dimensions that show effectiveness. The fact that evaluative research is often negative seems to inevitably create an atmosphere of hostility and fear. Wright and Hyman[136] believe that even under favorable conditions, action program people are not receptive to social science studies, and they conclude that conflict is more likely "if measurements threaten to reveal unfavorable information" [p. 123]. Ferman[43] states the matter succinctly:

Administrators and service staff of agencies rarely have anything good to say about evaluation studies, particularly by people from outside the agency. The common perspective is that 'no good can come of it,' or 'you can only be hurt,' because evaluation is organized fault finding, usually without adequate understanding or explanation of why the faults exist. There are strong feelings among the staff that the evaluator is concerned with negatives, neglects the positives, and gives little credit to the program for operating in the first place. At the core of these perspectives is a deep resentment at having one's behavior studied and judged by an outsider—a feeling that is common in American life. A number of considerations can intensify these antagonisms. One basic factor is the by-passing of local-agency expertise in favor of judgments by evaluators and the sponsors of the evaluation. The agency staff has little control over the criteria that are used in the evaluation study. There are frequently strong feelings among agency staff that performance of the program might look different if only other criteria were used to evaluate it. *The thrust of the argument is that a more balanced picture could be presented if the agency staff could participate in and designate some of the measuring instruments and outcomes to be observed in the evaluation.* . . . By far the most frequent source of hostility toward the evaluator stems from the threat that a negative evaluation can contribute to reducing an agency's resources [p. 147]. [Emphasis ours.]

Since negative outcomes of evaluative studies are distressingly frequent, these fears are somewhat understandable. Carol Weiss's[124] review of Elinson's catalog of "ten of the most competent and best known published evaluations" indicated that "none of them demonstrated much success," and concluded "the most serious political problem of all is that evaluative results, with dismaying frequency, turn out to be negative. Over the past several years, careful and competent studies have shown few positive effects from such varied programs as psychotherapy, probation services, casework, school desegregation, public housing, and compensatory education" [p. 51.]

Conflict over the fairness of evaluative strategies is common. Eysenck,[41] using a report of Teuber and Powers, describes how in the well known evaluation of the Cambridge-Somerville Youth Project, some of the counselors looked upon the control group concept as "slightly blasphemous" in contrast to the two evaluators who emphatically state that "the burden of proof is on anyone who claims specific results for a given form of therapy" [p. 14]. The inherent conflict, deriving from both sides, is obvious. According to Ferman, two frequent negative orientations among agency staffs make evaluation quite difficult when the research techniques and the evaluators are from outside the agency. The first of these he terms "conventional wisdom," the gist of which is that the reference points developed by practitioners from everyday experiences and practical judgments are far more realistic than evaluative results derived by outsiders' scientific methods. The second is that agency staffs tend to believe that "evaluation reveals little that people in the agency did not know before," implying that outsiders' evaluative strategies merely put into different words what they already know.

Caro[28] locates specific "basic tension" areas in the researcher-practitioner relation. Whereas the practitioner concerns himself with "immediate and specific application of knowledge," the evaluative researcher attempts to generate new knowledge and thinks in terms of "long-range problem solving," seeking out such items as "explicit statements of objectives and strategies" of action programs. Evaluative researchers are committed to seeking out how and where a program is ineffective and recommending program changes consistent with their findings; practitioners, however, tend to resist changes and defend the status quo. Out of practical experience, practitioners often attribute failure to inadequate resources, whereas evaluative researchers are apt to be academics who "are free to question program premises" and attribute program failure to "an inadequate understanding of the basic problem" [p. 96]. *In toto,* these dimensions add up to sharp ideological and practical discord.

Polak[92] also has described this incompatibility:

The clinician needs to be decisive and uncompulsive. He is placed in situations where important decisions must be made rapidly on the basis of what little information is available. . . . [T]he clinician feels he must have *faith* in what he is doing or his treatment will suffer. The researcher, on the other hand, is more likely to believe nothing and to question everything. He is unwilling to come to hasty conclusions and less willing to act on them, . . . and he may be looked on as a sort of prima donna. . . . [I]t usually takes [him] a great deal of time to gather, check, and recheck his data. . . . The clinician, dealing with everyday clinical cases, simply does not have the time the researcher has to solve the problems facing him [p. 337]. [Emphasis ours.]

Campbell[22] underscores the same point: "If the political and administrative system has committed itself in advance to the correctness and efficacy of its reforms, it cannot tolerate learning of failure" [p. 110].

The idea that evaluation is a threat naturally brings out defensive measures within the organization to protect it from unfavorable findings. We encountered one large social action program that informally trains its people in how to mislead, avoid, and manipulate evaluators. Another has deliberately set aside funds (under an innocuous category) to hire a research specialist to locate deficiencies in evaluation strategies as a means for attacking and discrediting the results. Carol Weiss[124] describes the startling reaction of a correctional institution to an evaluation study that revealed low effectiveness in a program: The agency expanded the program and threw out the researchers! Hyman and Wright[57] note that a program may go through cycles and warn that the time when an evaluator is invited may be manipulated: "Sometimes it helps simply to ask why he was called in on [this] cycle, since the answer may document the fact that some major turning point has occurred or suggest the suspicion that the cycle selected for evaluation was a hand-picked one" [p. 750].

Formal definitions of evaluation leave little doubt about what evaluators do. The authors of the classic *Four Studies of the Encampment for Citizenship*[56] attempted to define evaluation in a palatable fashion as the "procedure of fact finding about the results of planned social action" [p. 3]. Anderson's[3] definition is less euphemistic: evaluation is "measuring achievement of progress toward predetermined goals . . . [and] it is also concerned with whether the goals themselves are valid" [p. 7]. The Russell Sage Foundation's Program in Evaluation Research[98] introduces into its definition the highly tangible and instantly understood factor of money: Program evaluation "is to measure the benefits received from the program, particularly with respect to the costs incurred" [p. 3]. Costs can obviously include indexes other than money value, but it is difficult to leave monetary values out of evaluation. Ferman[43] also introduces the cost idea and explicitly includes a note of invidious comparison:

Evaluation activity may be either diagnostic or cost-effectiveness oriented. In diagnostic evaluation we seek to explain why some impact did or did not occur or why some goal or program was or was not achieved. . . . In cost-effectiveness evaluation, the emphasis is placed on the operating cost of the program *and particularly on how it compares in this respect with similar programs* [p. 144]. [Emphasis ours.]

Caro[28] cites Glass as stressing that "evaluation is an attempt to assess the worth or social utility of a thing." Glass argued that "since the desirability of announced program goals might be questioned, evaluation should include procedures for the evaluation of those goals" [p. 88]. Finally, Suchman[114] specifies evaluation as "the determination . . . of the results . . . attained by some activity designed to accomplish some valued goal or objective" [p. 32]. His specific evaluation categories are (1) assessment of the amount of "effort," (2) assessment of the effect or results of efforts, (3) assessment of process, i.e., how and why an effect was produced, and (4) efficiency or effects relative to cost [p. 68].

Even though practitioners deeply involved in change efforts may read few of these definitions, it is apparent that the most trusting of them easily "get the message" and become suspicious.[47] From most any standpoint, program evaluation carries the clear possibility of reviewing the program's parade and exclaiming, in the midst of practitioners' banner-waving, hand-clapping, and dramatic ceremony, "Look, the King has no clothes!"

The Potential for Change: Threat to Practitioners

In field interviews focused on how psychiatrists, social workers, and administrators in alcoholism organizations think about program evaluation, we encountered the common belief that evaluative research results would be used "to try to change us." And, of course, they were right. Not only does evaluation research focus on the degree to which desired results have been achieved, but it ideally emphasizes that these data be *used* for appropriate modification of existing programs, organizational structure, and guiding policy. This goal of "closing the circle" of the evaluation process[104] "has received little attention and even less use."[105] Nevertheless it is the ideal companion to assessing past action.

Thus a prominent objective of evaluators may set the stage for cutting off funds, changing goals, and altering policy. The Russell Sage Foundation lists as one of the four "minimum requirements for good evaluation studies . . . [the] means to communicate the findings of evaluation studies to those who have responsibility for expanding, modifying, or terminating the programs."[98] An example of policy implications of evaluative research on community treatment of psychiatric illness is Mechanic's[81] statement:

In summary the data indicate considerable social cost in keeping the patient in the community during the early periods of psychiatric illness; by 6 months the costs are low enough to make hospitalization the less reasonable alternative. The data support either of two policies: (1) emphasis on home care, with maximal services and community aids provided to help alleviate the strain on the family during the period when the costs are highest; or (2) short hospitalization during periods of greatest strain early in the illness, followed by speedy release. The choice of policy depends on the individual circumstances, the services available to relieve and aid the family in home care situations, and further data which define more specifically the costs and advantages of pursuing one policy rather than another [p. 84].

Other illustrations include the notions of "rapid feedback"[92] and "continual feedback."[78] Polak describes how variations in admission policy were evaluated within weeks so that disagreements between hospital and referral agency could be reduced. Marris and Rein insisted that demonstration projects were actually "explorations of the possibilities of reform" and that "immediate progress depends upon a continual feedback of information from the field of operation" [p. 206].

Ironically, those in the action program may originally accept the collection of evaluative data but later reject it, having discovered its potential feedback. Mann[76] projects such a possibility:

[Both evaluators and those in target systems] lack awareness as to what to expect. If such awareness can be attained before the research is initiated, its actual progress should prŏceed more smoothly. When such an awareness does not exist, the effects are unfortunate both in terms of the research itself, and for the institution in which it is conducted [p. 189].

In order to avoid such a development, Wright and Hyman[136] held "preliminary conferences between the educational and executive directors of the Encampment and ourselves." In these, the target group "quizzed" the evaluators "about what evaluation involves." Both sides became familiar with the orientations of the other before either made a final commitment [p. 124].

But even such preliminaries can be insufficient if practitioners discover that their work is far more difficult than they had originally anticipated, leading them to shy away from being studied. Weiss and Rein[129] describe a large-scale action program aimed at changing community institutions to be "more useful to citizens of the community, and especially to underprivileged youth." In the beginning, the administrators and action personnel had been attracted to evaluation because of "the promise of program impact." After two years of grappling with the difficulties in bringing about "significant changes," their ardor for evaluation had cooled considerably; they "knew that what they had been able to do was outweighed by what they had not been able to do" [p. 100].

As practitioners "live with" evaluation research they may come to realize that its influence can distinctively alter their desired goals. Weiss and Rein[128] note that "the problem is that the operationalization [of evaluation] may take on an importance far out of keeping with the program's actual, broader, goals. . ." [p. 141]. Etzioni[40] believes that eagerness to measure efficiency may encourage overemphasis, unduly concentrating organizational resources. When this occurs, alert and experienced program personnel can scarcely miss the gradual buildup of this effect, which they might rightly see as perverting program investments.

In addition to revealing shortcomings in achieving desired change, evaluation may highlight negative side-effects of program efforts. Suchman[114] states that "there is a constant concern with negative side-effects or contraindications" in drug evaluation studies and also speaks of the " 'boomerang' or negative side-ef-

fects which are almost inevitable consequences of any social action program."
Mechanic[81] also cautions that some mental health program services may harm
some types of patients.

Practitioners in action organizations often devise ways to counteract the risk of
negative results. For example, they may look at alternative interpretations of
evaluative data or develop rationalizations of negative results. Null results can be
interpreted as evidence that the program does not have enough "muscle" and
that the evaluative outcome calls for more resources. Or, practitioners may argue
that changes occurred that were not measured, e.g., mental patients kept with
their families may have adjusted well to job demands even though the family actively seeks rehospitalization because they cannot tolerate the patient's behavior;
if the evaluation used "return to hospital" as the principal criterion of program
success and ignored work adjustments, the criticism has foundation. Some become astute at ferreting out flaws in evaluative research. For example, practitioners can argue that the numerous individuals that made progress are buried
within group statistics. Other rationalizations are plentiful and may turn out to
be more than excuses. Borgatta[17] lists four common criticisms: (1) program effects are long range and cannot be measured immediately; (2) results are general,
not specific, so criteria are too limited to catch the positive results; (3) measuring
instruments are too crude and cannot detect small but important effects; and (4)
changes generated by the program are subtle and the research cannot penetrate
the complexity of the patient's situation. Williams and Evans[134] candidly
describe the kinds of methodological attacks that can be launched against
negative results. In their evaluation of Head Start, they encountered such cogent
criticisms as that the study was too narrow (it did not include outcomes in health
and nutrition); the study overlooked variations in programs (it lumped them all
together); the sample was too small (a larger, more representative sample might
have altered the findings); and the instruments used were discriminatory (they
were allegedly insensitive to changes occurring in disadvantaged children).

A less subtle way for the action organization to prevent damaging results is to
put direct pressure on the evaluator to obtain positive results. Mann[76] believes
that "most evaluative investigations are instituted to 'prove something' in which
people already believe. . . . The researcher is generally aware of how the study
is supposed to turn out" [p. 187]. In sum, the feedback feature of program
studies may be menacing to practitioners, and they often find ways of defense
against negative findings to reduce them to manageable proportions.

Questioning the Underlying Assumptions of Action Programs

An evaluative study may raise questions about the assumptions that openly or
subtly justify the action program, providing another potential for conflict. Although these assumptions may be reasonable, it is likely that some of them will
be difficult to support when scrutinized.

Underlying assumptions are "taken-for-granted" or "of course" statements.[74]
Since few community mental health programs are tightly formalized, evaluators

may be tempted to start with an examination of these "givens." Such an examination may offend practitioners by appearing to debunk emotionally laden notions and cherished beliefs. Even when done diplomatically, a critical review of assumptions sets the stage for more severe misunderstandings if and when actual evaluative research begins. The potential conflict inherent in questioning assumptions are best revealed by looking at some of the presuppositions currently underlying many of the efforts of community mental health programs:

1. *The program can actually reach its target population and, in so doing, raise the level of mental health to the benefit of the community at large.*[54] But Howe[54] notes that "the provision of extensive treatment services might engender such widespread preoccupation [with symptoms] that their incidence would actually increase faster than people could be relieved of them" [p. 252].

2. *Many community mental health assumptions are an extension of the concept of personal, individual pathology: in short, they define more and more problems in mental health terms.*[34] Actually, it is easily argued that many disordered behaviors are matters of *"social health* for which we will need drastic institutional change and reform."[47] Dinitz and Beran[34] argue that "one can conveniently ignore social problems by defining them as personal pathologies" [p. 106].

3. *A "catchment" area is synonymous with a "community."* Community psychiatry programs may operate under a community banner, but they use geographical units, even census tracts, which may or may not constitute or encompass communities.[109,94] (This issue is detailed by Preston in Chapter 3 of this volume.)

4. *Minor emotional disturbances are on a continuum with the severe, chronic psychoses, and so severe disorders will be prevented if minor disorders are "nipped in the bud."* Practically no extant evidence supports this belief; on the contrary, the oppositie seems to be more realistic: the two major categories of mental illness are largely unrelated.

5. *Immediate intervention will minimize chronicity and lengthy hospitalization of patients.* We gravely doubt that any early identification effort meets Hutchinson's[55] following criteria: "In order to predict benefit from early case finding, a disease must have the following characteristics in the population in which it is being studied: (1) there must be a known effective therapy; (2) there must be a diagnostic device capable of detecting the disease prior to its usual time of diagnosis in the community being studied; (3) there must be one or more critical points such that therapy instituted before the critical point is more effective in intervening with pathologic sequence than is therapy undertaken after that point; and (4) such a critical point must occur in the time sequence of the disease after the time when diagnosis first becomes possible and before the time when diagnosis is made under the usual disease pattern of the community" [p. 507].

6. *Remaining in community life is more constructive for the mentally ill than hospitalization.* The fact that retaining psychiatrically impaired soldiers in their

137

units during both World Wars revealed advantages appears to support such an assumption. Yet the comparison between military life and civilian community life is tenuous. Mechanic[81] holds that "family and community environments may have the same adverse effects on the patient's functioning and skills as a poor mental hospital" [p. 94]. Often hospitalized persons show a surprising decline of symptoms only to have them reappear upon returning home. While length of stay in the mental hospital has declined, readmission rates have increased. Freeman and Simmons[46] believe that "apart from the humanitarian issue, there actually is considerable grounds for arguing that the community may have been better off before the revolving door was installed in the hospital" [p. 23]. Moreover, both outpatients and inpatients in mental health centers may develop their own brand of dependency and a chronic recidivism that looks like that of state mental hospital patients.

7. *Mentally ill persons receive appropriate treatment and care.* Meehl,[83] however, estimates that ". . . present decision-making policies and procedures of therapists and agencies are so inefficient that selection results in at least half of patients currently in conventional psychotherapy being inappropriate. The literature suggests that at least 50 to 60 percent of persons seeking help will, if untreated, come to feel within the course of a year or so that they do not need it" [p. 58]. In contrast, Meehl believes that almost one quarter of persons currently in psychotherapy are "appropriate cases," the remainder being "schizo-types" who are "bad-outlook" cases and inappropriate for psychotherapy. Trice and Roman[121] developed data from a large alcoholism treatment unit showing that if certain types of persons had been given the specific therapies used, favorable outcomes would have risen sharply. Practically nothing is known about the effect of home care on various *types* of patients.

8. *It is viable for community psychiatry to actively seek out emotionally disturbed persons for treatment and, in so doing, both protect the community and relieve those who suffer.*[8] Such an assumption confers a degree of political power and environmental control to the psychiatrist that is unlikely to be accepted in American society. Even if this were not the case, it is quite difficult to spell out the methods available to mental health workers to accomplish these desirable goals. But such actions would smack of Orwellian regimentation to a degree visualized by Kenneth Keniston in his 1968 parody, "How Community Mental Health Stamped Out the Riots."[62] More realistic are the grave legal questions discussed by Cohen and Hollingshead in Chapters 4 and 5 of this volume; for example, the question of privileged information in relation to the public interest and the right to privacy.

9. *The goals of various types of prevention are realistic, and their achievement can be reasonably expected as a consequence of the community mental health movement.* Again, as laudable as such goals are, they readily collapse under critical scrutiny. Howe[54] has referred to the "promiscuous use of the 'prevention' slogan," and Dinitz and Beran[34] observe realistically that "mental health workers may urge people to resist undue stress, but people

continue to compete systematically and to generate all manner of disorders in the frantic race to succeed" [p. 106]. Dunham[37] reviews long-range efforts to prevent juvenile delinquency and finds extreme difficulty in deciding whether prevention has occurred or not. What solid evidence does exist is negative; and despite the genuine, well intended effort of child guidance clinics since 1922, in almost every state "juvenile delinquency remains a continuing problem" [p. 560]. Causal factors are largely unknown. Mechanic[81] pinpoints what is probably the major obstacle to prevention: "We should note that intervention when people have neither sought nor desired our assistance is a serious infringement on the public's privacy" [p. 101]. These and other obstacles to successful prevention are reviewed by us in Chapter 6 of this volume.

10. *The psychiatrist knows how to reorganize a community in order to increase the mental health of its population.* Although training about community dynamics is slowly entering psychiatric education, it is fitful and is without a body of tested knowledge. What are the approaches, techniques, and methods available to treat a "community" rather than individuals in it? Most social scientists and psychiatrists would agree that pathological forces exist in family, work, community, and racial conflict, but how can these pathogenic forces be reduced? Also, how can the psychiatrist gain rapport with community institutions and leaders in order to influence them?

11. *There has been some working resolution of the etiological debate.* Often scarcely noticed by many mental health workers, there remain unresolved deep-seated differences in opinion about causal forces. Bell and Spiegel[7] formulate the problem: "in its simplest terms the question can be stated in three forms: (1) are mental illnesses caused by stresses and strain in the social environment? (2) or are social problems caused by the psychological instabilities of individuals, instabilities that can be traced to essentially psychobiological causes? (3) or are both mental illnesses and social problems the result of interaction between social and psychobiological forces? . . . Obviously if answers are not available, there is little rational support for any type of practice whatsoever" [p. 66].

Avoiding Change: The Fantasy of Success

The term "evaluation" is widely used without any specific meaning. For example, an informative description of therapies for alcoholism has the added subtitle "An Evaluative Study,"[20] yet it is difficult to locate any explicit focus on evaluation of effectiveness in the book. In general, the literature on the "evaluation" of psychotherapy for alcoholics consists mainly of descriptions of therapy with little or no evaluative content. Our field experiences confirm the many-splendored usage of the term, ranging from the evaluation of patients for certain therapies to a site visit team's evaluation of an organization seeking funds.

Parsons[88] has delineated types of reactions produced by change or innovation within a social system, such as evaluation can potentially produce in a community mental health center: anxiety, fantasy, hostility, and defensive measures.

139

We have already noted aspects of anxiety, hostility, and organizations' means of defense. We now focus on fantasy.

One means of dealing with anxiety generated by evaluation is success by proclamation, i.e., proclamation of program success prior to or without any program testing at all. Examples abound of descriptions of programs as successful ("has been conducted successfully,"[101] "former patients . . . are far less likely to relapse,"[5] "the success of this undertaking,"[102] etc.) without even a gesture at evidence. The title of a 1969 reader[10] announced that "progress" had occurred in community mental health; unfortunately, the book does not demonstrate progress in any objective fashion. Many practitioners share the belief that "trying" means that reasonable results have occurred.

The assumed adequacy of success by proclamation is readily understandable in light of the intense socialization in omniscience experienced by many psychiatric professionals. Parsell[87] comments: "The program is being done; therefore it is good. All that is really required of evaluation is testimony to the professionals by the program operators, [documenting] their adherence to accepted principles and routines" [p. 3]. This is what MacMahon and his associates[75] term "evaluation of technique" as contrasted with "evaluation of accomplishment." Evaluation tends to be equated with a critical examination of the *process* by which a change program is performed, with little or no attention to *whether it produced desired results*. A reasonable amount of positive results tends to be assumed among practitioners, especially in community mental health programs where goals are quite intangible. Mann[76] puts it bluntly: "Most practitioners are fully convinced of the efficiency of their methods and do not require objective validation" [p. 11]. Carstairs[29] believes evaluation of impact may take place, but "one thing is quite clear: objective evaluations of the effectiveness of new procedures have seldom, if ever, preceded their gaining currency in psychiatric practice" [p. 46]. Finally, the sense of enthusiasm and hope, of excitement and faith in the "Third Psychiatric Revolution"[8] that has saturated community mental health programs is largely incompatible with the skeptical, "show me" attitude that prevails among evaluative researchers. Rather than look upon the Community Mental Health Centers Act as the Magna Carta of community mental health,[8] as many practitioners do, evaluators are more apt to see it as another example of untried social action programs that have waxed and waned in the United States since the 1930s.

Realizing that such success is fantasy is blurred by repeated calls by action personnel themselves for evaluative research.[33,14] Wilner[132] embellishes this plea: "These several considerations have led to what I can call only a colossal defensiveness on the part of the profession that has too long delayed the need to see *systematically* the outcome of what we are doing" [p. 13]. Sabshin[99] criticizes child guidance clinics because of "too much emphasis on pragmatics and too little emphasis on research." Smith and Hobbs[108] call for "active program evaluation" to be built into a program in order to promote sound development. They also spell out how the 1963 Community Mental Health Centers Act itself en-

140

courages research and evaluation as one of five services in a comprehensive community mental health program.

But the call for evaluation has gone largely unheeded. Mechanic[81] states that "one would anticipate that the consequences of this shift in mental health policy have been so vast that researchers would be flocking to study them. It is disillusioning, indeed, to find how underdeveloped this research area is and how blindly decision makers must grope in attempting to develop coherent policies and approaches" [p. 56]. Klein[63] insists that the need for evaluation is "apparent to most scientifically trained mental health specialists. Yet in practice even the most rudimentary efforts . . . are sometimes neglected by community mental health teams" [p. 55]. He attributes this unmet need to the complex and "fluid circumstances" involved. Phillips and Weiner[91] merely deplore the fact that "good followup data . . . are lacking, as they are on all forms of psychotherapy" [p. 55]. Others contend that evaluation research has received low priority because of the felt need to change deplorable mental hospital conditions as rapidly as possible, combined with zeal for the new therapeutic modalities.[29,46]

Anti-poverty programs also suffer from inadequate evaluation.[97, 7] To our knowledge none of the observers of this research lag have suggested the severe difficulty experienced by evaluators and practitioners in attempting to work together. This point can be expanded by examining contrasting professional values vis-a-vis evaluation studies.

Professional Styles and Evaluation

Upon reviewing the features of a "professional community" and the nature of a rigorous research design, Bergen[11] comments that "it would be hard to find conditions less suitable for working out a reasonable *modus vivendi*" [p. 128]. According to Bergen's analysis, a research design subjects the professional practitioner to public scrutiny, and the practitioner is apt to view this "as an open challenge to his sense of worth and self-esteem. This kind of challenge is not easily or lightly taken up." In contrast, the professional researcher is an advocate of science, with license to persistently inquire and question the validity of claims of program results. The evaluative researcher's identity and commitment are, of course, not involved in the success or failure of the programs. Rather his professional competence rests upon the adequacy and thoroughness of his research.

Major values of a professional practitioner derive from focusing on the "particular patient in his particular situation,"[11] making his clinical judgment a much valued reflection of his autonomy. The evaluator, however, is apt to view both the practitioner and his patients in an impersonal light, seeing both of them as variables in a research design. Evaluation research designs often subordinate the practioner to research procedures and call for a radical alteration in the relationship of the therapist to his patients, giving the sense to practitioners that they are subordinate to the evaluator. Such a relation violates the manner in which

141

professionals interrelate[53] and activates the practitioner's tendency to be jealous of his prerogatives. Nonpsychiatric professionals are especially vulnerable to challenges to their authority since they have only recently gained professional standing.[11] Moreover, there are numerous paraprofessional and semiprofessional community mental health workers whose authority is not firmly established. Consequently, the scrutiny of evaluative research may be more painful to community mental health workers than to professionals whose status as such has been socially validated.

Within the mental health team itself, variations in accepted legitimacy to engage in therapeutic activities generate rivalry for prestige and control that belies the notion of harmony. Rushing has been quoted[81] as contending that

> a community of equals is a fiction. . . . Despite their proclamations to the contrary, it is not likely that psychiatrists will accept their "ancillaries" as their status equals—at least most will not. . . . [I]n the new mental hospitals which have no clear precedents or traditions and whose structure does not so strongly support the medical profession's status as does that of the general hospital, . . . the basis of authority will become unclear; and it is not unlikely that the infighting will become more fierce [p. 105].

The evaluative researcher can be caught up in the confusion of emerging organizational and professional situations where boundaries are poorly defined and roles, tasks, and responsibilities are unspecified. But above all, the evaluator runs the risk that his work will be used in power struggles or that he will provide contending factions with a common enemy. In such circumstances, the evaluator's role may become very ambiguous.[59] He can be caught up in power struggles to the point that he is not conducting evaluative research at all, but instead acting as a minion for a powerful figure who is negotiating to sustain his power. We have seen sociologists in such a situation who lost all meaningful objectivity in their research.

Dunham[37] points out that in this confusion of occupations and professions negotiating for power, the psychiatrist may feel pressures to "learn new skills in order to provide the required leadership to the various professionals who are planning to work toward this new vision of maximizing treatment potential in the community for the mentally ill" [p. 565]. Such aspirations and attempts to develop charismatic leadership reinforce the practitioner's sensitivities to assessment already generated from a myriad of sources.

Evaluators as Sources of Practitioner Opposition

Majority opinion seems to support the practice of program testing by outsiders,[26] although it has potential shortcomings. External specialists employed as consultants may bias their work in order to maintain a lucrative contact or because they are friendly to the action program.[73] Nonetheless, these potential

142

problems appear to be outweighed by the barriers to objectivity encountered by "inside" evaluators, a pattern that has frequently been adopted in community mental health programs.

As an outsider, the evaluator must try to accommodate himself to a complex role that offers the potential of many double binds.[117] If the evaluator comes to identify closely with the organization, he will be influenced by many of its internal pressures; if he strictly maintains his "outsideness," he runs a considerable risk of being labeled a *prima donna*. Regardless of how he attempts to present himself, he represents an outside research community with values and skills that differ sharply from those of practitioners. As a representative of the scientific community, he may view practitioners in a patronizing manner and perceive his mission as bringing his "know how" to the aid of the uninformed. Evaluative researchers almost universally condemn practitioner's own efforts at evaluation. Rather, they, from the Olympian heights of academia or the consulting firm, bring in their superior methods of finding out if the ignorant are doing any good. Like a good dentist, they may try to assure their patients that "it won't hurt much," and like a good missionary, they may try to assure the natives that the esoteric research is "for the good of you and your people." Above all, the evaluator must try to convince practitioners that he is not a policeman or a spy.[72] Caro[28] urges that "the climate for evaluation might be improved if evaluators were to place more emphasis on educating administrators, practitioners, and client representatives regarding the role of evaluation in program development" [p. 111]. In sum, the evaluator brings in suspect "outsideness" in the form of relatively unknown devices for testing the practitioner's work, and he attempts to sell them on the virtue of his alien methods, all under the guise of helping them help their target populations.

There may be sources of resistance in the evaluation procedure that the evaluator cannot control. Oftentimes he is hired by the funding agency rather than by local program administrators, and the timing of the evaluation is predetermined, regardless of the progress of program development. Often the practitioners say, "We're not ready," knowing full well that an evaluation at a certain point in time will yield unimpressive results. Sometimes this is only a defense, but in many situations, especially with demonstration programs where progress cannot be accurately projected, this plea is valid. A recent example of this situation in our experience was with a funding agency with an end of the year budget surplus that they felt had to be spent. Evaluation seemed like a legitimate last-minute use of funds. Consequently, with little warning and little consideration of program progress, teams of evaluators were sent to a whole range of programs. There are milder variations of such a horror story, most of which revolve around poor communication between programs and funding agencies or a bull-headed agency attitude that a certain amount of program evaluation must be completed within a certain time, regardless of the progress of program development. Nonetheless, the evaluator must often forge ahead under his outside mandate and attempt to survive amidst the hostility.

A potent source of resistance is the practitioners' perception of whether the evaluator's background and credentials establish his prerogative to investigate their program. The evaluator can be aptly referred to as a *voyeur*. This position becomes a deeper source of conflict if the evaluator has had little or no direct experience with program activities and lacks empathy for program problems and needs. We obviously do not contend that program experience is necessary for good evaluation, but it is likely that the evaluator who has not experienced the realities of mounting program action will have greater difficulties in sustaining rapport, and perhaps respect, than the evaluator who has some program experience.

This raises the question of how evaluators are recruited in the first place. Why would a professional with research skills undertake such a potentially frustrating task? Evaluation can be the source of professional and disciplinary pay-offs, although priority to the testing of methodology or theory can cause major difficulties. Or, it may be that a particular type of personality is attracted to evaluation. While there is no evidence for such a contention, the repeated adjectives applied to evaluators of "hard-nosed" or "cold-blooded" may belie the attraction of particular kinds of people to these tasks, and this may be an underlying source of conflict—especially if it is true that program practitioners are likely to possess personality traits of an opposite type.

Finally, and aside from the preceding conjectures, the cynical observation that there is money to be made in evaluation research cannot be ignored. Often evaluation is carried out on a consultation basis whereby evaluators (especially academicians) receive income in addition to some other salary. This may attract entrepreneurial types of professionals who may have a style of interaction that may run contrary to the orientations of practitioners and contribute to conflict.

Overselling and Exploitation

Overselling stems from the evaluator's assumption that a sound assessment really can be done, coupled with his tendency to underestimate the complexity of the program setting in which he will work. A backlash occurs when practitioners discover that, despite the disruptive impacts on their program activities, the research does not provide the cogent results that were promised. Campbell[22] states: "We are in danger of pretentious scientism, which defensively claims more precision and control than has been achieved. . . . [N]ot all remedial programs that are worth undertaking can be meaningfully evaluated and this fact should not prevent the ameliorative effort from being made. . . . [B]road-aim interventions may be particularly likely to fall in this class" [p. 111]. For Mann,[76] "there is good reason to question whether evaluative studies ought to be performed except for highly specific and limited purposes" [p. 13].

Exploitation is at issue with the tendency of many evaluators, especially those who are academically based, to use a program to test research questions of significance to their academic discipline and to give short shrift to genuine evaluative research.[124] Marris and Rein[78] cite Melvin Herman to the effect that "researchers state that they are not primarily interested in program evaluation, but rather in basic research" [p. 200]. Weiss and Rein[128] have observed an administrator in a large scale community action program who came to believe "the research group was deeply committed to analyzing the baseline data and hoped through it to make a contribution to their field. . . ," while Freeman and Sherwood[45] speak of the basic importance of committment to the role of evaluator. Rossi[97] feels that even when such exploitation is not attempted, "it is part of the researcher's responsibility to impress on the practitioners that in most cases results are slight and that there is more than an off-chance that they will be unfavorable" [p. 52].

Purists Need Not Apply

The need for research compromises inevitably marks evaluative studies. The complexity, vagueness, and profusion of variables characterizing action programs typically forces adaptation of standard research approaches to local situations. Mann[76] screened over 600 evaluative reports and decided only 181 met the carefully selected research criteria of experimental design and methodology. He concluded that "evaluative research is generally formulated in the simplest possible terms, involving pre-post tests [and] one method and one control group" [p. 198]. Beyond doubt this reflects Borgatta's[17] view that "by its nature [evaluative research cannot] be as rigorous and strictly scientific as laboratory experiments." Binner[12] bluntly defends a research director in a large mental health center: "The unusual demands for precision in research design and measurement do not intimidate him. He knows full well the limitations of his data and reports them forthrightly, but proceeds to give the institution the benefit of the best empirical evidence that can be gathered in the existing time and circumstances" [p. 317].

Our experiences are marred by the give-and-take that inexorably confounds field problems: unevenness of amount and time of exposure to the program, exclusion of segments of a target population considered "sensitive" by administrators, the inevitably hostile refusal to cooperate by one or more of the program practitioners, and the sampling attrition that naturally follows. These factors open evaluation studies to attack and to alternative interpretation of the data, setting the stage for manipulative pressures from practitioners. Because evaluation often focus on controversial programs, they are destined to be a source of both political and professional troubles for the evaluator. In sum, research purists will be tempermentally repelled by involvement in an action program and the subsequent necessity of defending blemished data from a research design that is often badly compromised.

In this section, we have reviewed sources of conflict that reduce the probability of effective evaluation. To return to our introductory point, it is likely that these factors combine to prevent the feedback of evaluation results into program

145

design, a goal which usually has at least lip-service priority in evaluative activities. To a degree, this calls for more attention to the latent functions of evaluation and to unstated covert goals, inasmuch as the outcome of conflict can be on the evaluator's side more often than not ("they wouldn't cooperate"), fueling arguments to "cut them off." Rather than dwell further on this, we shall move toward a constructive evaluation of evaluation, where we suggest that goal attainment approaches and experimental designs need further consideration for adapting evaluation to community mental health programs. A recent comment by Mushkin[141] provides perspective:

> Surprisingly, analysts who have given new emphasis to the feedback consequences of public programs appear to have paid little heed to the feedback consequences of *their* evaluations. These analysts, whose major stock in trade is "questioning," have failed to be sensitive to how the results of their studies are impacting on policy. . . . It is my contention that evaluation is being used as a decision-making tool more than it warrants, especially in light of the present state of scientific understanding and of the expectations placed upon evaluations by the public and its officials. To use evaluation results for policy-making, we need to know what goes into the formulation of an evaluation study, what its limitations are, and what its findings really mean. We need to be able to separate fact from artifact. But above all, we need to refine our evaluation methods into as much a science as possible. . . . [I am concerned with] accountability, not through evaluation, but *of* evaluations that lead me to the label: "Evaluations: Use with Extreme Caution" [p. 31].

PROBLEMS WITH THE GOAL ATTAINMENT MODEL AND EXPERIMENTAL DESIGNS

Evaluators have shown a strong proclivity to approach program assessment with a "goal attainment model" and to employ its frequently called for research method, the experimental design.[6] Both have been widely described in the evaluative literature, suggesting evaluators' attraction and commitment to the combination. The rigor and elegance required approaches "the impossible dream" of evaluative studies. Nonetheless the approach is normative among evaluators; most try to come as close as possible to the goal attainment-experimental model. Caro[28] describes evaluators as preferring "some form of experimental design" to assure "that changes in measured behavior can be attributed exclusively to the program at hand" [p. 107]. But for practitioners in action organizations such as community mental health centers, the model can appear as rigid and time-limited and as locking them into a research pattern incompatible with their ongoing practice. A feature that causes great concern is the model's prescription of randomly assigning patients to treatment groups and to control groups in which they get either no treatment or some form of placebo. Many practitioners believe that this requirement approaches unethical behavior. Be-

146

cause this model is so deeply embedded in evaluators' thinking and is such a basic source of scorn and rejection among action personnel, we need to explore in some detail its nature and its defects.

The Goal Attainment Model

Practically all definitions of organizations are primarily in terms of goals. Much of the large research literature on productivity, morale, conformity, and adaptation is cast in a goal attainment framework. The goal attainment model defines organizational effectiveness in terms of accomplishment of goals, with specific criteria drawn from the content of these goals. Applying this to evaluation studies, Levenson[70] describes "people processing" within the goal model, beginning with "(1) an incoming group possessing certain population characteristics to whom (2) something is done which in turn produces (3) a desired change, assuming that (4) certain attitudinal and cognitive changes have previously occurred" [p. 76]. He uses the Work Experience Program of the Economic Opportunity Act as an example. The goal attainment model in this instance "assumed a sequential flow of time-related events such that at time 1 a population participating in a program during time 2 undergoes certain cognitive and normative changes at time 3 which result in employment at time 4" [p. 76]. In this example evaluation strategy would concentrate specifically on the stated goal of producing a person who can find and hold a job.

The model includes the assumption that specific goals can be evaluated in isolation from other goal-seeking subsystems within the organization. It is also assumed that the evaluation process is circular,[105] i.e., it "starts with initial goal setting, proceeds to determine measures of the goal, collects data and appraises the effect of the goal, and then modifies the initial goal on the basis of the collected data" [p. 565]. Here we find the "feedback" that was our basic concern in the previous section.

Despite the apparent simplicity of the goal attainment model, it has proven difficult to put into practice. Not only have many evaluators discovered that it is difficult to identify the "real goals,"[40] but the nature of real goals makes the use of the model much more complex than would appear on the surface. Perrow[90] points out that "official" goals often stand in sharp contrast to "operative" goals:

Official goals are the general purposes of the organization as put forth in the charter, annual reports, public statements by key executives and other authoritative pronouncements. For example, the goal of an employment agency may be to place job seekers in contact with firms seeking workers. The official goal of a hospital may be to promote the health of the community through curing the ills, and sometimes through preventing illness, teaching, and conducting research. . . . This level of analysis is inadequate in itself for a full understanding of organizational behavior. Official goals are purposely vague and

147

general and do not indicate two major factors which influence organizational behavior: the host of decisions that must be made among alternative ways of achieving official goals and the priority of multiple goals, and the many unofficial goals pursued by groups within the organization. The concept of "operative goals" will be used to cover these aspects. Operative goals designate the ends sought through the actual operating policies of the organization; they tell us actually what the organization is trying to do, regardless of what the official goals say are the aims [p. 855].

While it certainly makes sense, this distinction is insufficient for getting at the elusive goal-seeking features of an action program. Hyman and Wright[57] state: "Basic concepts and goals are often elusive and vague . . . ; [thus] a great deal of the initial labor in evaluation research consists of attempts to formulate in a clear and measurable fashion a list of goals which can serve as the basis for determining the program's relative success" [pp. 756-757]. Hyman, Wright, and Hopkins[56] add: "the breadth of the things assumed under a particular objective, the multiple objectives encompassed by many programs, the ambiguity inherent in any or all of the objectives as stated, and the disagreement as to the objectives—are characteristic of many programs and are enough to stagger the imagination of the evaluator" [p. 7]. Streuning and Peck[112] comment: "the scope and boundaries of [psychiatric programs] have generally been less well defined than the majority of its clinical neighbors . . ." [p. 167]. Freeman and Sherwood[45] provide this summation:

The researcher has three choices—he can follow Hyman's recommendation and try to guess the intermediate and overall goals, and later be told that the ones he selected were not relevant at all; he can insist that program persons provide them in which case he should bring lots of novels to the office to read while he waits; or he can participate or even take a major responsibility for the development of the action framework. There is little likelihood of developing evaluation designs for these massive programs by either second guessing the action people or by insisting upon their coming up with an appropriate and explicit flow chart. Indeed, if the researcher is going to act responsibly as an agent of social change through his evaluation research, it probably is mandatory for him to engage himself in program development [p. 17].

While one can make conceptual (and even measurable) distinctions between real and publicly stated goals, between operative and official goals, or between formal and informal goals, it is essential to understand the multiple nature of organizational goals if the goal attainment model is to be used properly: how goals come into being, their vulnerability to displacement and succession, their interrelatedness, and their specificity. Goals come into being as a result of a complicated interaction between power cliques, strong personalities, and forces impinging on the organization from the surrounding environment. Thus organizational goals

148

are dynamic; they cannot be conceived as stable features of organizational life. Their instability stems from the shifts that occur in bargaining power and negotiating effectiveness of occupational subgroups within organizations. Krause[65] describes a bargaining process between rehabilitation counselors, social workers, psychologists, and consultants, where those with professional status were pitted against those with control of funds. Both had some real power and had to negotiate which operative goals would guide their collective effort. Perrow[90] documents the shifts in goals of a general hospital that were closely related to shifts in the relative power positions of trustees, physicians, and administrators.

In the process of negotiation, subgoals tend to form, especially when there is a plethora of specialized groups brought together under a single organizational canopy.[106] Whether subgoals arise from different occupational commitments and identities or from formal organizational assignment, an exclusive orientation toward the subgoal without regard for its consequences for the organization as a whole tends to follow.[77]

The problem of instability of goals for the evaluative researcher is illustrated by Ferman's[43] description of an evaluative effort in a manpower training program. At first, the evaluator used the number of training-related job placements as a criteria of program effectiveness. Months later, however, the goal was redefined by practitioners as the placement of graduates in practically any kind of work. Some months later, the agency began emphasizing the therapeutic value of training as a fundamental index of effectiveness. In each of these instances, the evaluator had to be aware of the shift to make the drastic changes necessary in the measures of effectiveness used.

Not only are organizational goals unstable, they also tend to be multiple and complexly interrelated. Goss[51] found that hospitals often have multiple goals and that a certain combination of goals were most likely to produce good medical care, i.e., formally recognized teaching, research, specialized service, and the absence of profit. Other observers have defined an organization as having a multiplicity of goals, often arranged in a hierarchy.[84] The evaluative researcher must come to grips with this multiplicity of goals, each with related subgoals, when he is using the goal attainment model. Since it is impossible to bring all goals and subgoals under the scrutiny of the research effort, he must make some selections.

This raises a problem of primary importance. The goal attainment model contains the assumption that a particular goal can be selected out and evaluated singly without concern for its interrelatedness with other goals. This appears to be unsupportable. One study[104] has shown that in a large state hospital a sharp alteration in the treatment program for the aged and the alteration of organizational goals to support the change brought about widespread resistance among many residents and in the overall teaching program. Although much of the literature concerning organizational behavior tends to underscore the interrelated nature of goals and the extent to which the modification of one results in an alteration in other goals, most applications of the goal attainment model in evaluation have ignored this point. The basic question for evaluative research is how it can focus upon a single goal and its evaluation when this separation is unnatural and artificial. Secondly, if the feedback of evaluative data alter one organizational goal, what will be the effects on interrelated goals? Can they still be maintained and achieved?

Organizational goals are vulnerable to diversion, original objectives being supplanted by alternative ones, and to goal displacement or what is called "means-ends inversion," the neglect of the claimed goals in favor of the means as ends in themselves.[122] Blau and Scott[142] state that in goal diversion there may be a "retreat from the original goal to more modest objectives, as exemplified by the history of the Tennessee Valley Authority and by the tendencies in socialist parties and unions in imperial Germany" [p. 231]. Warner and Havens[122] argue persuasively that "the greater the intangibility of the organizational goals, the greater the tendency for the goals to be displaced." Examples of intangible goals are: "helping people become better citizens, developing a greater community integration or stronger community spirit, developing attitudes and skills of cooperation, helping people help themselves solve a problem, educating people and changing their attitudes, developing human resources, increasing the dignity of human life, improving society, improving the well being of people."[122] Such goals are readily subject to displacement because organizations are expected to produce tangible results, particularly when faced by evaluation; the organization has to coordinate and control specific member behavior, and intangible goals produce uncertainty, anxiety, frustration, and feelings of insecurity in members.

The analyses of Warner and Havens also suggest that claimed goals are neglected in favor of the means as ends in themselves. When record keeping, report making, and thorough program planning join with this necessity to act, there is a high likelihood of goal displacement. Consequently, the evaluative researcher may unwittingly concentrate upon a highly intangible goal, attempting to operationalize it by a specific criterion and to attach a tight research design. He may not detect a substantial goal displacement within the organization and that there is only minimal focus on what the researcher assumes to be the chief objective. This probability increases when organizations develop specific rewards and punishments to secure appropriate behavior from individual members. In a situation with highly intangible goals, sanctions often tend to be directed towards what can be evaluated, namely, what is visible, tangible, and measurable.

The instability of goals can be further understood by considering goal conflict among organization members, the development of goal consensus, and the subsequent diffusion of goals. There are variations in the sharing of organizational goals among organization members. Even where intangible goals prevail, strong sentiments of acceptance of the goal may be widely diffused. On the other hand, conflict and subgoal formation may leave initial goals weakened and badly dilated. Furthermore, new goals may emerge which may or may not conflict with original ones. One axiom seems to emerge. Lack of specificity of objectives and intangible reference points for organizational goals mean that evaluative re-

150

searchers using the goal attainment model must spend an inordinate amount of time specifying the actual aims and objectives of an organization.

Certain additional cautions regarding the goal attainment model should be noted. Because goals are often ultra-idealistic, when an organization's performance is measured against them, low effectiveness is typically shown.[39] This may well lead to disillusionment among practitioners, recipients of services, and the program's sponsors, creating barriers to evaluation feedback. Also, the fact that measuring tends to encourage over-emphasis on the measurable goals and neglect of those less measurable[22] makes it clear that use of the goal attainment model of evaluation may have an intense "Hawthorne effect," i.e., the organization may be changed by the research process itself. It may particularly alter the broader, intangible, ideal aspects of program goals.

Experimental Designs

A typical accompaniment of the goal attainment model is the experimental method. This methodology needs to be examined in terms of its legion of technical problems and its failures and successes.

Suchman[114] summarizes the range of experimental designs designated by Campbell. They are deceptively simple in graphic portrayal: X indicates exposure of a group to an alleged change agent; O stands for the observation of the desired effect (criterion). Xs and Os "in a given row refer to the same specific persons, while parallel rows represent equivalent or matched samples of persons" [p. 93]. Time sequence goes from left to right. Four examples of experimental design follow:

1. XO, or, the "one-shot case study." Observations are made on the target group *only* after they have experienced the program. There is no comparison group. In strict terms, this does not involve an experiment, but is often referred to as a simple experimental design.

2. $O_1 X O_2$. Here O_1 represents base line measures of a target group before they experience the program; O_2 represents taking the same measures of the group after they experience the program. Again, no comparison group is used.

3. $\frac{XO_1}{O_2}$. This design involves the comparison of measurements of a group that has experienced the program (O_1) with measurements of a group that has not experienced the program (O_2).

4. $\frac{O_1 X O_2}{O_3 O_4}$. This design calls for two groups with membership characteristics as identical as possible. This is typically achieved by randomization in the assignment to groups. The similarities in starting points are determined by measurements (O_1 and O_3) before the program. Then one of these groups experiences the program (X) and the other does not. Both are again measured after the program is over (O_2 and O_4) and results compared.

The Solomon 4-way design[110] adds two additional study groups to ascertain the effects of administering the measurements (the Hawthorne effect). Other extensions of these patterns have been proposed.[21] The four designs above, however, provide the basics.

We have been struck by the many reports that describe the near impossibility of using experimental designs that involve comparison groups (numbers 3 and 4 above). Schulberg and his co-workers[105] report that "one is hard pressed to uncover any successfully completed studies of this type in the health field." Regarding studies of psychotherapy, Eysenck[41] observes that practically all studies in the field have neglected to provide control groups. Kandel and Williams,[59] reporting on a conference of representatives of 49 psychiatric research projects, indicate a consensus against the establishment of control groups in psychiatric research because such research is very difficult to execute. Borgatta[17] simply observes that "a true experimental design is in the nature of things impossible." Hyman and associates[56] concur: "The ideal is hard to achieve." One observer,[24] however, suggests a source of these formidable technical problems: "The researcher depends upon the actionist in nearly every stage of the research process, while the actionist likely considers the presence of the evaluation researcher as a necessary evil at best" [p. 139]. We believe that a breakthrough in evaluative studies will occur when researchers refocus their attention on the relationship between themselves and practitioners, seeking ways to effectively work within it with integrity.

Establishing and maintaining control subjects is problematic. Beyond doubt, practitioners' concern becomes most intense regarding controls, the very heart of experimentation. Random assignments of patients to treatment and comparison groups can assure a high degree of legitimacy of comparisons because it tends to assure that all salient characteristics are evenly distributed, but the notion of a group which receives no treatment or partial treatment is unacceptable to most practitioners. Social circumstances within action programs can change control groups as much, if not more, than treatment can affect the experimental group, particularly when ethical concerns are sharpened. The equalizing effects of randomization can be eroded by a multitude of other factors: relatives can intervene, a patient can use influence to get shifted to the treatment group, members of either group may become physically sick or drop out for a numerous other reasons. The same factors mar "matching" as a device for developing a control group. Inevitably, a series of forces produce uncontrolled attrition.[38] Not only does matching require an extremely large pool of candidates for its legitimate execution, but also usually calls for the withholding of treatment.

Equally frustrating is the ever-present conflict over what constitutes "success" or "favorable outcome," an issue that is highlighted in experimental designs. The problem of criterion haunts practically every effort at program assessment, setting the stage for confrontations between researchers and practitioners. Practitioners are apt to be satisfied with practical criteria, such as, for an alcoholic, remaining sober for a set period of time, whereas researchers are apt to set up more complex criteria, like multi-faceted community adjustment among those who have undergone treatment.[6] Especially confusing to practitioners is the tendency for evaluators to use attitude change, rather than behavior change, as evaluative criteria. Practitioners are oriented to tangible results and doubt the validity of paper and pencil tests of subjective feelings, attitudes, personality, and beliefs. Even if such changes are shown, their value is difficult to communicate to practitioners. Indexes of actual behavior are conspicuously infrequent among the 181 superior evaluation studies analyzed by Mann,[76] suggesting methodological difficulties in their use. Results on attitude change relative to behavior change tend to support practitioner skepticism.[61, 95] In any event, the criterion problem cuts across *all* experimental designs: They abound, for example, in nonexperimental devices such as simple questionnaires administered to patients or relatives of patients. But they are especially acute in what Weiss and Rein[129] term broad and intangible aim programs such as those in community mental health centers.

An experimental design demands standardization and uniformity. If no "before" criterion measures are used, how can "starting points" be estimated? "Baseline" problems are forever plaguing experimentalists.[91] The practitioner is usually depended upon for assuring standardization. Uniformity of exposure to the program is often in his hands. Can the practitioner assure that *all* those in the treatment group get the *same* therapist, for the *same* amount of time, the *same* type of therapy, *ad infinitum?* It is nearly impossible for the researcher to gain control over the manifold sources of contamination.

Measurement devices may interact with the actual program effects to produce an "interaction effect," and the design usually does not separate out results due to the research instruments (the Hawthorne effect) from those due to the program action. To avoid this, the program administrator may be asked to provide more groups to add to the design in order to filter out interactive effects.[6] Even if he cooperates with this request, the administrator faces the high likelihood of negative results from the study, but no identification of specific shortcomings in the program. Experimental studies are often purely mechanical techniques to ascertain if change took place and do not identify factors to aid in replanning and regrouping the program forces. The practitioners are left with barren, dry-as-dust data that say the program works, that it works moderately, or that it doesn't work at all. The *why* is beyond the design. It is small wonder that evaluation generates defensive, hostile, and anxious reactions.

The previously mentioned problem of the timing of evaluative studies can be accentuated by experimental designs. The evaluator can find that program action shifts sharply in the midst of his data collection, rendering its results useless. Furthermore, even if he takes care to include significant "why" variables in the design and some sound reasons for failure or success emerge from the data, they may come very late in the program, having provided little guidance for operating decisions that continually arose in program management. As we have seen, organizational goals are dynamic, but experimental design is necessarily statis. For example, during the year or two probably needed to complete an experimental design, very basic shifts in goals may have made the variables included in the design irrelevant.

Many of these points are reflected in analyses of evaluative research studies. Of the 181 studies selected as the best out of the hundreds of studies analyzed by Mann,[76] only 23 per cent satisfied randomization standards, while 80 per cent had pre-post measures, and 74 per cent tested one change method with one type of control group. But 96 per cent of these studies had no control for the "interaction effect" between research devices and the change methods used. Mann concludes that the vast majority of evaluative studies "use the simplest possible experimental design, substituting simplicity for efficiency" [p. 204].

To a degree, this point is exemplified by the evaluators of Head Start programs in public schools. Called in after the program was well underway, the evaluators had to opt for an *ex post facto* design (number 3 above) and concentrate only on one aspect of the program. Despite an admirable defense,[134] the evaluators remain plagued by such basic questions as similarity of starting points between control and experimental subjects, wide variations in how and by whom the program was executed, and attrition in the sampling. Certainly they could not get to the question of interaction effects between measuring devices and the program with such a design, even though they proudly designate it as a "respected and widely used scientific procedure." Undoubtedly community mental health programs are being subject to rather similar evaluation. An example is the study by Lefton and co-workers[68] that sustained a design that compared female, urban, hospitalized, functionally impaired mental patients with "normal" neighbors living within ten house numbers, using criteria of role performances. But uniformity of treatment exposure remains a question, particularly within a program as diffuse as a community mental health program.

Certainly these points do not exhaust the list of technical problems that will plague the researcher and disrupt the practitioner; they do, however, underscore the central deficiency of evaluative research: the inherent difference between the research world and the world of social action of which community mental health centers are a part. But goal attainment models of evaluation and experimental designs seem poorly adapted to the inevitable contingencies that arise in action programs. Furthermore, these strategies contain inevitable sources of conflict that can exacerbate the basic relational problems between evaluators and practitioners.

So far our profile of evaluation in programs such as community mental health has tended to be dismal. In the next and final section, we turn to some reasons for optimism, based on some potential means for adapting evaluation to community mental health programs and some notable instances of success.

SUGGESTIONS FOR IMPROVING EVALUATION

Despite our emphasis on the quasi-enemy nature of practitioner-researcher relations, instances of successful collective effort in evaluation have been reported. Schulberg and Baker[104] note "sufficient examples [that] research and evaluation directly affecting clinical practice can be harmonious. . . ." Meyer and Borgatta[85] seemed to have had excellent practitioner acceptance of their randomized design, although they could not carry it to completion because of patient unwillingness. Since few evaluations are reported in the professional literature, there may be many unreported instances of joint evaluation efforts with successful outcomes. In this section we pursue this positive note and advance some suggestions for reducing resentments and rejections of evaluative research.

Adapting the Experimental Approach

Although less powerful than a classical design with a control group and before and after measurements, there are variations on the experimental theme that retain significant testing power and are more acceptable to practitioners. Closest to the ideal is the $\frac{XO_1}{O_2}$ design in which one group is exposed to the program techniques and the other is not. Neither receive "before" measures, thus avoiding potential research effects and subsequent interaction effects. But, as Suchman[114] points out, "this design affords no way of knowing that the two groups were equivalent *before* the program . . ." [p. 95]. Possible differences in starting points between the two groups can, however, be reduced sharply under two conditions: (1) the availability of a large number of subjects (200 or more) at a common starting time for program testing, and (2) the availability of information about group members that goes beyond simple demographic data such as sex, age, and marital status. While simple random assignment is acceptable when very large numbers of cases are involved, most circumstances require that the overall study population be stratified on variables believed to be related to different starting points (e.g., chronicity or prior treatment experience). Using such strata along with standard demographic variables in the sampling strategy will probably yield two groups with highly similar baseline points. These two ingredients maximize the probability of identical group composition and similar starting points, thereby sidestepping the need for "before" measurement, and provide for legitimate comparison of the "after" scores of groups that have and have not been exposed to treatment. Furthermore, specific therapeutic efforts lasting a relatively short period of time (e.g., operant conditioning, brief therapies, and group therapies), are likely to remain stable for long enough to use this simple design. In other words, when brief treatments are evaluated, the disruptive possibilities of program change in the midst of data collection are minimized.

Yet the emotionally charged problem of withholding treatment for the control group remains. This can be managed when the therapy is relatively brief, there is a high demand for service, and the number of available treatment personnel precludes simultaneous administration of the treatment anyway. Under such conditions, the control group remains untreated only for a short time, and its members can be included in the next wave of treatment after the evaluative data have been collected.

Needless to say, brief treatments are only one target for evaluation, and even this simple design does not eliminate the "control problem." Ways of minimizing negative sentiments associated with withholding treatment while preserving some means of legitimate comparison are badly needed. One solution is to use the population studied, over time, as its own control group. Brandon and Gruenberg,[18] using as a criterion the annual incidence of the chronic social breakdown syndrome among a group of patients believed to be vulnerable, were able to show that the incidence was "perhaps twice as high" in 1960 than at the end of 1962 after a community mental health program was introduced in Dutchess County, New York. Hyman and his associates[56] support this method and describe how Carl Rogers and his associates developed an "own-control" group. Rogers attempted to control for maturation processes among the subjects. These processes are described by Campbell[22] as factors "within the respondents producing changes as a function of the passage of time *per se,* such as growth, fatigue, secular trends, etc." [p. 111]. Rogers delayed therapy in a sampled group for 60 days during which he attempted to establish "the magnitude of change due to natural events and growth, against which the effects of subsequent therapy could be appraised" [Hyman *et al.,* p. 43]. Campbell refined this approach into what he calls an "interrupted time-series design." By using a "speed crackdown" program aimed at reducing traffic accidents as an example, he examined the various errors, i.e., maturation, history, instability, selection, etc., that plague the method, but suggested how to track these variables to make use of the method feasible.[22] An anti-smoking campaign in England used a variation of this strategy by drawing two carefully stratified, random samples of the target population, one before the campaign, one after it, and then comparing them.[69]

It is also possible to gain some degree of control by comparing rates of specific behavior disorders (e.g., depression) in a uniformly treated group with the probability rate in a given time period within the general population from which the treatment group emerged. Thus in a limited, high risk population, the expected rate of depression would be worked out from a retrospective analysis of data from sources such as a psychiatric register. The comparison is made after a program directed toward the limited population has been underway. We are not aware of research efforts using this strategy, but since evaluative studies tend to be under-reported, it probably has been employed.

Another strategy involves replications, which Hyman and his associates[56] feel "are peculiarly suitable to evaluations in solving the problem of a control-group design. . . . Notable is the problem of excluding eligible subjects from treatment. The replication provides the answer. All subjects receive the full treatment, yet they still serve as controls" [p. 53]. Furthermore, replication makes possible "estimates of the influence of events, natural stability, and unreliability of instruments on the gross changes observed" [p. 52]. Thus, if results vary from repeated use of the treatment strategy in different groups, the possibility of tracing the factors contributing to success or failure within the treatment groups emerges, perhaps setting the stage for "selection for treatment."[121] As

Weiss[126] points out, "Repetition of results is the basis of scientific generalization. And through repeated investigation, we can increasingly specify the conditions under which programs succeed or fail and the processes by which success and failure come about" [p. 84].

Constant intervening factors cannot be noted by replication. Also, replication calls for extremely precise repetition of the treatment intervention with identical techniques, setting, personnel, and resources input. This may be very difficult from an administrative viewpoint; on the other hand, there probably are mature community mental health programs where a specific subprogram is stable and uniform enough for a close approximation of three or four replications. Apparently this strategy has rarely been used; Mann[76] reports 93 per cent of his superior evaluative studies made no use of replication.

Comparison Group Strategy: A Viable Substitute for Controls

Aside from these strategies that use the control group in some form, there appears to be much wider acceptance and understanding of legitimate comparison, using a common criterion, of markedly different programs whose content, strategy, and philosophy are distinctive. Instead of experimental or control groups, two distinct change efforts directed toward the same outcome are compared. The need for common starting points calls for randomized assignment of patients into the different treatments. Organizing such randomization may be particularly difficult in community mental health programs where there is an abundance of therapeutic strategies to compare. Wilner[132] sees the community mental health center concept placing inpatient, outpatient, and partial hospitalization care "under a single umbrella, if not actually at the same site. . . . This has the potential of putting several branches of treatment in close touch with one another. . . . Enough treatment variants will be available to permit in the long run assessment of different treatment modalities" [pp. 20, 22]. Phillips and Wiener[91] cull from their experiences and from reported evaluation studies comparisons of structured and unstructured therapies, of different approaches to structured short term therapies, and comparisons of short term and long term therapy. There is clearly the possibility of natural comparison groups developing in community mental health programs, needing only the systematic input of the evaluator. Weiss[124] comments: "Many government programs . . . are not so much unitary programs as a congeries of diverse efforts addressed to the same problem. Within the programs there are different emphases and different content and procedures. The evaluator is able to identify the different theories that underlie the different emphases, categorize them—and the program activities— along a number of significant dimensions, then relate the type of program to program outcome" [p. 63].

But randomization still "locks in" patient assignment and makes for potential conflict with practitioners' clinical judgment. At the same time, no one is denied treatment. Projected results can make sense to the practitioner as they help

157

answer the question of what kind of patient benefits most from what therapeutic regimen. The evaluator, however, must be fully familiar with the actual experience of all the groups he is comparing, and he must exhibit as much neutrality as he can muster. A prominent problem is formulating a realistic and fair criterion for gauging successful outcome across a range of treatments. This may be a potent source of disagreement.

A number of good comparison group studies are available. We will give five summary examples:

1. Pasamanick and his associates[89] assessed the relative merit of hospital versus home treatment for schizophrenics. The researchers randomized 152 patients originally referred to a state hospital into three groups: a hospitalized group, a home care group receiving medication, and a home care group receiving placebos. Those treated at home received regular visits from public health nurses and occasional visits from a psychologist, a social worker, and a psychiatrist. Unfortunately the time of treatment exposure varied sharply, ranging from 6 to 30 months. One of the measures of success used, the number of times the patient was hospitalized, raised other questions. Those treated in the hospital required returns to the hospital more often than those treated at home with medication, but this may reflect "institutionalism" more than specific treatment effects. In the home care group receiving medication, over 77 per cent remained constantly at home, contrasted to 34 per cent of the group receiving placebos. A second criterion, social functioning, was used after 6, 18, and 24 months. After 6 months no one form of treatment had any superiority over another on this measure. The data did, however, clearly suggest that home treatment can reduce hospitalization, and that social costs to home and community are about equal after 6 months; prior to that time, home care constituted a substantial burden for relatives and friends.

Followup of this landmark study continued, with a "wash-out" being revealed after five years.[143] "A gradual erosion of the original significant differences [was found] when only usual clinic and aftercare services were available. By the end of five years, no differences in social or psychological functioning could be found among the three groups."[144]

2. Fairweather[42] conducted a carefully designed study for comparison between patient behavior in hospital wards and in the community following two types of treatment. He randomized a population of patients into a small group ward and a traditional ward. "Task group" ward housekeeping, ward meeting hour, and autonomous meetings of task groups were introduced in the small group ward, in contrast to traditional ward regimen, all of which was designed to facilitate return to community life. Sampling for participation in the two wards was refined and a procedure set up for each staff member to spend equal amounts of time in both. Followup time for both groups was six months from the day they left the hospital. Fairweather indicated that "overall followup results have demonstrated that the small group treatment reduced hospitalization sig-

nificantly and brought about more employment and active involvement with others. Nonetheless, when viewed as a total problem, approximately 50 percent of the non-psychotics and long term psychotics returned to the hospital within 6 months" [p. 168].

3. A comparison group study in England[52] broadened the units compared: two cities that appeared to be demographically and environmentally similar were used. In 1958, a program of community care for the mentally ill was introduced in one city; the other continued with a hospital based service. "To evaluate these differing policies, a random sample of all patients referred in each area in the year 1960-61 was followed up for two years. The success of each policy was examined . . . by measuring the help it gave the community in reducing the burden of mental illness to families, and . . . the help it gave to individual patients in reducing the clinical signs and symptoms of their illness" [p. 430]. On all the ratings of family burden of work performance used, the hospital based service produced superior results.

4. Also in England, Wing[135] and his research group compared the quality of care and style of administration in three mental hospitals. They concluded that it was not hospitalization *per se* that brought on the clinical impression of deterioration, but rather the quantity and quality of care that chronically ill patients receive.

5. Lazarus[66] compared highly specific therapies—traditional group therapy and behavior therapy (desensitization)—in terms of their effectiveness in altering phobic behaviors. Patients studied were matched on sex, age, and the type and observed severity of the phobic disorder. Lazarus tossed a coin to determine which one of the matched pair would be treated by desensitization and which by group therapy. The same therapist conducted all the groups. Desensitization was clearly superior.

A Break With Traditional Patterns: The Systems Model

All the evaluative procedures discussed so far fall within the goal attainment paradigm, i.e., attention is focused exclusively on the organization's goals. Recently this singularity of focus has been broadened into a "systems model" that represents a break with the traditional goal oriented approach, although still including goals as a prominent dimension.[103] The perspective includes "multiple goals, many of which are not relevant to fulfillment of explicitly stated objectives."[120] This model grows directly out of systems theory in sociology that views component activities as organized into systemic relationships. Thus a collectivity has emergent properties that are usually not present in its discrete parts.[15, 19] It cannot be assumed that social collectivities automatically constitute systems.[19] Advocates of this model do assume, however, that an action program and its encompassing organization are a multifunctional unit in which some of its basic resources serve non-goal functions, i.e., they maintain the functioning of the organization itself.[39, 105] This model conceives of all variables within the organization as being reciprocally dependent upon one another. Over-concentration on any single activity, including the formal goals, is a mark of ineffectiveness; other necessary functions within the organization are being neglected. Thus an evaluation using this model assesses the coordination of subunits, maintenance of resources, and adaptation to internal and environmental demands in addition to the basic issue of goal attainment.[104, 105]

The approach is divided into "closed system" and "open system" strategies of organizational analysis. Closed systems are relatively self-contained structures that can be analyzed by focusing upon the system's internal functioning independent of external factors. The closed system approach assumes that the variables and relationships involved are few enough to comprehend and control. If closure is not complete, it is assumed that outside forces acting on the organization are predictable.[116] By ignoring or minimizing the environmental forces that influence the organization, it is possible to focus upon performance or efficiency; this, Thompson states, "results in everything being functional—making a positive, indeed an optimum, contribution to the overall results. All resources are appropriate resources and their allocation fits a master plan. All action is appropriate action, and its outcomes are predictable" [p. 6]. The model attempts to maximize what Thompson describes as "the search for certainty."

In the open systems frame of reference, it is assumed there are forces and variables operating that cannot be brought under rational planning and control. It is assumed that the organization is dependent not only upon its interactions with the external environment, but also on internal forces that cannot be neatly subsumed under the highly rational approach characteristic of traditional administrative management. Thompson has labeled the open systems approach a "natural-systems model" in contrast to the rational assumptions that underlie the closed systems analysis.

Katz and Kahn[60] place less emphasis upon "managing uncertainty" in systems analysis. They imply, however, that evaluation of organizational effectiveness must start with its dynamic relationships with the environment, "including the importation of energy from the environment, the through-put or transformation of the imported energy into some product which is characteristic of the system, the exporting of that product into the environment, and the re-energizing of the system from sources in the environment" [p. 28].

While each of these approaches may be useful in analysis, neither alone affords an adequate understanding of complex organizations.[116] Complex organizations manifest sizeable success in planning and controlling inputs, transforming these resources into products, and manipulating the social and political environment in order to sustain itself. But there is a sizeable amount of caprice operating in the external environment with which the organization must interact as well as within the formal internal structure of the organization.

An integration of the closed and open system orientations has developed a more realistic systems model. It focuses on the natural processes within the organization in the effort to achieve goals, but includes an emphasis upon limited rationality in gathering and processing information and in predicting consequences of alternative courses of action.[32,77] Thompson[116] summarizes this conception of complex organizations as "open systems, hence indeterminant and faced with uncertainty, but at the same time as subject to criteria of rationality and hence needing determinateness and certainty" [p. 10].

In regard to evaluative research, these concepts call for the evaluation of activities aimed at organizational survival as well as assessment of goal achievement. Schulberg and Baker[104] outline the functions that pertain to survival: "the effective coordination of organizational subunits, the acquisition and maintenance of necessary sources, and the adaptation of the organization to the environment and to its own internal demands" [p. 1252]. The model calls first for the evaluation of organizational functions that must be performed effectively before goal achievement is possible. These "vital functions" include personnel recruitment, personal growth among the organization's personnel, the organization's development and expansion, and the individual's desire for control of organizational resources and of personal influence and status.[105] Etzioni[39] formulates criteria for determining effectiveness within this model as: "how close the organizational allocation of resources approaches an optimum distribution. . . . [W]hat counts is a balanced distribution of resources among the various organizational needs, not maximal satisfaction of one activity, even of goal activities" [p. 259].

Katz and Kahn[60] suggest that organizational effectiveness can be viewed from the standpoint of the individual member, "defining as most effective that organization which offers the greatest aggregate return to the member." In addition, systems analysis could be utilized within the frame of reference of the "transactions between the organization and other agencies in society [and] would be judged effective to the degree that the organization provided maximal return to the society for the energetic demands which it made on the society. The test of effectiveness . . . would be applied at the next higher level of social organization. In doing so, the prosperity and survival of the organization becomes secondary" [p. 166].

Robert Weiss[127] adds another way in which the systems model might be utilized to measure organizational effectiveness. He believes that the clients of the organization, especially health organizations, can first be viewed as clients who are involved in larger systems: "The clients are enmeshed in relationships with other individuals in other programs which then interrelate with the way in which the clients respond to the services of the program." An alternate frame of reference which is also cliented-oriented conceptualizes the clients themselves as "embodying systems of needs, motivations, perceptions, attitudes, and beliefs which affect the use they make of the services of the program." In sum, there are numerous subsystems functioning in any organization that can serve as the focal point for systems assessment. This variety of frames of reference contrasts with the goal attainment model which frequently singles out the most prominent operationalized goal and concentrates upon it exclusively.

A systems model of evaluation is much more difficult than a goal attainment model to put into operation. The evaluator must know much more about the organization's history and its diverse activities and functions. He will thus generate a great deal of data for analysis. As he tries to encompass the total action system and its continuously changing processes, he will find it very difficult to locate objective criteria for codifying this information. The model demands much more of the evaluator's time and energy in direct observation and interaction with all parts of the organization than the goal attainment model. Because of these difficulties, the systems model seems to be more discussed than applied.[124]

An example of the use of the systems model is a study of organizational effectiveness by Georgopoulas and Tannenbaum.[50] They constructed three indexes, each measuring a basic element of the system: *organizational flexibility,* the ability to adjust to external or internal change; *strain within the organization,* as evidenced by incidences of tension and conflict among subgroups; and *station productivity.* A total score of effectiveness was computed for each of the 32 delivery service stations. These were correlated with the ratings on effectiveness that various experts and "insiders" assigned to each station. These ratings and the effectiveness scores were significantly correlated.

Schulberg and Baker[104] describe an almost classic instance of the greater ability of the systems model than the goal attainment model to offer the program director sufficient guidance for implementing change, i.e., the work of the Cummings[31] regarding the effectiveness of mental health education:

[The Cummings] started out to study to what extent and what directions attitudes toward mental illness could be changed through an intensive education program. After completing the six months program, the Cummings found virtually no change in the population's general orientation, either toward the social problem of mental illness or toward the mentally ill themselves. If the goal attainment model had been pursued, the researchers might simply have concluded that mental health education is ineffective and that the program should be dropped. Instead the Cummings shifted to a systems model of evaluation and considered their data within the context of the functions, both manifest and latent, that traditional attitudes toward mental health play for the community as a social system. From this perspective, the researchers were able to formulate several hypotheses explaining the failure of their mental health education effort and to suggest possible concrete avenues for bringing about future change [p. 1253].

As an example of a systems approach viewing an action program as a component of a larger social system, Robert Weiss[127] describes Thernstrom's work with Action for Boston Community Development (ABCD). This program, entirely dependent on sponsor approval, in Thernstrom's view, had to respond "opportunistically" to the whims of its sponsors. It was a new program and had developed no political support of its own. The ABCD Program personnel wanted to introduce change in the scope of interests of existing community agencies such as the school board. "However, the representatives of the other agencies acted first and foremost to further the policies of their home agencies and not to further the program of ABCD." Finally, not having developed its own supporters among the poor within the urban complex, it had no specific support from its target population nor did it possess power vis-a-vis other agencies in the "helping" field. Weiss concludes that the ABCD Programs were, as a result, bland and conventional.

Weiss also supplies intriguing examples of systems analysis by using the program itself as the frame of reference and by focusing upon the client as a part of a larger system. For the first instance, he uses an analysis by Schon showing how programs serving the blind have remained concentrated upon cases resulting from industrial accidents, diseases of childhood, and other causes affecting younger age groups. Presently, however, blindness is increasingly an affliction of the aged, when it is often coupled with numerous other handicaps. Programs serving the blind have not, however, changed their tactics. They continue to provide their traditional services, avoiding a disruption of organizational structures and the careers of the people within them. The various agencies offering such services compete among themselves for the decreasing number of younger clients by sharply augmenting the quality and quantity of their services. The net effect is neglect of the aged blind and a showering of new services upon the younger blind client. The system of agency services can thus be judged as relatively ineffective from the standpoint of this type of evaluation.

For his second example, Weiss describes[127] an English study by Marsden that focused upon women who are raising children alone while receiving public assistance. Marsden's analysis delineated two types of household arrangements within this population, the first where relatives are available and the other where the woman must develop her household strictly from her own resources. Women fortunate enough to be in a kinship system received presents for children, incidental material help, emotional support, and small loans with no repayment date or interest. In contrast, the woman who was alone was faced with the fact that her public assistance limited the income she could get from working, even if she could find a way to care for her small children while she worked. She might receive covert forms of support from male friends, but she had to be sensitive to a charge of co-habitation, which would reduce the amount of public assistance support. Women in this situation were forced to survive on such slim resources that they often deprived themselves of both food and clothing so that their children could be better sustained. This type of system analysis clearly indicates that the system of public assistance is not effective for a woman with children who is outside a kinship network.

Another example of a systems approach to program evaluation is research

163

based on a psychiatric case register, a central file to which all persons with a diagnosed mental illness and all contacts with a group of psychiatric services are reported. The case register aims at (a) identification of persons with a mental disorder who reside in a specific geographical area and are seen in local psychiatric facilities, and (b) maintenance of cumulative statistical records on the psychiatric care these individuals receive.[48] The use of the information so gathered is, in Gardner's[48] opinion,

> indispensible in evaluating the impact of a mental health center on the psychiatric network . We can observe the number and geographic distribution of persons admitted to psychiatric care for the year and compare it with an extrapolation from previous years. The register is also indispensible if we wish to study the movement of patients between services and how this will be affected by the pattern of movement between the community services and the public mental hospital, with particular references to such factors as diagnosis, age, sex, area of residency, private versus public care, facility of first contact, number of contacts. We may then judge the effect of the new mental health center on the case load of the public mental hospital [p. 259].

In order to assess the impact of a new mental health center, Gardner made various assumptions about the psychiatric population such as "the number of persons, ages 15 and over, admitted to all psychiatric services will also continue to increase at the same rate in 1964 to 1967 as in the period 1961 to 1964." He then attempted to estimate the changes that might occur within the psychiatric network with the initiation of a new mental health center. Thus, for example, "if the same number of patients were to seek care directly in the clinic of the new mental health center as estimated for the clinic of the University Medical Center (1,300 in 1967), then we would expect a range of 1,475 to 1,630 patients to be seen in the clinic . . . . [C]onsidering the limited staff that would be available, we might reasonably estimate that 1,000 patients would be seen in the clinic of the new mental health center" [p. 269]. Central to the evaluation of the community mental health program concept is the projection of the flow of patients to the state hospital. Assuming that a new mental health center was designed to alter the flow of patients to such a treatment facility, Gardner estimated that the case load of the new mental health center would be increased by almost 25 per cent and the personnel for such an increase would be necessary. By implication, he is providing an evaluative base from which the organization can judge whether there are sufficient personnel within the system to manage such an increase. He cautions that even with the vast amount of data available in the psychiatric case register, many unknown factors remain and the projections are necessarily rough estimates.

Gardner and his associates[49] also used the case register for specific evaluations of various kinds of psychiatric activities within the entire network. For example,

164

focusing upon the patient pattern in two major hospitals, they report that "about one half of all received patients subsequently received out-patient psychiatric care from either a clinic or a private psychiatrist. About one third received such care without further hospitalization. The rate of rehospitalization for schizophrenic patients who received out-patient care was 38 percent, and for those who did not the rate was 23 percent. *These rates were about the same for both hospitals. It appears that out-patient care did not reduce the rate of readmission of the schizophrenic patients*" [p. 425].

Research methods compatible with the systems model, sometimes called "qualitative methodologies,"[44] contrast with experimental methods in that they involve (a) process-oriented qualitative research, (b) historical research, or (c) case study research.[129] Emphasis on process contrasts with most experimental methods since the latter require that the program "hold still" while it implements its design. A process focus is much more descriptive and inductive. According to Weiss and Rein,[128] "It is concerned with describing the unfolding form of the intervention, the reactions of individuals and instructions subjected to its impact. . ." [p. 142]. Historical research refers to the development of program events through time, while the case study aims at a "nearly complete description of the relevant community systems before the [program] intervention, of the form taken by the intervention and of the new systems which develop incorporating the intervention as a dynamic constituent" [p. 105].[129]

Research methods that complement these approaches would be interviewing in depth, systematic field observations, use of program documents, and even participant observations. Regarding the latter, Whyte[130] writes: "I think I can even see that almost forgotten figure, the participant observer, coming back into view. In my service on the Research Advisory Committee to the National Manpower Administration of the Department of Labor, I have been arguing that before-and-after measures of the effects of given governmental programs are not good enough. We need to know what went on within the program that may be presumed to account for the differences, if any, in our before-and-after measures" [p. 12].

Constructive typology can also be used to implement the systems model through the formulation of types of community mental health programs, thereby facilitating reliable comparative studies between programs. McKinney[79] notes: "The constructed type is a special kind of concept especially developed for descriptive, comparative, and predictive purposes. . . . [I]t orders the concrete data so that they may be described in terms that make them comparable, so that the experience had in one case, despite its uniqueness, may be made to reveal with some degree of probability what may be expected in others" [p. 11]. Data from a combination of these methods can provide the materials from which to form an inductive assessment of the program's consequences.[128]

A Radical Departure: The Indigenous Model

The people engaged in program development activities are not likely to come from, or particularly value, the social science frontier. Nor, on their side, are social scientists doing much applied research on the development of programs. Little is done to apply existing theory and knowledge to program development, to study means for securing acceptance of new programs, or to analyze alternative methods. . . . *On no side does there seem to be encouragement for radical departures from the past"* [p. 66].[124]

Here we advance a new model for evaluative studies, both in community mental health programs and in other action organizations. The indigenous model emphasizes the natural sociological processes in action organizations, seeks ways to accommodate outside methods and evaluative specialists, and involves the use of whatever indices of effectiveness are generated by the organization itself.

The individual perceptions of the members of mental health organizations are the basis for their continual evaluation of what goes on around them.[107] Whyte[131] uses the term "sentiments" to describe "the mental and emotional reactions we have to people and physical objects." Sentiments act as a "personal frame of reference, through which the individual perceives, interprets, and evaluates the world around him and his place in it" [p. 128]. Sentiments emerge from self-concepts, evaluation of activities, personal identification, and ranking. It is the evaluation of activities that primarily concerns us here. According to Whyte's scheme, self evaluation involves assessment of "personal worth"; i.e., the individual generates his own evaluations of activities at which he is good and those at which he is relatively inferior, or "what things are good to do and what are bad, what activities have high prestige and what are looked down upon" [p. 144]. Likewise, organizational life contains a "native" or indigenous evaluative process that grows out of the perceptions and sentiments of its individual members. Warner and Havens[122] conclude that "to ascertain both the progress toward the goals and the contribution of the role incumbents to the group activity, role performance is evaluated, either formally or informally, and sanctioned both to induce role performance and to control the quantity and quality of the performance" [p. 551]. At a more abstract level, Parsons[88] indicates that "cognitive mapping has alternatives of judgment or interpretation as to what objects are or what they 'mean.' There must be ordered selection among such alternatives. The term 'evaluation' will be given to this process of ordered selection. There is, therefore, an *evaluative* aspect of all concrete action orientation" [p. 7].

Values of American society reinforce native tendencies toward self evaluation. Williams[133] states: "In this culture the individual tends to 'face outward'—to be interested in making things happen in the external world. In ideal type, he seeks to dominate the world of nature, to subdue and exploit the physical world around him" [p. 458]. Such an ideal is closely aligned with the valuation of suc-

166

cess that permeates American culture. Williams emphasizes that this is not merely a gross emphasis upon acquisitive and materialistic power: "the theme of achievement unlimited is not limited to economic prowess or acquisition. In hundreds of complex forms it is pervasive in American *expressive* culture, where emphasis on the vision of the future produces impatience with the imperfect present and striving towards a salvation yet to be attained" [p. 457].

Americans also value efficiency, practicality, and humanitarianism. Williams[133] writes that "efficient is a word of high praise in a society that has long emphasized adaptability, technological innovation, economic expansion, up-to-dateness, practicality, expediency, 'getting things done' " [p. 462]. Although there are forces that may partially blunt the thrust of these cultural supports, progress is a basic theme in American culture. Thus, "our rich vocabulary of epithets ('backward,' 'out-moded,' 'old-fashioned,' 'stagnant,' and the like) can be understood *as epithets* only against the unquestioning assumption that the new is the better—that 'forward' is better than 'backward' " [p. 468]. All of these factors support ongoing evaluation of one's own activities as well as the activities of the organizations in which one has responsibilities. These beliefs and values contrast sharply with fatalistic views that nature and society are not subject to change or improvement.

The indigenous model of evaluation is oriented to learning as much as possible about indigenous, subjective evaluative processes at work in the organization. Its fundamental purpose is to strengthen and supplement these processes rather than replace them with imposed designs and models. This contrasts sharply with traditional approaches such as that expressed by Suchman[114] for whom "the task for the development of evaluative research as a 'scientific' process is to 'control' intrinsic subjectivity, since it cannot be eliminated" [p. 11]. Suchman does, however, agree that evaluation is a process natural to organizational members and the structure of organizations: "Evaluation is a continuous social process, rarely stopping to challenge assumptions or to bring the values into the open." The indigenous model attempts to articulate methods native to the organization with "outside" strategies such as sampling and experimental design. An example might be the improvement of questionnaire and survey techniques should these be found to be the dominant indigenous approach to evaluating organizational effectiveness.

The literature on evaluative research seems to have ignored this model. There are two basic types of evaluation: that by "imported" methods and that by methods natural to the organization itself. The indigenous model involves a combination of these in which the evaluator's first task is the careful delineation of evaluation methods functioning within the organization.

Although this model has never been used in a specific evaluative study, it has been suggested that it is highly unreliable. Williams and Evans,[134] following a detailed description of an experimental design in which the Head Start Program was evaluated, conclude that "self evaluation is an almost impossible task for a manager who has strong convictions about the value of his programs" [p. 131].

167

Eysenck[41] specifically warns that "the psychiatrist in charge of the patient must always be suspected of favoring the positive outcome compared with the negative one" [p. 13]. Eysenck summarizes the Cambridge-Somerville Youth Study, showing that the counselors who were carrying out the program

> were asked on several different occasions to list all treatment boys who were thought to have "substantially benefited" by their contact with the study. About two thirds of the boys were so listed. About half of these were reported by the counselors as having been "outstanding" in respect of benefit received. . . . The picture changes dramatically when the control group is brought into the picture. The total number of court appearances from the beginning of treatment was recorded, and it was found that 96 treatment boys and 92 control boys were involved, the number of offenses being 264 for the treatment group and 218 for the control group. A similar picture is given by the number of appearances before the court prevention bureau [p. 13].

Thus Eysenck regards therapists' self evaluation as largely misleading.

On the other hand, we have emphasized in this chapter the numerous dimensions of hostility, resistance, and opposition to imposed evaluation schemes. This suggests that evaluative research must incorporate natural evaluative processes if destructive hostility is to be minimized. This model calls for the evaluator to search his armamentarium for objective strategies that "fit" those that have arisen naturally within the organization. In this way the evaluator may reduce negative self-fulfilling prophecies about evaluation and tap natural tendencies within the organization and among individual practitioners to see their efforts as effective. This model also offers some hope for reducing resistance to translating evaluation results into changed behavior, practices, and procedures. Since constructive feedback is the ultimate goal, evaluative research, organizational practices, and internal belief systems should be as harmonious as possible.

What is the organizational nature of indigenous evaluative processes? Thompson[116] raises the question of how organizations "keep score":

> Even if we concede that organizations sometimes maximize, the organizational question is whether the organization has any way of knowing that it has done so. . . . There is nothing automatic about standards of desirability nor is knowledge of effects always easily come by. Thus both of these characteristics of assessing organizational effectiveness by those within the organization are variables. Consequently the standard of desirability or criteria of effectiveness will vary from "crystallized" to "ambiguous" and the understanding of cause-effect relations will vary from "complete" to "incomplete" [p. 85].

Thus members of one organization attempting to activate a specific mental health program may use a relatively uniform series of indices as yardsticks for assessment of effectiveness, while another organization may be characterized by low consensus among its members regarding the standards of desirability "against which actual or conceivable effects of causal actions can be evaluated" [p. 84]. In much the same way, organizations will vary in the extent to which "some consequences of action may be known, some suspected but not proved, and still others unnoticed. So, the individual or organization engaged in assessment may *believe* that its understanding of cause-effect is complete or incomplete" [p. 84]. In sum, the indigenous model requires the evaluator to develop three starting points: First, he needs to get a clear picture of the specific indexes that organization members use to judge their effectiveness. Second, he needs to determine the extent to which these have crystallized. Third, he needs to assess the extent to which organization members believe that their efforts are related to specific results.

The routine data collected within the organization can bring to light the natural evaluative processes within the organization. Carstairs[29] points out that these data may provide a "systematic scrutiny of the operation, in terms of patient flow through different treatment modalities. . . . Efficient systematic record keeping also demonstrates changes in the operation of a service through time, and is the basis of what Cumming and Rudolph have termed 'quality control,' following the analogy of the self scrutiny practiced by all modern large scale industrial concerns" [p. 49].

The psychiatric case register can provide a rapid summary of accumulated patient records. If such a register covers the program to be evaluated and is systematically updated, the evaluator has internal records that can help him operationalize the indigenous model. Such registers may have built-in criteria of effectiveness that are widely accepted within the organization. The known existence of such data and the way they are used may throw light on the extent to which organization members believe there is a relationship between their efforts and particular results.

Examples from recent exploratory research by the senior author provide insight into how the indigenous model might operate. Research interviews were conducted with 40 administrators and therapists in 25 alcoholism treatment units in New York and Pennsylvania. The guiding questions used in the open-ended interviews were: "How do you identify desirable effects of your program on your patients?" "What do you do with these assessments?" "To what extent would formal research techniques such as before-after measures, the use of control groups that are randomized, and questionnaire survey techniques fit with how you 'keep score' on the effectiveness of your efforts?" Analysis of the responses suggested typologies of respondents. One group tended to "keep score" by focusing upon "changes in attitude towards self" among their patients. By clinical observation they felt they could detect when the patient was less egocentric and more willing to accept responsibility; by behavioral observation, they noted when he was more punctual for appointments, more neat in physical appearance, and more poised in his posture as well as walking gait. Interestingly, numerous respondents emphasized telephone behavior, i.e., the extent to which the patient sounded less depressed and more self-respecting when appointments for visits were made.

A second type of score-keeping emerged that we labeled "the grapevine approach." This pattern tended to concentrate among administrators who worked closely with therapists rather than among therapists themselves. The strategy consisted of developing a series of informal and formal contracts throughout the community from whom information was garnered about the behavior of a patient following discharge. One respondent described an informal network he regularly tapped for information about former patients which consisted of workers in other treatment agencies in the vicinity, other former patients, Alcoholics Anonymous, and police. Persons using this type of score-keeping clearly indicated that systematic techniques such as sampling and questionnaire construction would fit harmoniously with their indigenous technique.

A third type of score-keeping focused on changes in patients' interactions with others, including behavior in the therapeutic situation and interactions with significant others outside of therapy. The therapists would keep a mental record of increased interaction, change in voice tone reflecting less emotional affect, and decreased hostility toward authority, including the therapists themselves and administrative personnel in the treatment setting.

Concerning the actual use of these observations, two patterns emerged. In the first, observations about program effectiveness were in no way shared or fed back into the organization. In the second, staff members regularly used their observations about program effectiveness in staff meetings, making suggestions about change in tactics and procedure.

Finally, two types of reaction emerged to the suggestion that formal evaluative techniques might articulate their own native way of keeping score. First, there were those who really did not understand the implications of before-after designs with comparison groups and randomization. At first they reacted negatively to explanations, i.e., they saw randomization as cheating those patients who were not a part of referral network and appeared at the clinic in some haphazard fashion. Some respondents clearly exhibited hostility and fear of formal evaluation devices; one respondent felt such devices were used only to "see what we are doing wrong." Second, there were frequent positive reactions to the suggestion of followup devices and an expressed desire to use such techniques. Here was a clear-cut opportunity for an evaluator to build on an already accepted idea for evaluation. With acceptance of the followup idea, there is the possibility of a timely introduction of sampling, such as the easily performed "systematic" type. After refining the practitioner's native system, some of the pitfalls in simple followups could be explored with him, e.g., cycles of favorable response may be historically present, and followups may tap a favorable or unfavorable period. In turn, this could lead to the refinement of adding a past dimension to the followup, making possible an interrupted time series evaluative design. Upon exploring with the practitioner how to interpret simple followup data, the evaluator may discover the many intervening factors that may be influencing behavior of patients after their completion of therapy. This could be a propitious point at which to introduce the notion of comparison groups.

Some time ago, the senior author sat in on the design of a program for the ghetto alcoholic in a large, urban alcoholism treatment center. The practitioners spoke openly of training alcoholism workers from the target population and "experimenting" to see if their introduction would decrease dropouts and increase length of sobriety (their native criteria). Here was an excellent chance to introduce comparison group strategy and perhaps even discuss randomization. This situation represents the hallmark of the indigenous model: it starts with what practitioners already do to keep score. If the evaluator is a secure professional in his own discipline, he can maintain his own identity while slowly but surely introducing somewhat alien methods that are compatible with and improve the indigenous system. By starting with the action program's system and firming up initial rapport, there is a much higher likelihood that acceptable feedback of results will take place, the *raison d'etre* for evaluative studies.

There is no doubt that the indigenous model sets the stage for a totally different relationship between the evaluator and the target organization than usually obtains when outside methods are directly imposed. By no means is the evaluator limited to the techniques that are native to the target system. The indigenous approach can get the evaluative foot in the door. There is reason to believe that a highly sophisticated evaluative design can emerge as long as the target practitioners participate in building the design and are accepted by the evaluator as equal participants in the work of evaluation.

It is likely that a thorough evaluation could include the indigenous, the systems, and the goal attainment approaches. They are indeed complementary, particularly when employed in this sequence. The indigenous model is an excellent means of gaining both admittance to the system and developing a broad acquaintance with it. When this is done, the evaluator is in a more realistic position to understand goals, and may well have the rapport for implementing a sophisticated goal attainment design for data collection. By this time he should have collected a range of other data that can make the outcome of evaluation more than just "it doesn't work" or "it works." Such broad data coupled with a sound foundation of rapport should maximize the potential of meaningful feedback. Obviously this is an idealized sequence, for there are many potential pitfalls along this route to successful evaluation. But we believe that much evaluation will be improved with the recognition that there is much more to the process than simply formulating program goals and setting up an experimental design.

CONCLUSION

In this chapter we have explored the numerous problems affecting program evaluation, with particular concern for the evaluation of community mental health. We have attempted to temper some necessarily pessimistic observations of the current scene with constructive suggestions for adapting evaluation to program realities. Our basic theme is that there are many improvements in evaluative research that can be brought about by a closer look at the sociology of evaluation. Sociology and behavioral science generally have a series of approaches to research that do not often find their way into evaluative studies. The shortcomings may be summarized as follows:

1. Evaluators frequently lack a feeling for the program action they are to evaluate. With the range of activities included under the umbrella of community mental health as the target, such knowledge is fundamental.

2. Evaluators too often neglect the ultimate goal of feedback into program functioning, seeing their work as a mechanical "job to be done" with little concern for the avenues of feedback.

3. Evaluators frequently neglect the social psychology of rapport and the potential conflict inherent in insider-outsider relationships. They see themselves as technical experts rather than as researchers with the broad tasks of understanding and compromise in dealing with the practitioners' subculture, which sharply differs from their own. The "care and feeding" of rapport needs much greater attention.

4. Evaluators have neglected organizational dynamics and have unrealistically clung to rational models of organizational functioning. Thus they impose a narrow goal attainment model, neglecting the possibilities of broader approaches such as the systems model. Moreover, adaptations of goal attainment models and experimental designs that will render them less abrasive deserve wider use.

5. Evaluators usually approach target systems with only one research strategy, neglecting the fruitful possibilities of "multiple triangulation,"[145] where data are collected with a variety of strategies to form a composite picture of program action in terms of both its advantages and deficiencies.

6. Evaluators have almost entirely neglected the anthropological technique of learning about "the natives" and their techniques of evaluation. The successful diffusion and adoption of evaluative results most certainly depends upon linkages with existing practices and beliefs in target systems.

There are presently many ongoing evaluations of community mental health programs, and there will be many more in the future. If evaluators approach their assessment of "Psychiatry's Third Revolution" with broad and flexible strategies, perhaps they will create Evaluation's First Revolution.

REFERENCES

1. ALBRECHT, GARY L,: "Review of Arthur Bindman and Allen D. Spiegel (eds.), *Perspectives in Community Mental Health;* and Leopold Bellak and Harvey Barten (eds.), *Progress in Community Mental Health." Journal of Health and Social Behavior* 11:336-339, 1970.
2. ANDERSEN, STIG: "Operations Research in Public Health," in Herbert Schulberg, Alan Sheldon, and Frank Baker (eds.): *Program Evaluation in the Health Fields,* pp. 254-267. New York: Behavioral Publications, 1969.
3. ANDERSON, OTIS: Report of the First National Conference on Evaluation in Public Health. Ann Arbor: University of Michigan, School of Public Health, 1955, p. 7.

4. BARTEN, HARVEY: "The Coming of Age of the Brief Psychotherapies," in Leopold Bellak and Harvey Barten (eds.): *Progress in Community Mental Health,* pp. 93-123. New York: Grune and Stratton, 1969.
5. BECKER, ALVIN, MURPHY, N. MICHAEL, AND GREENBLATT, MILTON: "Recent Advances in Community Mental Health," in Arthur J. Bindman and Allen D. Spiegel (eds.): *Perspectives in Community Mental Health,* pp. 201-323. Chicago: Aldine Publishing Company, 1969.
6. BELASCO, JAMES, AND TRICE, HARRISON M.: *The Assessment of Change in Training and Therapy.* New York: McGraw-Hill, 1969.
7. BELL, NORMAN, AND SPIEGEL, JOHN: "Social Psychiatry: Vagaries of a Term," in Ari Kiev (ed.): *Social Psychiatry,* pp. 52-70. New York: Science House, 1966.
8. BELLAK, LEOPOLD: "Introduction." in Leopold Bellak (ed.): *Handbook of Community Psychiatry,* pp. 1-12 and 156. New York: Grune and Stratton, 1964.
9. BELLAK, LEOPOLD (ed.): *Handbook of Community Psychiatry.* New York: Grune and Stratton, 1964.
10. BELLAK, LEOPOLD, AND BARTEN, HARVEY (eds.): *Progress in Community Mental Health.* New York: Grune and Stratton, 1969.
11. BERGEN, BERNARD: "Professional Communities on the Evaluation of Demonstration Projects in Community Mental Health," in Herbert Schulberg, Alan Sheldon, and Frank Baker (eds.): *Program Evaluations in the Health Fields,* pp. 121-138. New York: Behavioral Publications, 1969.
12. BINNER, PAUL R.: "Development of the Research Department," in Ernest Gruenberg (ed.): *Evaluating the Effectiveness of Mental Health Services. Milbank Memorial Fund Quarterly* XLIV:313-320, 1966.
13. BLOOM, B. L.: *Mental Health Program Evaluation.* Washington: U.S. Public Health Service (mimeographed), 1965.
14. BOBBITT, JOSEPH M.: "Community Mental Health Research," in Arthur Bindman and Allan Spiegel (eds.): *Perspectives in Community Mental Health,* pp. 659-661. Chicago: Aldine Publishing Company, 1969.
15. BOGUSLAW, ROBERT: *The New Utopians: A Study of System Design and Social Change.* Englewood Cliffs, N.J.: Prentice-Hall, 1965.
16. BORGATTA, EDGAR: *An Experiment in Mental Patient Rehabilitation: Evaluating a Social Agency Program.* New York: Russell Sage Foundation, 1965.
17. BORGATTA, EDGAR: "Research Problems in Evaluation of Health Service Demonstration." *Milbank Memorial Fund Quarterly* LXIV:182-201, 1966.
18. BRANDON, SYDNEY, AND GRUENBERG, ERNEST: "Measurements of the Incidence of Chronic Severe Social Breakdown," in Ernest Gruenberg (ed.): *Evaluating the Effectiveness of Mental Health Services. Milbank Memorial Fund Quarterly* XLIV:129-150, 1966.
19. BUCKLEY, WALTER: *Sociology and Modern Systems Theory.* Englewood Cliffs, N.J.: Prentice-Hall, 1967.
20. CAHN, SIDNEY: *The Treatment of Alcoholics: An Evaluative Study.* New York: Oxford University Press, 1970.
21. CAMPBELL, DONALD, AND STANLEY, JULIAN: *Experimental and Quasi-Experimental Designs for Research.* Chicago: Rand McNally and Company, 1966.
22. CAMPBELL, DONALD: "Considering the Case against Experimental Evaluations of Social Innovations." *Administrative Science Quarterly* 15:110-113, 1970.
23. CAMPBELL, DONALD: "Reforms as Experiments," in Francis G. Caro (ed.): *Readings in Evaluative Research,* pp. 233-261. New York: Russell Sage Foundation, 1971.
24. CAPLAN, ELEANOR: "Evaluation of a Program involving Multiple Community Agencies." *International Journal of Comparative Sociology* 9:137-142, 1968.
25. CAPLAN, GERALD: *Principles of Preventive Psychiatry.* New York: Basic Books, 1964.
26. CARO, FRANCIS: "Approaches to Evaluative Research." *Human Organization* 28:87-99, 1969.
27. CARO, FRANCIS: "Evaluation Research: An Overview," in Francis Caro (ed.): *Readings in Evaluative Research,* pp. 1-34. New York: Russell Sage Foundation, 1971.
28. CARO, FRANCIS: "Issues in the Evaluation of Social Programs." *Review of Educational Research* 41:87-114, 1971.
29. CARSTAIRS, G. M.: "Problems of Evaluative Research," in Richard H. Williams and Lucy Ozarin (eds.): *Community Mental Health: An International Perspective,* pp. 44-62. San Francisco: Jossey-Bass, 1968.

173

30. COLLINS, JEROME: "Evaluative Research in Community Psychiatry." *Hospital and Community Psychiatry* 19:97-102, 1968.

31. CUMMING, ELAINE, AND CUMMING, JOHN: *Closed Ranks—An Experiment in Mental Health Education.* Cambridge, Mass.: Harvard University Press, 1957.

32. CYERT, RICHARD, AND MARCH, JAMES G.: *A Behavioral Theory of the Firm.* Englewood Cliffs, N.J.: Prentice-Hall, 1963.

33. DANIELS, ROBERT S.: "Community Psychiatry—A New Profession, A Developing Subspecialty, or Effective Clinical Psychiatry?" *Community Mental Health Journal* 2:47-54, 1966.

34. DINITZ, SIMON, AND BERAN, NANCY: "Community Mental Health as a Boundaryless and Boundary-Busting System." *Journal of Health and Social Behavior* 12:99-108, 1971.

35. DOLE, VINCENT, AND WARNER, ALAN: "Evaluation of Narcotics Treatment Programs." *American Journal of Public Health* 57:2000-2006, 1967.

36. DUMONT, MATTHEW: *The Absurd Healer: Perspectives of a Community Psychiatry.* New York: Science House, 1968.

37. DUNHAM, WARREN: "Community Psychiatry: The Newest Therapeutic Bandwagon." *International Journal of Psychiatry* 1:553-584, 1965.

38. ENGLEHARDT, DAVID, AND FRIEDMAN, NORBERT: "Maintenance Drug Therapy: The Schizophrenic Patient in the Community," in Ari Kiev (ed.): *Social Psychiatry,* Volume 1, pp. 256-282. New York: Science House, 1969.

39. ETZIONI, AMITAI: "Two Approaches to Organizational Analysis." *Administrative Science Quarterly* 5:257-278, 1960.

40. ETZIONI, AMITAI: *Modern Organizations.* Englewood Cliffs, N.J.: Prentice-Hall, 1964.

41. EYSENCK, HANS J.: *The Effects of Psychotherapy.* New York: International Science Press, 1966.

42. FAIRWEATHER, GEORGE: *Social Psychology in Treating Mental Illness: An Experimental Approach.* New York: John Wiley and Sons, 1964.

43. FERMAN, LOUIS: "Some Perspectives on Evaluating Social Welfare Programs." *Annals of the American Academy of Political and Social Science* 385:143-156, 1969.

44. FILSTEAD, WILLIAM (ed.): *Qualitative Methodology.* Chicago: Markham Publishing Company, 1970.

45. FREEMAN, HOWARD, AND SHERWOOD, CLARENCE: "Research in Large-Scale Intervention Programs." *Journal of Social Issues* 21:11-28, 1965.

46. FREEMAN, HOWARD, AND SIMMONS, OZZIE: *The Mental Patient Comes Home.* New York: John Wiley and Sons, 1963.

47. FORT, JOEL: "The Persecution and Assassination of the Inmates of the Asylum of the United States as Performed by the Community Mental Health Movement." *Psychiatry and Social Science Review* 5:14-17, 1971.

48. GARDNER, ELMER A.: "The Use of a Psychiatric Case Register in the Planning and Evaluation of a Mental Health Program," in R. Monroe, G. Klee, and E. Brody (eds.): *Psychiatric Epidemiology and Mental Health Planning,* pp. 259-281. Washington: American Psychiatric Association, 1967.

49. GARDNER, ELMER, BAHN, ANITA K., AND MILES, HAROLD: "Patient Experience in Psychiatric Units of General and State Mental Hospitals," in Herbert C. Schulberg, Alan Sheldon, and Frank Baker (eds.): *Program Evaluation in the Health Fields,* pp. 416-437. New York: Behavioral Publications, 1969.

50. GEORGOPOULOUS, BASIL S., AND TANNENBAUM, ARNOLD S.: "A Study of Organizational Effectiveness." *American Sociological Review* 22:534-541, 1957.

51. GOSS, MARY E. W.: "Organizational Goals and Quality of Medical Care: Evidence from Comparative Research on Hospitals." *Journal of Health and Social Behavior* 11:255-268, 1970.

52. GRAD, JACQUELINE: "A Two-Year Follow-Up," in Richard Williams and Lucy Ozarin (eds.): *Community Mental Health: An International Perspective,* pp. 429-454. San Francisco: Jossey-Bass, 1968.

53. GREENWOOD, ERNEST: "Attributes of a Profession." *Social Work* 2:44-55, 1957.

54. HOWE, LOUISA: "Problems in the Evaluations of Mental Health Programs," in R. Katinsky (ed.): *Community Programs for Mental Health,* pp. 127-145. New York: Harvard University Press, 1955.

55. HUTCHINSON, GEORGE B.: "Evaluation of Preventive Services." *Journal of Chronic Diseases* 11:497-508, 1960.
56. HYMAN, HERBERT, WRIGHT, CHARLES, R., AND HOPKINS, TERENCE: *Application of Methods of Evaluation: Four Studies of the Encampment for Citizenship.* Berkeley: University of California Press, 1962.
57. HYMAN, HERBERT, AND WRIGHT, CHARLES: "Evaluating Social Action Programs," in Paul Lazarsfeld, William Sewell, and Harold Wilensky (eds.): *The Uses of Sociology,* pp. 741-782. New York: Basic Books, 1967.
58. KAHN, J. H.: "Evolution of a Community Mental Health Service." in Richard Williams and Lucy Ozarin (eds.): *Community Mental Health: An International Perspective,* pp. 140-157. San Francisco: Jossey-Bass, 1968.
59. KANDEL, DENISE, AND WILLIAMS, RICHARD: *Psychiatric Rehabilitation: Some Problems in Research.* New York: Atherton Press, 1964.
60. KATZ, DANIEL, AND KAHN, ROBERT: *The Social Psychology of Organizations.* New York: John Wiley and Sons, 1966.
61. KEGELES, STEPHAN: "A Field Experimental Attempt to Change Beliefs and Behaviors of Women in an Urban Ghetto." *Journal of Health and Social Behavior* 10:115-124, 1969.
62. KENISTON, KENNETH: "How Community Mental Health Stamped Out the Riots (1968-78)." *Transaction* 6:21-29, 1968.
63. KLEIN, DONALD C.: *Community Dynamics and Mental Health.* New York: John Wiley and Sons, 1968.
64. KRAFT, ALAN: "The Fort Logan Mental Health Center," in Ernest Gruenberg (ed.): *Evaluating the Effectiveness of Mental Health Services. Milbank Memorial Fund Quarterly* XLIV:10-28, 1966.
65. KRAUSE, ELLIOTT: "After the Rehabilitation Center." *Social Problems* 14:197-206, 1966.
66. LAZARUS, A. A.: "Group Therapy of Phobic Disorders by Systematic Desensitization." *Journal of Abnormal and Social Psychology* 63:504-510, 1961.
67. LEEDY, JACK (ed.): *Poetry Therapy.* Philadelphia: J. B. Lippincott Company, 1969.
68. LEFTON, MARK, DINITZ, SIMON, ANGRIST, SHIRLEY S., AND PASAMANICK, BENJAMIN: "Former Mental Patients and Their Neighbors," in S. Kirson Weinberg (ed.): *The Sociology of Mental Disorders,* pp. 255-266. Chicago: Aldine Publishing Company, 1967.
69. LEVENTHAL, HOWARD: "Experimental Studies of Anti-Smoking Communications," in Edgar Borgatta and Robert Evans (eds.): *Smoking, Health, and Behavior,* pp. 95-122. Chicago: Aldine Publishing Company, 1968.
70. LEVENSON, ALAN: "Organizational Patterns of Community Mental Health," in Leopold Bellak and Harvey Barten (eds.): *Progress in Community Mental Health,* pp. 67-93. New York: Grune and Stratton, 1969.
71. LEVINSON, PERRY: "Evaluation of Social Welfare Programs: Two Research Models." *Welfare in Review* 4:5-12, 1966.
72. LIKERT, R., AND LIPPITT, R.: "Utilization of Social Science," in L. Festinger and D. Katz (eds.): *Research Methods in the Behavioral Sciences,* pp. 48-61. New York: Holt and Company, 1953.
73. LUCHTERHAND, ELMER: "Research and the Dilemmas in Developing Social Programs," in Paul Lazarfeld, William Sewell, and Harold Wilensky (eds.): *The Uses of Sociology,* pp. 506-521. New York: Basic Books, 1967.
74. LYND, ROBERT S., AND LYND, HELEN M.: *Middletown in Transition.* New York: Harcourt, Brace and World, 1937.
75. MACMAHON, BRIAN, PUGH, THOMAS, AND HUTCHINSON, GEORGE: "Principles in the Evaluation of Community Mental Health Programs," in Herbert Schulberg, Alan Sheldon, and Frank Baker (eds.): *Program Evaluation in the Health Fields,* pp. 51-59. New York: Behavioral Publications, 1969.
76. MANN, JOHN: *Changing Human Behavior.* New York: Charles Scribner's Sons, 1965.
77. MARCH, JAMES, AND SIMON, HERBERT: *Organizations.* New York: John Wiley and Sons, 1958.
78. MARRIS, PETER, AND REIN, MARTIN: *Dilemmas of Social Reform.* New York: Atherton Press, 1967.
79. MCKINNEY, JOHN C.: *Constructive Typology and Social Theory.* New York: Appleton-Century-Crofts, 1966.

175

80. MECHANIC, DAVID: "Community Psychiatry: Some Sociological Perspectives and Implications," in Leigh Roberts, Seymour Halleck, and Martin Loeb (eds.): *Community Psychiatry,* pp. 201-222. Madison: University of Wisconsin Press, 1966.

81. MECHANIC, DAVID: *Mental Health and Social Policy.* Englewood Cliffs, N.J.: Prentice-Hall, 1969.

82. MECHANIC, DAVID: "Social Issues in Mental Health," in Leopold Bellak and Harvey Barten (eds.): *Progress in Community Mental Health,* pp. 43-66. New York: Grune and Stratton, 1969.

83. MEEHL, PAUL: "Discussion," in Hans J. Eysenck (ed.): *The Effects of Psychotherapy,* pp. 58-59. New York: International Science Press, 1966.

84. MESAROVIC, M. B., *et al.:* "An Axiomatic Approach to Organizations from a General Systems Viewpoint," in William Cooper *et al.* (eds.): *New Perspectives in Organization Research,* pp. 220-244. New York: John Wiley and Sons, 1964.

85. MEYER, HENRY, AND BORGATTA, EDGAR: *An Experiment in Mental Patient Rehabilitation.* New York: Russell Sage Foundation, 1959.

86. OZARIN, LUCY: "Introduction to Part II," in Richard Williams and Lucy Ozarin (eds.): *Community Mental Health: An International Perspective,* pp. 69-96. San Francisco: Jossey-Bass, 1968.

87. PARSELL, ALFRED: "Dynamic Evaluation: The Systems Approach to Action Research." Paper presented to the 61st Annual Meeting of the American Sociological Society, Miami Beach, September, 1966.

88. PARSONS, TALCOTT: *The Social System.* New York: The Free Press, 1951.

89. PASAMANICK, BENJAMIN, SCARPITTI, FRANK, AND DINITZ, SIMON: *Schizophrenics in the Community.* New York: Appleton-Century-Crofts, 1967.

90. PERROW, CHARLES: "The Analysis of Goals in Complex Organizations." *American Sociological Review* 26:854-866, 1961.

91. PHILLIPS, E. LAKIN, AND WIENER, DANIEL: *Short-Term Psychotherapy and Structured Behavior Change.* New York: McGraw-Hill, 1966.

92. POLAK, PAUL: "Unclean Research and Clinical Change," in Ernest Gruenberg (ed.): *Evaluating the Effectiveness of Mental Health Services. Milbank Memorial Fund Quarterly* XLIV:237-345, 1966.

93. PRICE, JAMES L.: *Organizational Effectiveness: An Inventory of Propositions.* Homewood, Ill.: Richard D. Irwin, Inc., 1968.

94. ROBERTS, LEIGH M.: "Introduction," in Leigh M. Roberts, Seymour Halleck, and Martin Loeb (eds.): *Community Psychiatry,* pp. 3-11. Madison: University of Wisconsin Press, 1966.

95. ROKEACH, MILTON: "Attitude Change and Behavior Change." *Public Opinion Quarterly* XXX:529-550, 1966.

96. ROME, HOWARD: "Barriers to the Establishment of Comprehensive Community Mental Health Centers," in Leigh Roberts, Seymour Halleck, and Martin Loeb (eds.): *Community Psychiatry,* pp. 31-57. Madison: University of Wisconsin Press, 1966.

97. ROSSI, PETER: "Evaluating Social Action Programs." *Transaction* 5:51-53, 1967.

98. *Russell Sage Foundation Program in Evaluation Research.* New York: Russell Sage Foundation (mimeographed), 1970.

99. SABSHIN, MELVIN: "Theoretical Models in Community and Social Psychiatry," in Leigh Roberts, Seymour Halleck, and Martin Loeb (eds.): *Community Psychiatry,* pp. 15-30. Madison: University of Wisconsin Press, 1966.

100. SAGER, CLIFFORD, WASENBERG, SHELDON, BRAYBOY, THOMAS, SLIPP, SAMUEL, AND WAXENBERG, BARBARA: "Dimensions of Family Therapy," in Leopold Bellak and Harvey Barten (eds.): *Progress in Community Mental Health,* pp. 137-167. New York: Grune and Stratton, 1969.

101. SATA, LINDBERGH: "Epidemiology: Prerequisite for Planning," in Leopold Bellak and Harvey Barten (eds.): *Progress in Community Mental Health,* pp. 24-43. New York: Grune and Stratton, 1969.

102. SCHEIDLINGER, SAUL: "Innovative Group Approaches," in Leopold Bellak and Harvey Barten (eds.): *Progress in Community Mental Health,* pp. 123-136. New York: Grune and Stratton, 1969.

103. SCHLIEWEN, ROLF: "Organizational Effectiveness and Its Relation to Power and Efficiency."

176

Paper presented to the Canadian Sociology/Anthropology Association, June, 1971. (Mimeographed.)

104. SCHULBERG, HERBERT, AND BAKER, FRANK: "Program Evaluation Models and the Implementation of Research Findings." *American Journal of Public Health* 58:1248-1255, 1968.

105. SCHULBERG, HERBERT, SHELDON, ALAN, AND BAKER, FRANK: "Introduction," in Herbert Schulberg, Alan Sheldon, and Frank Baker (eds.): *Program Evaluation in the Health Fields,* p. 308. New York: Behavioral Publications, 1969.

106. SCOTT, W. RICHARD: *Social Processes and Social Structures: An Introduction to Sociology.* New York: Holt, Rinehart and Winston, 1970.

107. SECORD, PAUL, AND BACKMAN, CARL: *Social Psychology.* New York: McGraw-Hill Book Company, 1964.

108. SMITH, M. BREWSTER, AND HOBBS, NICHOLAS: "The Community and the Community Mental Health Center." *American Psychologist* 21:499-509, 1966.

109. SNOW, HERMAN: "The Dutchess County Project after Five Years," in Ernest Gruenberg (ed.): *Evaluating the Effectiveness of Mental Health Services. Milbank Memorial Fund Quarterly* XLIV:57-79, 1966.

110. SOLOMON, RICHARD: "Extension of Control Group Design." *Psychological Reports* 46:137-150, 1949.

111. STRAUSS, ANSELM, SCHATZMAN, LEONARD, BUCHER, RUE, EHRLICH, DANUTA, AND SABSHIN, MELVIN: *Psychiatric Ideologies and Institutions.* Glencoe: Free Press, 1964.

112. STREUNING, ELMER, AND PECK, HARRIS: "The Role of Research in Evaluation," in Richard Williams and Lucy Ozarin (eds.): *Community Mental Health: An International Perspective,* pp. 167-197. San Francisco: Jossey-Bass, 1968.

113. SUCHMAN, EDWARD: "A Model for Research and Evaluation on Rehabilitation," in Marvin Sussman (ed.): *Sociology and Rehabilitation,* pp. 52-70. Washington: American Sociological Association, 1966.

114. SUCHMAN, EDWIN: *Evaluative Research.* New York: Russell Sage Foundation, 1967.

115. SUSSER, MERVYN: *Community Psychiatry: Epidemiologic and Social Themes.* New York: Random House, 1968.

116. THOMPSON, JAMES D.: *Organizations in Action.* New York: McGraw-Hill, 1967.

117. TRICE, HARRISON M.: "The 'Outsiders' Role in Field Study." *Sociology and Social Research* 41:27-32, 1956.

118. TRICE, HARRISON M.: *Report on Alcoholism in the State of Maryland.* Baltimore, Maryland: Commission on Alcoholism, February 10, 1961.

119. TRICE, HARRISON M., AND BELASCO, JAMES: "Supervisory Training about Alcoholics and Other Problem Employees: A Controlled Evaluation." *Quarterly Journal of Studies on Alcohol* 29:382-398, 1968.

120. TRICE, HARRISON M., BELASCO, JAMES, AND ALUTTO, JOSEPH: "The Role of Ceremonials in Organizational Behavior." *Industrial and Labor Relations Review* 23:40-52, 1969.

121. TRICE, HARRISON M., ROMAN, PAUL M., AND BELASCO, JAMES: "Selection for Treatment: A Predictive Evaluation of an Alcoholism Treatment Regimen." *International Journal of the Addictions* 4:303-317, 1969.

122. WARNER, W. KEITH, AND HAVENS, A. EUGENE: "Goal Displacement and the Intangibility of Organizational Goals." *Administrative Science Quarterly* 12:539-555, 1968.

123. WEISS, CAROL: "Utilization of Evaluation: Toward Comparative Study." Paper presented at the American Sociological Meeting, Miami Beach, September, 1966 (mimeographed).

124. WEISS, CAROL: "Politicization of Evaluative Research." *Journal of Social Issues* 26:57-68, 1970.

125. WEISS, CAROL: Personal correspondence, January 4, 1971.

126. WEISS, CAROL: *Evaluation Research.* Englewood Cliffs, N.J.: Prentice-Hall, 1972.

127. WEISS, ROBERT S.: *Evaluation Research.* Unpublished manuscript, 1970.

128. WEISS, ROBERT, AND REIN, MARTIN: "The Evaluation of Broad-Aim Programs: A Cautionary Case and a Moral." *Annals of the American Academy of Political and Social Science* 385:133-142, 1969.

129. WEISS, ROBERT, AND REIN, MARTIN: "The Evaluation of Broad-Aim Programs." *Administrative Science Quarterly* 15:97-109, 1970.

130. WHYTE, WILLIAM F.: "Reflections on My Work." *American Behavioral Scientist* XII:9-13, 1968.

177

131. WHYTE, WILLIAM F.: *Organizational Behavior: Theory and Application*. Homewood, Ill.: Richard D. Irwin and the Dorsey Press, 1969.
132. WILNER, D. M.: "Research and Evaluation in Social Psychiatry." Paper presented to the American Psychopathological Association, New York, February, 1967.
133. WILLIAMS, ROBIN: *American Society* (3rd ed.). New York: Alfred A. Knopf, 1970.
134. WILLIAMS, WALTER, AND EVANS, JOHN: "The Politics of Evaluation: The Case of Head Start." *Annals of the American Academy of Political and Social Science* 385:118-132, 1969.
135. WING, J. K.: "Evaluating Community Care for Schizophrenic Patients," in Leigh Roberts, Seymour Halleck, and Martin Loeb (eds.): *Community Psychiatry*, pp. 133-165. Madison: University of Wisconsin Press, 1966.
136. WRIGHT, CHARLES, AND HYMAN, HERBERT: "The Evaluators," in Phillip Hammong (ed.): *Sociologists at Work*, pp. 121-141. New York: Basic Books, 1964.
137. YATES, AUBREY: *Behavior Therapy*. New York: John Wiley and Sons, 1970.
138. BERNARD, VIOLA: "Education for Community Psychiatry in a University Medical Center," in Bellak, Leopold (ed.): *Handbook of Community Psychiatry*, pp. 82-122. New York: Grune and Stratton, 1964.
139. TRICE, H. M., AND ROMAN, P. M.: "Sociopsychological Predictors of Affiliation with Alcoholics Anonymous." *Social Psychiatry* 5:51-59, 1970.
140. MERTON, ROBERT K.: *Social Theory and Social Structure*. Glencoe, Ill.: The Free Press, 1957.
141. KUSHKIN, SELMA: "Evaluations: Use with Caution." *Evaluation* 1:31-35, 1973.
142. BLAU, PETER, AND SCOTT, W. R.: *Formal Organizations*. San Francisco: Chandler, 1962.
143. DAVIS, ANN, DINITE, S., AND PASAMANICK, B.: "The Prevention of Hospitalization in Schizophrenia." *American Journal of Orthopsychiatry* 42:375-388, 1972.
144. MOSHER, L. R., AND GUNDERSON, J. G.: "Special Report: Schizophrenia." *Schizophrenia Bulletin* 7:12-52, 1973.
145. DENZIN, NORMAN: *The Research Act*. Chicago: Aldine, 1971.

CHAPTER 8

Organizational Adaptation to Community Mental Health: A Case Study

DAVID L. ELLISON, PATRICIA RIEKER, AND JOHN H. MARX

INTRODUCTION

The national mental health program established by the 1963 Community Mental Health Centers Act committed the Federal government to recognize mental health and illness as social issues (or problems) requiring rational social planning and public policy. Furthermore, the decision to allocate resources for mental health services through community mental health centers explicitly indicated acceptance of several controversial assumptions: (1) the treatment of psychological problems should be engaged in their natural setting (i.e., the community, the family, the school, etc.); and (2) society or the community, as well as the individual, can be both the locus and focus of treatment.

The social significance of the 1963 Community Mental Health Centers Act derives from two considerations: first, the innovative legislation was a consequence of changes and developments in both governmental policy and the mental health field; second, the Act had important ramifications for the future direction of public policy and for the mental health field. These authors have discussed the first set of issues in Chapter 1 of this volume. This discussion will focus on the second consideration. Specifically, the present paper will be a description of the ramifications of the 1963 Act for the organizational, professional, and treatment aspects of an existing psychiatric institution.

Federal intervention into the mental health field underscored several problematic issues. Foremost were those involved in developing public policy in a substantive area like community and social psychiatry which had no clear boundaries, tasks, or goals. Another set of issues involved government sponsorship of a program which appeared to promote change in the way mental health services were organized and delivered.

In an attempt to reconcile conflicts between those practitioners traditionally responsible for established mental health practices and those attempting to implement the innovative program, the Federal government designed ambiguous legislation with flexible implementing guidelines. In fact, a recent study[10] of two community mental health centers showed that the guidelines are so flexible that nearly any function, new or old, can be carried out in the name of community mental health. In addition, the legislation is subject to radical change depending on the attitudes and financial allocations of both Congress and the President. Although unclear about their official mandate,[3] nearly 400 community mental health centers are operating.[8] The guidelines stress community-based programs incorporating the vague directives of prevention, treatment, and rehabilitation organized around the principle of "continuity of care." However, only five services are specified as essential in a program to qualify for funds as a community mental health center: (1) inpatient services; (2) outpatient services; (3) partial hospitalization, including day, night, and week end care; (4) 24-hour emergency service; and (5) consultation and education. The only features shared by every mental health center are the activities performed to fulfill these essential services—although the nature of these activities vary considerably from center to center. Even the word center can refer to a physical structure or to a cluster of activities and human beings. Examples of the arrangements possible under the term community mental health center are numerous: (1) an entirely new physical structure can be build, such as Maimonides Community Mental Health Center in New York; (2) part of an already existing clinic or hospital can be used, such as Western Psychiatric Institute and Clinic in Pittsburgh; (3) in the absence of an actual physical structure, individuals or agencies can be hired to perform any of the required services, such as is generally characteristic of programs in rural areas; (4) Federal grants can be awarded to either an institution or a group of incorporated citizens; (5) a community mental health center can serve as part of a teaching/training program for future mental health personnel, such as at Lincoln Hospital, or it can be entirely service oriented, as in St. Francis Hospital's Community Mental Health Center in Pittsburgh; (6) personnel can be hired on a full or part time basis, the latter being more frequent because of the shortage of mental health personnel, particularly psychiatrists; (7) centers can be staffed by formally trained individuals and individuals without formal training who are generally referred to as community workers. Western Psychiatric Institute utilizes community workers; St. Francis does not. The West Philadelphia Community Mental Health Center hires and trains community workers to do psychotherapy.

In order to analyze and discuss the consequences and implications of community mental health centers for those professional specialties and institutions which deal with mental health and illness, it is necessary to clarify the meaning of certain basic terms.

We view social psychiatry as a theoretical frame of reference and as an area of research, rather than as a unique treatment approach in the mental health field. In contrast, community psychiatry includes those medically trained mental health therapists concerned with the development and direction of service programs, intervening into community structures and processes for purposes of promoting psychosocial functioning, and preventing or ameliorating community processes inimical to individual or collective well-being. In addition to community psychiatrists, there are nonmedical personnel, both professional and nonprofessional as well as therapeutic and nontherapeutic, working in the area of community mental health. As yet, however, they have not coalesced into a distinct profession or professional speciality with a distinct, common sub-culture or esoteric knowledge base and body of theory.[4, 13] It is for this reason that we view community mental health as a social movement rather than as a professional specialty. Within this framework, the following discussion will examine one community mental health center that emerged from a university affiliated psychiatric hospital and clinic. In keeping with the perspective developed in this paper, we suggest the effects of introducing a community mental health center will vary according to the pre-existing organizational context. Consequently, the conclusions of this paper are not necessarily generalizable to dissimilar organizational settings.

ORGANIZATIONAL SETTING

The original organizational setting was a 180-bed psychiatric hospital and clinic largely supported by state funds and run by the Department of Psychiatry of the University Medical School for the purpose of training medical students and psychiatrists. The regional Institute for Psychoanalysis is based in the hospital and exercises a pervasive influence over all aspects of training and treatment. As a result, the entire hospital staff was primarily psychoanalytically oriented and stressed the traditional one-to-one relationship as a means of understanding and treating intrapsychic conflicts. This orientation generated an elaborate screening and referral system in which the dominant criteria for selecting patients were compatibility with analytic treatment and their potential value as teaching material. This resulted in such highly selective recruitment of patients that over 90 per cent of the inpatients paid for treatment and were White.

The community mental health center began operation within this university affiliated psychiatric hospital and clinic in the summer of 1967. Prior to that time, there had been little attempt to work with the community, except for the psychiatrist who applied for and now directs the center. Although only one component of the psychiatric hospital, the center employs 150 people (24 per cent of the entire staff, but a larger proportion of the professional staff). However, of the 20 psychiatrists presently employed by the center, only two, the director of the center and the director of the inpatient unit, work on a fulltime basis. Other personnel include social workers, community workers,

181

psychologists, nurses, occupational and recreational therapists, anthropologists, and sociologists. In contrast to the dominant individual approach of the parent institution, the center focuses on the community, its institutions, and their effect on individuals and collectivities.

This section describes some of the consequences of the introduction of this program into the pre-existing institution. The most fruitful way to describe the effect of a community mental health center on the organizational structure of an existing psychiatric facility is to examine separately the influence of each unit of service on the overall institution. The following discussion covers: (1) new or existing services; (2) the primary function of the mental health center in contrast to the existing institutions; and (3) changes in the criteria for selecting patients. Besides the five required community mental health services, one additional unit, the base service unit, will be described.

Inpatient Service

The community mental health center inpatient service occupies one of the university psychiatric hospital's newly remodeled wards and contains 36 beds, in single and double rooms. Although there are similarities between this ward and conventional wards, there are several important differences. In contrast to the usual teaching ward operation, where rotating residents report to the clinical director of the hospital, the permanent fulltime psychiatrist responsible for the center's ward reports only to the director of the center. The center's inpatients are not part of the hospital training program and hence are not treated by psychiatric residents. This policy emerged after residents elected not to treat community mental health center inpatients.* These inpatients are seen by psychiatrists and community workers from the center's staff. Eight community workers refer persons to the center, work with the family, and attempt to alleviate social reality problems impinging upon the patient. Twenty-eight fulltime personnel, including 12 nurses and 10 nurses aides, are assigned to this ward.

The center's inpatient unit staffed by one fulltime and several parttime psychiatrists accounts for almost 40 per cent of inpatients. The remaining 60 per cent are covered by residents and about six fulltime staff psychiatrists. This unbalanced division of labor has generated strains and tensions between mental health center and non-center psychiatrists. This situation, however, has strengthened the center's bargaining power and legitimated its structural importance.

Outpatient Service

The University affiliated Psychiatric Hospital has always offered outpatient services staffed by psychiatrists, residents, and medical students. Source of refer-

---

*This refusal represents a significant departure from the traditional pattern of cooperative compliance which characterizes resident behavior and is symptomatic of the conflict engendered by the introduction of this psychiatric innovation.[11]

ral was the main criterion for selection, with usefulness for teaching purposes the second criterion. The primary form of treatment was individual psychotherapy.

In contrast, the community mental health center outpatient service consists of individual therapy, group therapy, family therapy, and home visits. Therapy is conducted by psychiatrists, psychologists, social workers, nurses, and college graduates but not by psychiatric residents. Unlike the traditional screening mechanism for selecting patients, with its attendant six-month waiting list, mental health center patients can walk in, be referred from within the center, or be referred by anyone outside the center. Thus, the only criterion for selection is residence in the catchment area and the wait is comparatively short.

Twenty-Four Hour Emergency Service

Prior to the inception of the 24-hour emergency service, all psychiatric emergencies were taken to a general hospital outside the catchment area, whereas they are now taken to the emergency room of the university general hospital across the street from the center. This unit sees all psychiatric emergencies, but only initiates followup for catchment area residents. Originally, psychiatric residents covered this service on a rotating basis, but a shortage of residents forced the center's psychiatrists to take over this responsibility. Disposition of patients is reviewed weekly by an immediate care committee of psychiatrists, nurses, social workers, and community workers. In contrast to referral patterns elsewhere, the existence of this service encourages walk-in patients, many of whom refer themselves.

Partial Hospitalization

Another new and unique community mental health service is partial hospitalization. The purpose of this service is to provide alternatives to patients for whom hospitalization is unnecessary and conventional outpatient services are inadequate. Patients are presumably free to use this service on a day, night, or week end basis. This unit functions mostly as a day hospital and has never reached the enrollment for which it was designed (50 patients). The usual number ranges between 25 and 35. No unusual mode of treatment is offered in this tightly structured, conventionally run new service. Patients can be referred from within the center or by individuals or agencies in the community. Criteria for selection limit the number of patients admitted. Specifically, the service will not admit patients who are addicts, suicidal, chronic, under 16 years old, cannot travel, do not have a supportive home or family, and do not have a potential for improvement. Nontraditional mental health personnel do not work in this unit. The program is geared to four patient types:

1. Those who have been fully hospitalized and released but still need support.
2. Those never hospitalized and getting "sick."

3. People in crises (including students).
4. Patients to be oriented for hospital admission.

Base Service Unit

Though not one of the five required services, the base service unit was organized to provide continuity of care within the mental health center and to offer direct outpatient services. In addition to operating a walk-in clinic, personnel in the base service unit offer family therapy, group therapy, individual therapy, followup care, and home visits. In contrast, the psychiatric hospital has rarely offered family therapy, after care, home care, or walk-in services.

The various treatment approaches are practiced by nonpsychiatric personnel such as psychologists, social workers, nurses, and college graduates; psychiatrists function in a supervisory capacity. Once again, the only criterion for patient selection is area of residence. Patients already receiving one service have priority over new patients for additional services. Prevention is carried out through the principle of comprehensive care. For example, it is possible for members of a single family to receive individual therapy, attend the day hospital, have children in group therapy, receive home visits, and be seen as a three-generational family system. More importantly, all of these services change the focus of treatment from intrapsychic conflicts to family and community contexts.

Education and Consultation

Education and consultation is the least traditional and clearly defined of all the community mental health services. Approximately one third of the total center staff is organized into education and consultation teams assigned to specific geographical sections (usually an identifiable neighborhood) of the catchment area. There is no set format for the organization and composition of the teams nor operating guidelines for their activities. Prevention of mental illness and promotion of positive mental health is the common long-range objective. The teams focus almost entirely on the community and its institutions, and thus deal mainly with a nonpatient population. Due to the newness and ill-defined nature of the prevention approach, there are no established general patterns. We will therefore describe specific activities and composition.

The center gives each team the freedom to initiate and develop the course of action and activities most relevant to the needs and characteristics of a particular neighborhood. In practice, it allows the team leader (generally a psychiatrist) maximum flexibility in determining objectives, utilizing and hiring staff, and devising ways of interpreting and implementing the preventive approach. In addition, most of the unorthodox activities are not constrained because they occur in the community outside the physical structure and supervision of the psychiatric hospital. Team positions and functions permit a range of new professional roles and relationships for center personnel, especially psychiatrists.

Three teams are currently staffed and operating. In order of length of operation they are: the Steel Mill Neighborhood Team, the Black Neighborhood Team, and the Upper Income Neighborhood Team. (A fourth team in a university neighborhood consists of one staff member, a social worker who concentrates on youth activities.)

The Steel Mill Neighborhood Team: This team was designed as a community laboratory where persons from various disciplines could collaborate to study relationships between individual behavior and the environment. The disciplines involved include psychiatry, child psychiatry, psychology, sociology, anthropology, history, political science, economics, nursing, social work, and public health. The rationale for this cross-disciplinary participation was that each *specialist* would use his own observational and research skills to study the community and its residents. This team attempted to clarify and work out problems attending an inter-disciplinary approach.[1,2] It did not follow through with its overall plan, nor were agreed upon goals and professional distinctions maintained. The result has been the interaction of diverse professionals whose goals, philosophy, and operating procedures are quite distinct and unmeshed. In addition to its research, the team provides consultation to anyone in the community. Recipients include clergymen, physicians, nurses, anti-poverty workers, public housing managers, school personnel, and individual citizens.

The Black Neighborhood Team: For two years after its inception the Black Neighborhood Team was led by a White psychiatrist. The other team members included Black social workers and eight Black community workers (community residents without formal training). The current team leader is a Black psychiatrist. Each member of this team engages in activities aimed at social system modification. Although they also refer, help, and follow up individual patients, the bulk of energy is focused on organized collectivities such as schools, community groups, agencies, and economic enterprises. All team members initiate, plan, administer, consult, and educate in response to community demands. This is the largest community team, boasting 13 members. The predominant techniques utilized by this team are community organization and sensitivity training. For example, following riots after the assassination of Dr. Martin Luther King, the team organized groups for the distribution of clothing, food, medical, and transportation services. Much later, they developed an organization known as the United Black Front, an umbrella agency for restoring human dignity to Black people through economic and political ventures. Sensitivity training led by selected team members has included diverse groups of individuals, including university administrators such as the Chancellor, Vice-Chancellors, and Deans. The subject matter revolved around civil rights and racism. The team served to interpret and promote statements of Black power in a mental health context. Team members also deal with the referral, in-hospital care, and followup of Black patients. The university affiliated psychiatric hospital had never before employed community residents, Black or White, in this capacity.

Upper Middle Class Neighborhood Team: The psychiatrist that formed and directs this team previously directed the Black Neighborhood Team for two years, that experience providing his apprenticeship in community psychiatry. This second team includes a psychologist, a community organizer, a group worker, a college graduate, and a sociologist. Other center personnel, such as a nurse who does family therapy and a community worker from the Black Neighborhood Team, occasionally augment the staff for specific tasks. The team's major focus is the community and the effect of its various institutions on individuals and families. In particular, the team focuses on assisting young people with the developmental tasks of adolescence. Initially, all team members undertook a five-month study of the major youth activities in the upper middle class neighborhood. The informal contacts and the data gathered provided the basis for planning and implementing a prevention program. The team also established working relationships with schools, church-related youth groups, commercial groups, the police, citizens' committees, and the young people. As part of its program, the team established headquarters in a 15-room mansion donated by a church in the community. This extension of the center into the community functions as a center for intergroup youth activities, parent-child discussions, sensitivity groups, and creative expression groups. Another service provided at the headquarters is psychological and career counseling by neighborhood residents screened and trained by the team. The team observes, consults, and occasionally intervenes in the neighborhood high school, which is experiencing wide spread intergroup conflicts. In this situation, the unit of intervention is a collectivity, the school system. In initiating and implementing these activities, professional distinctions and hierarchical relations among team members are ignored, and roles are determined by expertise and availability.

This section has described the organizational innovations resulting from the introduction of a community mental health center into a university affiliated psychiatric hospital. The following section discusses professional roles, tasks, and responsibilities associated with these organizational changes.

ROLES, TASKS, AND RESPONSIBILITIES

The mental health field is going through inevitable changes, both from general societal pressures and from the funding of community mental health centers. Personnel affiliated with the community mental health center, regardless of their professional background and training, belong to an emergent profession that has ill-defined boundaries—unspecified roles, tasks, and responsibilities. Moreover, present professional labels do not adequately describe the new roles, tasks, and responsibilities of the staff, especially for nonprofessionals, and are therefore less significant and salient for the effective functioning of the staff. A wide range of roles, tasks, and responsibilities characterize the various professionals and nonprofessionals on the center staff. For example, traditionally-oriented professionals as well as professionals whose activities are uniquely innovative implement community mental health approaches. For these reasons, the following discussion acknowledges the importance of professional designations, but emphasizes roles, tasks, and responsibilities as more significant for differentiating among community mental health personnel and comparing them with non-center personnel. Specifically, we examine differences among psychiatrists in the mental health center and compare them to psychiatrists in the sponsoring psychiatric hospital.

The organizational structures of the psychiatric hospital and the center provide a framework for illustrating differences. The emphasis on formal professional designations within the psychiatric hospital perpetuates traditional lines of authority and prestige, which in turn influence the practices of individual professionals, the settings for task performance, and the patterns of interprofessional and intraprofessional relations. For example, hiring a psychiatrist to treat outpatients (nonmedical personnel could *not* be hired for this function) circumscribes his role as a Freudian psychotherapist, defines his task as one-to-one psychoanalysis with patients screened as suitable for treatment, makes him responsible only for this treatment approach, and prescribes the private office as the setting for treatment. Treatment focuses on intrapsychic conflicts in individual patients. The psychiatrist is accountable largely to himself and may on occasion report to a psychiatric administrator or supervisor. The only differences between private and institutional psychotherapists stem from the fact that the latter are salaried and have less freedom in selecting patients. Professional training and socialization of psychiatrists at this psychiatric hospital is controlled by psychiatrists who adhere to these traditional approaches and practices.

In contrast to this traditional adherence to professional distinction, community mental health center psychiatrists are frequently hired to perform the same functions as both formally and informally trained nonmedical personnel. For example, psychiatrists, psychologists, and college graduates in the base service unit all treat outpatients, utilizing individual and family therapy. Thus, professional affiliation alone does *not* determine the individual's roles, tasks, responsibilities, work setting, or colleague relations. Within the center's organizational structure, these are determined by professional and personal abilities and experiences as well as the unit or program in which the practitioner works. Furthermore, the degree to which a unit or program is traditional as well as functionally and organizationally specified affects the degree to which the practitioner adopts established or innovative roles, tasks, and responsibilities.

To illustrate this proposition, we will examine the center's inpatient unit, the 24-hour emergency unit, and the education and consultation teams in greater detail. In regard to the center's inpatient unit, hospitalizing the mentally ill is both traditional and functionally specified. Psychiatrists hired to serve this function find their professional training as Freudian analysts provides a role and orientation appropriate to the unit. Their primary task is one-to-one psychoanalysis for patients screened solely on the basis of residence. This means that psychiatrists are sometimes confronted with patients whose sociocultural and socioeconomic characteristics make them less suitable for analytically-oriented forms of treatment. Consequently, they may be forced to try other techniques, such as milieu or behavior therapy. The hospital ward remains the circumscribed setting of professional activities in this unit.

Most treatment in the center's inpatient unit remains focused on the intrapsychic conflicts of the individual. However, the presence of Black community workers assigned to Black patients frequently imposes constraints on the psychiatrists by forcing them to consider the realities of the patients' social world. In such cases, psychiatrists must develop working relationships with unfamiliar colleagues on either a hierarchial or egalitarian basis in order to formulate treatment plans. These psychiatrists are accountable not only to the center's administration, but also to representatives of the community. In sum, although some of their roles, tasks, and responsibilities have altered, psychiatrists on the center's inpatient unit continue to function in a manner similar to psychiatrists hired for conventional inpatient services.

The 24-hour emergency unit, although a new service, alters the psychiatrists' roles, tasks, and responsibilities in only one important way. The psychiatrists are confronted with many persons who have *defined themselves* as in need of mental health services and, consequently, have not been referred or screened by any of the existing systems. Under the traditional screening system, patients are defined as in need of psychiatric care and tentatively diagnosed by other professionals. In the 24-hour emergency unit, diagnosis and disposition are not predetermined and must be made for the first time, subject to review by family, neighbors, and a professional committee within the center. This unit offers traditional services and is functionally specified. Only one feature modifies psychiatrists' tasks and responsibilities, even though these are still circumscribed by the hospital setting.

The education and consultation unit is least traditional, most unspecified, and most open to individual interpretation. More than any other community mental health service, this unit defines treatment as prevention. The psychiatrists hired to organize and lead neighborhood teams that are located in and focusing on the community and its institutions must respond more directly to community demands. Moreover, because of their greater visibility, they are more directly accountable to the community for their actions. This, in turn, means that psychiatrists are less visible to their hospital colleagues and less constrained by them.

In this unit, psychiatrists also work largely with nonpatient populations, which forces them to imagine new roles, tasks, and responsibilities instead of merely exercising old ones. It increasingly puts them in unprecedented contact and collaboration with three new groups. The first group is other professionals with whom collaboration in the past has been minimal or under highly structured situations with clearly drawn lines of authority. The second group is "new patients," particularly those who are not labeled mentally ill, dealt with in natural settings such as home, school, or neighborhood. The third group consists of the various kinds of nonprofessionals who have direct and partially independent roles in both prevention and treatment.

Responsibility for promoting positive mental health among whole communities and groups within them forces psychiatrists to examine the social structure and environment to determine their effect on the well-being of individuals and groups. This often puts psychiatrists in the role of social change agents seeking social system modifications. They also take on the task of actively intervening in the lives of individuals as well as in complex organizational processes. In terms of the definitions proposed in this paper, they are functioning as community psychiatrists: that is, psychiatrists for the community.

Not every psychiatrist hired for the education and consultation unit adopts the same new roles, tasks, responsibilities, settings, and patterns of collaboration. The descriptions of the Steel Mill Team leader and the Upper Middle Class Neighborhood Team leader illustrate two psychiatrists hired for the same unit and functions who adopted quite different roles, tasks, and responsibilities.

Apart from the center's inpatient ward, from which psychiatric residents withdrew, the efforts of community psychiatry occur in the community. Thus, few professionals operating within the traditional hospital structure really know the scope, objectives, and content of the center's programs and services. By withdrawing from internal involvement with the center and lacking knowledge of the center's external activities, existing institutional patterns perpetuate themselves relatively unhampered.

Many issues require attention from both mental health professionals and researchers. For example, what are the scope and boundaries of community psychiatry? What professional education, experiences, and titles are appropriate for medical and nonmedical practitioners of community psychiatry? How far beyond the individual mentally ill patient does responsibility extend—to a disfunctional family system, to a disfunctional school system, or perhaps even to a disfunctional municipal governing system? According to what models should training and certification programs be developed? If all professional lines are blurred, how are responsibilities to be determined and allocated, especially in linked open systems like communities? We do not really know nearly enough about the professionals and nonprofessionals working in community mental health centers or about their roles, tasks, and responsibilities.

In order to better understand selected effects of the 1963 Community Mental Health Center Act, we have described organizational and professional changes that have occurred in one psychiatric institution. However, it is clear that the central objective of the legislation, as of any center established to implement it, concerns changes in patient populations treated as well as in the locus for treatment. We now turn to a discussion of these issues.

CHANGES IN PATIENT POPULATION

Prior to the inception of the community mental health center, patients were sifted through an elaborate screening and referral process which selected them without regard for area of residence, but largely because they were interesting teaching cases. But the community mental health center is obligated to provide care for all the residents of a specific catchment area. Education and consultation are particularly oriented toward serving the community. The inevitable result is that patients with a broader range of demographic and psychopathological characteristics are admitted and treated.[9] These changes in the patient population affect the sponsoring institution.

As in most psychiatric facilities, first admissions of inpatients to the psychiatric hospital have increased in the last decade, but most considerably since 1967, when the community mental health center began. The pattern of referrals to inpatient care began to change prior to the center's inception. Since 1965 there has been a steady decrease in the proportion of referrals from private psychiatrists. Correspondingly, there has been a steady increase in the proportion of referrals from clinics in other parts of the health center and, more recently, from the emergency room of the university general hospital where the center's psychiatric emergency service is located. One of the first effects of the center was that criteria for patient selection changed. In addition to being selected for teaching purposes, patients are now selected on the basis of their need for treatment. This change in criteria has altered the characteristics of inpatients. From 1960 to 1966, the proportion of schizophrenics admitted as inpatients steadily decreased. Since 1967, the proportion of schizophrenic inpatients has increased, more markedly since 1968. That this has posed greater management problems is reflected by the fact that the number of patients secluded has increased at a rate parallel to the increase in schizophrenics. Perhaps another indicator of increased management problems has been an increased rate of turnover among nursing personnel.

If the center is functioning properly, patients with mental disorders with more favorable prognoses should be treated in the center and those with more severe prognoses should be referred to the state mental hospital. By comparing the percentage of first admissions to the state mental hospital by diagnosis from the community mental health center catchment area with a comparable area having no community mental health center, it is possible to note certain changes. One change is that the percentage of persons admitted to the state hospital with functional disorders has decreased, while the percentage of persons admitted with organic disorders has increased. In other words, those mental diseases with a definable and probably chronic disease process in operation (organic disorders) are increasingly more likely to be sent to the state mental hospital from the center's catchment area than from an area without a center. On the other hand, the functional disorders, which tend to have no identifiable organic disease process, are increasingly less likely to be sent to the state hospital from the area with the mental health center. These data, along with the data indicating increased ad-

190

missions of schizophrenics, suggest that the functional disorders are increasingly being treated in the community mental health center.

Making services available to the Black neighborhood has had a marked effect upon the racial composition of inpatients. The proportion of non-White patients was 3 per cent in 1966. After 1967, this proportion began to increase until the end of 1969, when the proportion was 27 per cent, which approached the proportion of Blacks in the catchment area. The study by Hollingshead and Redlich[5] suggests that an increased proportion of Black patients in the psychiatric hospital would lead to a greater proportion of Blacks referred to the state mental hospital. Comparison of state hospital first admissions from the center's catchment area with a comparable area having no center reveals no corresponding increase in referrals of Blacks to the state mental hospital. In other words, the center brought more Blacks into the psychiatric hospital and treated them there, contrary to what Hollingshead and Redlich would have predicted.

The inception of the community mental health center legitimated a change in the criteria for patient selection, and as a result, the sociocultural and psychopathological characteristics of patients changed. The effect of this is to force a traditional psychiatric hospital to confront and treat a much broader spectrum of patients and social categories than before. These changes in the patient population are a constant and persistent catalyst for a dramatic changes in traditional psychiatry, which have so far been minimal. Other than bringing more Black people into the center for treatment and having many more Black staff members participating in institutional activities, the center has not in this short period extensively modified the organizational structure, primary objectives, or operational procedures of the university affiliated psychiatric hospital. As long as the center remains non-threatening and its activities are out of sight, it is tolerated by the parent institution. Just how much longer the centers can remain invisible and avoid direct confrontations with their sponsoring institutions is uncertain.

CONCLUDING REMARKS

It is important to emphasize the fact that none of the essential services or concepts specified in the 1963 Federal legislation or actually found in the various community mental health centers is entirely new. However, the combination and integration of these services and concepts into a single institutional framework and setting represents a significant innovative departure from traditional arrangements. What is most clearly new is the charge, placed upon community mental health centers by the legislation of social policy, to assume responsibilities for the community and the society-at-large never before considered the professional domain of the mental health establishment. This charge and its attendant responsibility involves determining how to discover the unmet needs of citizens and how to adapt or develop theories, techniques, organizational forms, and procedures for anticipating and meeting those needs. Stated in this fashion, one of the crucial implications of the social policy underlying the 1963 Act becomes clear: the new social mandate placed upon community mental health centers (in addition to preventing mental disorder) is to discover not who will most benefit by therapeutic techniques that are already known and utilized, but how to help those who need help, regardless of whether they are fit subjects for these present approaches and techniques. This implication underlies the existence, composition, and operation of all these centers and is the basis of their social significance. The radical restructuring and reorientation of the mental health field implied are also the source of some of the professional opposition to the original Federal legislation and subsequent resistance to the general approaches and organizational arrangements designed to implement it.

In the most general and ideal sense, community mental health centers were designed to provide certain necessary facilities and services seen as appropriate to an unprecedentedly broad concept of mental health care. This conception of mental health services to citizens of all ages and backgrounds shifted the emphasis from treatment and care as being the purchasable right of the appropriate few to being an inalienable right of or necessary service to all citizens. More concretely, the social mandate implied that the unmet needs of citizens, rather than the professional techniques, concepts, approaches, and responsibilities of mental health practitioners, are the crucial determinants of who needs help and of the appropriate techniques and approaches. In brief, existing unmet mental health care needs of the populace were made the defining and guiding focus of the community mental health center.

The significance and uniqueness of this superficially innocuous shift in the basis for determining mental health needs is related to the nature of professional service and practice in all highly professionalized occupational fields, including mental health. A crucial characteristic of all highly professionalized occupations is that practitioners must undergo an intensive professional socialization which transcends the acquisition of specialized technical skills and procedures. The purpose of this socialization is to insure the internalization of common models of professional practice, traditional definitions of appropriate problems or clients, and shared conceptions of professional responsibility on the part of future practitioners. In the mental health professions, practitioners have been (and still are being) trained and socialized into the traditional medical disease model of professional responsibility which has the objective of bettering the patient, but clearly also has the aim of doing so under conditions which the professional has come to believe are necessary for that very betterment. These conditions tend to maximize the ability of the professional to perform the specific services he has learned and is committed to. In short, the professional believes that only certain types of problems are appropriate to his specialty and that only certain types of patients will benefit from it, and he treats only those patients who have these psychosocial and symptomatic characteristics. Thus, the professional practitioner determines who shall receive his specialized professional services.

But this is the very antithesis of the perspective and the mandate contained in the 1963 legislation. The social policy underlying that legislation implicitly gave the power to define and determine mental health needs to lay citizens. For example, the concepts of 24-hour emergency services and walk-in clinics implicitly assume that individual citizens can and will define mental health and illness in terms of their own (community based) criteria and are able to determine whether they actually need help. This assumption derives from (and increases) skepticism concerning professional omniscience and omnipotence. Since the institutionalized prerogative to define problems and patients as appropriate to specialized skills, techniques, and procedures lies at the very core of professional authority and expertise, the community mental health policy and legislation implicitly threatened the legitimacy and prestige of professional mental health practitioners.

A comparative study of two Pittsburgh community mental health centers,[10] which describes in detail the responses of the sponsoring psychiatric organization, suggested three dimensions along which conflicts arise. These are:

1. training vs. service as an emphasis;
2. individual vs. community as a focus;
3. old vs. new roles for psychiatrists.

These dimensions provided the framework for organizing the data characterizing the differences between the center and existing patterns. The study concluded that some conflicts could be reconciled through negotiating and compromise, but the dominant response of the existing organization was to constrain the day-to-day operations of the center that sharply departed from well established patterns.

It is important to emphasize that the government sought to avoid such conflict at all costs. The very ambiguity and inconsistencies in the Federal legislation testify to that. The government attempted to produce and then influence the direction of social change in the mental health field without explicitly affecting the status quo. Yet the radical implications of the 1963 legislation, the widespread professional opposition (particularly from the AMA) to it, and the subsequent professional resistance to attempts to implement these policies indicate that the government did not totally succeed.

The basic conflict between the perspective, assumptions, and implications of the original community mental health legislation and those underlying the highly professionalized occupational groups has had diverse, pervasive, and significant ramifications. One consequence has been the partial breakdown of formerly impenetrable professional boundaries. Inter- and cross-professional contact and collaboration in the mental health field had been minimal: it occurred in highly structured situations where roles, responsibilities, and lines of prestige and authority were sharply drawn. The interpretations in this paper and in other studies indicate that professional boundaries, distinctions, and differences take on less actual, operational significance and are less salient to professionals themselves in the context of a community mental health program. Thus, in one sense, the centers may be said to engender interprofessional relationships, similarity, and homogeneity. In the long run, however, there can be little doubt but that the most significant and unique profession relevant change introduced by community mental health centers involves a breakdown in the distinction between professionals and nonprofessionals. Some of the center's operational units (specifically, some of the education and consultation teams) described in this paper bear testimony to the gradual and partial blurring of professional-nonprofessional lines. The general point, however, is that the public policy and legislation establishing the community mental health centers has weakened the power and legitimacy of traditional professional distinctions—both interprofessional and nonprofessional-professional distinctions—as a function of the implicit decision to remove definitions of mental health care needs from exclusive professional control.

REFERENCES

1. CAUDILL, WILLIAM, AND ROBERTS, B. H.: "Pitfalls in the Organization of Interdisciplinary Research." *Human Organization*. Winter: 12-15, 1951.
2. ELLISON, DAVID L., et al.: "Problems in Developing a Community Based Research Component for a Mental Health Center." *Mental Hygiene* 43:168-179, 1972.
3. GLASSCOTE, R., SUSSEX, J., CUMMING, E., AND SMITH, L.: *The Community Mental Health Center: An Interim Appraisal.* Baltimore: Garamond/Pridemark Press and the Joint Information Service of the American Psychiatric Association and the National Association for Mental Health, 1969.
4. GREENWOOD, ERNEST: "Attributes of a Profession." *Social Work* 2:44-55, 1957.
5. HOLLINGSHEAD, AUGUST B., AND REDLICH, FREDRICK C.: *Social Class and Mental Illness: A Community Study.* New York: John Wiley and Sons, 1958.
6. KELLER, DOROTHY S.: *Annual Report,* Western Psychiatric Institute and Clinic, Division of Medical Records. Pittsburgh, Pennsylvania, 1964.
7. KELLER, DOROTHY S.: *Annual Report,* Western Psychiatric Institute and Clinic, Division of Medical Records. Pittsburgh, Pennsylvania, 1969.
8. KISSICK, WILLIAM L.: "Health Policy Directions for the 1970s." *The New England Journal of Medicine* 282:1343-1354, 1970.
9. MESNIKOFF, ALVIN M.: "The Effects of a Community Mental Health Service on Residency Training." *Journal of Medical Education* 43: 1059-1067, 1968.
10. RIEKER, PATRICIA: "A Comparative Study of Two Pittsburgh Community Mental Health Centers." Unpublished Department of Sociology Preliminary Paper. University of Pittsburgh, 1970.
11. SCHULMAN, JAY: *Remaking an Organization.* Albany: State University of New York Press, 1969.
12. UNIVERSITY OF PITTSBURGH: Annual Report, Western Psychiatric Institute and Clinic, 1969.
13. WILENSKY, HAROLD L.: "The Professionalization of Everyone?" *American Journal of Sociology* LXX:137-158, 1964.

CHAPTER 9

Conflict and Cooperation in a Community Mental Health Program

NANCY BERAN AND SIMON DINITZ

INTRODUCTION, METHOD, AND BACKGROUND

Despite considerable professional interest in the transition from conventional psychiatric facilities to community mental health centers, few studies have attempted to document the nature and consequences of such change for staff and patient functioning. This paper describes and analyzes the ideological and practical problems encountered in implementing the policies and practices of community mental health.

Data were collected during a three and one-half month period of participant observation in an Ohio psychiatric hospital. This institution was unique in that it operated within a single physical facility and under the same superintendency two separate and distinct psychiatric programs: a traditionally oriented receiving hospital and a modern community mental health center. The receiving hospital had been in operation since 1946 and was designed in line with the ideology and method of operation characteristic of the traditional "medical model" orientation to mental illness. This approach is characterized by an emphasis on the supremacy of psychiatric expertise and decision-making authority in diagnosis, treatment, and disposition, a heavy reliance on organic therapies in treatment regimens, and the perpetuation of custodial ward atmospheres.

On August 1, 1968, a mental health center began operations within the same physical facility and alongside the receiving hospital. The institution (although still directed by a single superintendent) at that time became divided in program philosophy, structure, function, and personnel between the receiving hospital and the mental health center. The mental health center was designed to implement the principles and practices of community mental health as outlined in

195

the 1963 Federal Community Mental Health Centers Act, and was partially funded by Federal agencies. In contrast to traditional mental health systems (as exemplified by the receiving hospital), community mental health emphasizes comprehensiveness and continuity of patient care and therefore insists on the provision of multiple services including inpatient, outpatient, partial hospitalization, 24-hour emergency, consultation and education, training, and research and evaluation. More importantly, community mental health incorporates the talents of paramedical and nonmedical personnel in diagnosis, treatment, and disposition; it replaces psychiatric dominance with team decision-making; it emphasizes nonmedically-based treatment modalities; and it seeks to replace custodial ward atmospheres and routines with milieu therapy or therapeutic communities.

When the receiving hospital and mental health center began conjunctive operations, six treatment teams were established, three per division. Each of the teams was composed of a staff psychiatrist, an MA psychologist, a BA social worker, a registered nurse, and a psychiatric aide. Each team member was officially designated as a "case manager" and was therefore to assume primary responsibility (excepting the medical-legal responsibility) for the management of all patients assigned to him. Inpatient treatment services were distributed among the six teams on the four 28-bed male-female wards in the following manner: two mental health center teams conducted their inpatient activities on one ward; one mental health center team and one receiving hospital team shared the facilities of a second ward; and the remaining two receiving hospital teams each operated their own separate wards. Patients were assigned to teams on the basis of residential location: the mental health center served a part of the home county, which includes about one third of that county's population, and the receiving hospital served the balance of the home county plus four adjoining counties.

The above anatomical sketch describes the approximate state of affairs at the institution when the participant observation began, about 10 months after the dual program was initiated. A large part of the researcher's time during the study period was devoted to direct observation of and interaction with the staff and patients at the hospital. An attempt was made to become well acquainted with all aspects of life at the institution and therefore included exposure to a large variety of activities: formal and informal meetings of both treatment teams and patients, administrative staff meetings, daily ward activities, and many other varied and sundry affairs.

A CASE STUDY OF ADAPTATION TO CHANGE

The most obvious conclusion derived from 14 weeks of participant observation is that the receiving hospital and the mental health center constituted two distinct psychiatric systems representing often gross differences in the definition and management of the mentally ill. This contrast was indeed evident on every ideological and procedural dimension examined. The two divisions were clearly distinguishable in terms of the following variables: the status of the treatment team and case manager concepts; the frequency and interactional pattern of general team meetings; the format and tenor of interviews with patients; the distribution of decision-making power within teams; the methods of treatment developed and employed; and the conduct and atmosphere of inpatient wards. On all of these dimensions, the receiving hospital displayed a traditional mental health orientation which stood in noticeable contrast to the community mental health approach more typical of the mental health center.

Furthermore, observations for three and one-half months consistently revealed an absence of affection and, at times, overt hostility between the personnel in the receiving hospital and the mental health center. The philosophy, staff, and procedures of the receiving hospital teams were often the target of derision of the mental health center teams, and the response on the part of the receiving hospital teams was no less negative. Members of the mental health center teams despairingly described the receiving hospital as old-fashioned, unenlightened, custodial, and as oriented solely to the traditional medical model. In retaliation, members of the receiving hospital teams characterized the mental health center as grossly naive and unrealistic in its aims, nonprofessional and chaotic in operation, neglectful of organic therapies, and an insult and injustice to the psychiatrists' medical expertise and superiority. As only one example of typical exchanges: a mental health center psychiatrist criticized a receiving hospital colleague for attempting to retain total treatment control over all the patients on his ward—"he can't see 20 patients for an hour a day." The receiving hospital psychiatrist in turn ridiculed his mental health center colleague for attempting to solve social problems—"you can't treat an unhappy marriage in a hospital setting."

But despite all the observations supporting this conclusion of difference between the receiving hospital and the mental health center, other equally convincing evidence led to a second conclusion which stands in qualification of the first: various philosophies and practices of the traditional mental health system persisted in the otherwise enlightened program of the mental health center. This became particularly clear in the wake of organizational changes that took place during the course of the study period itself and were therefore directly witnessed by the researcher in a kind of "natural experiment."

On July 1, 1969, two weeks after the researcher's arrival, the mental health center staff psychiatrists left their individual treatment teams and one of them assumed the role of Coordinator of Clinical Services for all three teams. This constituted a significant transformation in team structure. Since the opening of the mental health center almost one year earlier, each of the mental health center teams had been under the team leadership of their own staff psychiatrist. Though one of the teams had indeed been functioning without the services of a staff psychiatrist for a few months prior to July, this exception was apparently one less of administrative choice than of administrative inability to retain the employment of the psychiatrist's services. Moreover, this particular team was reportedly displeased with the loss of their staff psychiatrist.

In any event, one of the two remaining mental health center team psychiatrists left his post to assume the position of Director of the Residency Program. The other psychiatrist became the Coordinator of Clinical Services, or sole consultant and supervisor for all three mental health center teams. Though each of the teams had both a first and second year resident as fulltime team members, they began to share the services of this single staff psychiatrist as consultant and supervisor in patient diagnosis, treatment, and disposition.

This mental health center program alteration represented a realization of the community mental health system's "case manager," nonmedical-model ideal. The removal of the staff psychiatrist from the team constituted a redefinition of his role in the team enterprise and a reinforcement of community mental health's contention that paramedical and nonmedical personnel are competent agents in managing the mentally ill. Over and above this, the researcher would have predicted an enthusiastic response to this program change on the basis of two observations during the first few weeks of the study: (1) a number of mental health center staff were heard to complain about the fact that "the doctor too often has the final word around here," and (2) the members of one team who felt they really had ultimate authority over the treatment of their own patients expressed satisfaction and even delight with their team psychiatrist's respect for their roles as case managers. Indeed, one would have expected mental health center team members to applaud the change as an implementation of the community mental health system's philosophy above and beyond that originally hoped for by the Superintendent of the institution in 1967, at which time he wrote the following:

The most important variable is that of power—overt, explicit power. It is my view that, given competence, if the team psychologist, the team nurse or any other competent person on the team does not have the clear option of making decisions concerning the patients assigned to him, then no real team exists. Here I refer to decisions traditionally reserved for the physician— passes, privileges, and the like. The final test or the proof of the existence of such a team comes when the doctor-leader disagrees with the decision of another team member. If he simply countermands the decision the other team members quickly learn that their decision-making power is only illusory and they make no more meaningful decisions.

It is clear from the above that I consider the shared-power team superior to the more traditionally organized team. The major reason for this is my belief that if responsibility for patient care is not shared, the skills, talents and humanity of the other team members are not fully utilized. We are being wasteful with our already limited resources. A corollary of this concerns motivation. To the extent that an individual has a stake in a given task, to that extent will he perform. There is no more powerful way to motivate human beings than to give them responsibility—more responsibility and the power of making decisions. Admittedly the shortage of professional mental health workers has given a powerful incentive to this type of organization. It must be emphasized, however, that given a hundred-fold increase in the availability of psychiatrists, the organization directions herein outlined would remain the same.

Developments surrounding the July 1 program change cast very serious doubts on the validity of both the researcher's original expectations and the Superintendent's notion of the relationships among motivation, responsibility, and decision-making power. From the time the proposed change was officially discussed with the teams to its implementation a week or so later, team members were often heard expressing reservations about the wisdom of the new plan. Their less-than-enthusiastic initial response developed into a generalized negative reaction. Thus, the researcher's daily log contains numerous references to case manager ambivalence, case manager concern that the Coordinator could not possibly attend all meetings of all three teams, case manager fear that the Coordinator would not be available for many patient admission interviews (at which time the diagnosis is typically made and the treatment plan formulated), case manager separation anxiety from former team psychiatrists, and overall, pervasive low morale on teams. (It will be recalled that one of the teams had been functioning without the services of a staff psychiatrist for a period of time. Even though there was no change for this team, the researcher had a number of indications that the team members disliked the absence of a staff psychiatrist—though perhaps not as intensely as the other two teams.)

Many case managers seemed genuinely ambivalent in their response to the program alteration, experiencing simultaneous pleasure and apprehension. On the one hand, they appeared to appreciate the freedom from psychiatric dominance and to enjoy the ego-boosting vote of confidence the hospital administration implied in executing the change. They were certainly acutely aware that the structural alterations were an enhancement, in the hospital's actual operation, of the community mental health system's philosophy. On the other hand, they appeared to feel deeply insecure about their own abilities to function effectively without direct psychiatric guidance. Complaints about the unavailability of such guidance were particularly common among those team members who voiced flat disapproval of the new method of operation, a response overrepresented among residents and aides—two groups obviously comfortably entrenched in the traditional medical model organizational structure. Outright opponents of the program change made such comments as:

"The doctor really does know best."
"The doctor is better qualified to make decisions of a certain type or magnitude."
"The doctor should be around to handle such touchy matters as discussions

with lawyers about patients. I (aide) am not competent to do this; a lawyer could run me around in circles, make a fool out of me, and perhaps cause me professional damage."

"The doctor is invaluable on the team—after all, it's mental illness we're working with, and that's a medical matter."

"The team leader will become an impotent position—a nonpsychiatric leader will just be a figurehead, because he'll have no power."

"The psychiatrist is critical on the team as a teacher to other team members not as well trained or versed in psychiatric matters."

Thus evolved the rather ironic situation in which the greatest threat to an implementation of community mental health principles in practice appeared to be the insecurity-based resistance of some mental health center team members themselves. No one—the staff psychiatrists included—seemed to believe less in the competency of paramedical and nonmedical personnel to function independently of constant psychiatric assistance than some of these personnel themselves.

By the end of the month after the withdrawal of the psychiatrists from the individual teams, the problem of low morale was a central topic of conversation around the institution. One member of a mental health center team told the researcher that: "Morale is at an all-time low . . . the place is just functioning and nothing more . . . everyone just seems to have given up." Many members of the mental health center teams felt the new program was working poorly and were disenchanted with the course of events; a number indicated they were thinking of changing positions—either within or outside the mental health center. A common complaint was that the community mental health system's notion of continuity of care was being rendered ludicrous by continuous changes in program and personnel. But whatever the basis of dissatisfaction, it appeared certain that many of the mental health center staff agreed with one of their members who stated: "If they don't do something quickly, this whole hospital is just going to go up in smoke."

Thus, within one and one-half months, the researcher witnessed antagonism between the mental health center and the receiving hospital become coupled with a deepening disenchantment among mental health center personnel with the concept of community mental health, at least in so far as this concept was being implemented in the research institution. The articulation of these two somewhat contradictory yet simultaneously held attitudes posed serious dilemmas to both staff and researcher. Confusion was in no way lessened by events surrounding another development transpiring during the study period: the institution had recently been awarded a grant earmarked for refashioning the three receiving hospital teams in the image of the three mental health center teams. It is perhaps redundant to mention that few treatment team staff members were very optimistic about the possibility of such an eventual outcome. The prevailing opinion among mental health center staff that "it will never work" was based on contentions that receiving hospital staff were "too entrenched in their traditional ways," and "the traditional philosophy is so engrained in them that their resistance will be insurmountable." This pessimistic attitude was widely expressed even before the mental health center program revision. But in the wake of the negative reactions to that program change, the pessimism about redesigning the receiving hospital in the mental health center's image began to take on some intriguing nuances as members of the mental health center teams themselves became disenchanted with the community mental health concept.

An excellent example of the interplay of both these strands—that is, both the basic contrast between the "traditional" receiving hospital and the "enlightened" mental health center, and the growing disillusionment with the community mental health concept—was found in the attitudes of the mental health center psychiatric aides. All three of these aides (one per mental health center team) had functioned as receiving hospital aides prior to the introduction of the mental health center into the institution and thus were well acquainted with both divisions of the hospital. All three of these aides were, at least prior to the mid-study period decline in morale if not consistently throughout the research period, committed to the mental health center ideal. On numerous occasions these individuals drew comparisons between the receiving hospital and the mental health center for the researcher's edification, and often praised the "new way" as vastly improved over the "old way." But there is equally little doubt that some of the deepest disenchantment with the mental health center concept existed within this group and was articulated to the researcher with increasing frequency in the latter stages of the study period. To state some of their most common complaints:

"Under the new system we may have gone a little overboard in delegating responsibility to nonmedical personnel; case managers have to perform a number of duties that could be better handled by the doctors."

"We may have a lot more doctors running around this hospital now, but we used to get better service when only two doctors ran the whole place."

"I don't like to see patients so drugged up they look like zombies, but now we use such low doses that some very sick patients are much more miserable than they need be, and they also disturb the entire ward."

"I don't think we should revert to the old system—the new one is a vast improvement—but under the old system life on the ward was not so lenient that one patient could drink cleaning fluid and another set her bed on fire while in restraints." (Both of these incidents occurred during the study period.)

To further highlight the ambivalence among this group: One of the aides informed the researcher that the Superintendent had decided to ask all three of the mental health center aides to switch back to the receiving hospital under the new grant for the purpose of serving as links between the receiving hospital and the mental health center in efforts to transform the former division. Her response to this proposal was totally negative. She said: "I wouldn't do it for *ten* step raises; it would only be a big headache."

Eventually, the hospital administration and upper-level treatment staff felt it necessary to meet with each of the three mental health center teams respectively to discuss the problems which developed in the wake of the program change. A variety of attitudes were expressed by the mental health center team members— some were solemnly resigned to what they perceived as a hopeless situation, others were openly angry about the state of affairs, and some suggested that the whole issue had been blown out of proportion and that their team had no major problems or complaints. The administration apparently perceived the majority of opinions to be negative, for at one of the last administrative "planning committee" meetings held during the research period, the Superintendent proposed that three staff psychiatrists each devote one-fourth time to each of the three mental health center teams. To quote from the minutes of that meeting:

Dr. A suggested that Dr. B work one-fourth time on Team I and Dr. C. spend one-fourth time on Team II and Dr. D spend one-fourth of his time on Team III. There seems to be a breakdown in organizational structure and some morale problems on Teams I, II, and III because of a lack of leadership. . . . Mr. X expressed some apprehension about re-introducing the medical model to the Center treatment teams (Teams I, II, III). NIMH would prefer that a non-medical model be followed on these teams. Dr. A suggested that this would only be a temporary measure until the psychiatric residents and the team professionals have reached a level of training which would allow them to handle the situation. A brief discussion of Dr. C's qualifications followed. Dr. E wished to know if Dr. C had a community mental health approach to his treatment of patients. Several members gave negative responses. The morale on Teams I, II, and III was discussed for a short period of time. It is felt that the psychiatric residents feel uncomfortable when they are placed on teams where the Chairman is a non-medical person. Mrs. Z suggested that team members are often afraid to make decisions for fear that they will not be supported by the psychiatric residents. Mr. Y suggested that the weakness in team leadership by the nonmedical team chairman might be negatively reinforced if a psychiatrist was once again placed in charge. It was suggested by Mr. X that Dr. F devote one-fourth of his time to Team II. A counter proposal was made by Dr. A that Dr. B be assigned on a one-fourth basis to Team I, Dr. F on a one-fourth basis to Team II, and Dr. D to Team III on a one-fourth time basis. This is a stop gap or emergency measure and would be temporary in nature. Dr. A suggested that the Planning Committee consider this proposal and discuss it at the next meeting.

This proposal was still under consideration at the termination of the research period.

202

Perhaps no summary could better reflect the atmosphere of this institution undergoing change than a few quotations from staff members themselves. With reference to the operation of the mental health center, a mental health center staff psychiatrist suggested:

> The trouble with all this is that the role prescriptions are completely vague—nobody knows what he's supposed to be doing anytime, and nobody has anybody above him to answer to. The whole thing is supposed to be so democratic, but then nobody knows what to do, people just go their own way doing as they wish, and nothing gets done.

With reference to remaking the receiving hospital teams in the image of the mental health center, this same psychiatrist added:

> They'll just have to get new people to staff the receiving hospital teams, because nobody here will take on that job. But new people will be at a disadvantage in not being acquainted with the set-up. And the old people just won't do it the new way if they're not watched.

Said a psychiatric aide:

> There must be a middle of the road somewhere, between the old system and the new. There was a lot wrong with the old approach; the new approach is on the right track and is a vast improvement over the old. But there's a lot wrong with the new system too; there's a lot more to be done.

The psychiatrist who was Superintendent of the institution during most of the research period resigned from this position two months after the change. The researcher had been informed of his decision *prior to* the beginning of the study period. Throughout the summer, various staff members expressed the opinion that the Superintendent's decision to leave was heavily influenced by the numerous problems in the institution and by various negative evaluations of the mental health center program on the part of the National Institute of Mental Health. A representative of NIMH had visited the mental health center and was reportedly harshly critical of certain aspects of the operations he observed. With reference to this evaluation, one mental health center staff psychiatrist suggested to the researcher:

> I think [the Superintendent] should not have taken the criticisms so much to heart. He should not have expected the Center to be working perfectly during its first nine months of operation. But the mental health center grant was his baby—other people may have helped him write it, but it was all his idea, he got the ball rolling, and he pushed it through.

DISCUSSION

It is clear that the institution under study experienced impressive resistance to the shift from the ideologies and methods of the traditional mental health system to those of the recently developed community mental health system. The traditional status relationships and their accompanying role prescriptions were found to be deeply entrenched in the subculture and social system of the hospital, while the tenets of community mental health call for a radical alteration in the social organization of traditional mental health services. Indeed, the mental health center under study, even as it functioned with psychiatrists as team leaders for the first 11 months of operation, constituted a significant departure from the philosophies and practices of its companion division, the receiving hospital. In light of this, it is perhaps not surprising that many mental health center case managers reacted ambivalently if not adversely to the complete removal of staff psychiatrists from individual treatment teams. These team members had already been struggling through 11 months of rigorous desocialization and resocialization which was sufficiently incomplete that some felt the removal of psychiatrists from the teams represented, if not "the straw that broke the camel's back," at best a move "from the frying pan into the fire."

The lesson in all this, according to some students of social organization, is to provide a greater number of less radically different steps or stages in the change process, plus a longer period of time to evolve through these stages to the final organizational system desired. Certainly behavioral scientists have long been aware of the significance of the passage of time and incremental modifications in adjustment to change.

But other students of the problem would object and suggest that gradual evolutionary change encourages the survival of residual characteristics. From this perspective, programmed change should be sudden and complete, perhaps even removing the need for desocialization and resocialization by employing an entirely new set of system participants unindoctrinated in the ways and means of the traditional system.

Whatever one's attitudes towards the dilemmas of organizational change, one thing is clear: the community mental health system is pressuring its participants to think and act in a manner to which they are unaccustomed and for which they are often unprepared. Perhaps all radically new programs pose this problem. In any event, as presently formulated, the ideology of the community mental health system contends that all manner of paramedical and nonmedical personnel—from clinical psychologists to psychiatric aides—are authorized to function as "case managers." The role of case manager is defined to include not only an equal voice in team decision-making relative to diagnosis, treatment, and disposition, but, more importantly, competence in the performance of all but the most organically-based therapies (e.g., electroshock treatment). Indeed, the community mental health system maintains that, although each team member is to function as the "team expert" in his respective field of specialization (be it medical, paramedical, or nonmedical), every team member is in fact basically capable of acting as a therapist, and is in fact assigned this responsibility, in execution of the most preferred treatment modalities—psychotherapy, group therapy, milieu therapy, and other psychodynamic and environmental techniques. This approach constitutes a radical alteration for all system participants, and the strains to be expected were evident in the institution under study as the status of psychiatric aides was raised from custodians to therapists and that of psychiatrists lowered from chiefs to consultants.

If this approach, as embodied in community mental health, is to survive as a viable system in the management of the mentally ill, it seems essential that action be immediately taken on two fronts:

(1) Clinical psychologists, psychiatric social workers, registered nurses, and other paramedical and nonmedical personnel sanctioned as case managers in the community mental health system must be more adequately trained to accept, assume, and appropriately manage more complete responsibility for patient diagnosis and treatment. As matters now stand, the insecurity of these personnel about their own professional abilities to function adequately without psychiatric guidance seriously undermines the community mental health system. There were indications in the present study that the self-fulfilling prophecy of ineptness was beginning to take its toll in the actual therapeutic effectiveness of paramedical and nonmedical personnel; a self-fulfilling prophecy of confidence in case managers could promote therapeutic competency. Furthermore, it seems advisable that such training begin prior to actual employment as case managers so that inservice or on the job training become reinforcements rather than baptisms by fire.

(2) This task will likely be dwarfed by the magnitude of effort community mental health will need to alter the role of the medical professional in the mental health field. Psychiatrists are not unlike the rest of us in disvaluing status demotion; indeed, the best evidence is that they resist such loss of position and power more vociferously and effectively than most other social groups. The fact remains, however, that community mental health rejects the therapeutic omnipotence of psychiatrists, and the implications for power redistribution are clear. Most importantly, if, as community mental health seems to imply, the rights and responsibilities of practitioners in the disciplines of psychiatry, clinical psychology, and perhaps even psychiatric social work are going to be redefined so that present boundaries are torn down and power is more widely diffused— both among these disciplines and between them and other paramedical and nonmedical fields—legislative reforms relative to patient responsibility seem imperative. The vesting of legal responsibility solely in the psychiatric profession is hardly in accord with community mental health's broad definition of therapeutically competent case managers; indeed, this policy functions to undermine the basic ideologies and operations of community mental health.

The power of the psychiatrist, moreover, is not just legal; it is social-psychological as well. The "mystique of medicine" is strong in American society.

205

Some would suggest that as the scientific pursuit of health has become the "new religion" in our society, the physician has become the new apostolic delegate— "the healer." Those distraught over the fear that "God is dead" can reassure themselves that the psychiatrist is very much alive. Furthermore, medicine is assumed to be, by definition, both humanitarian and scientific. The physician, dedicated to the health of his patient and pursuing this goal by the application of concrete empirical knowledge, is therefore considered a highly qualified authority with impressive expertise. Moreover, the medical profession has built a firm foundation of faith in medical practice and research in effecting cures. The definition of mental health problems as medical entitles these forms of deviance to a share of the faith in the progress of medical science. Designation of mental illness as a disease—and therefore primarily in the province of the medical professions—casts it in the framework of being treatable and perhaps curable.

In light of all this, the community mental health system would seem well advised to launch a program of public education in the new ideology of community mental health. In the present investigation, the case manager concept was often challenged by the medically oriented attitudes of the patients and their families. The researcher often observed patients subverting the mental health center approach by attempting to sidestep their assigned case managers and demanding to "see the doctor." Case managers were acutely aware of their subordinate role definitions among the patient population. And as far as patients' families were concerned, the Superintendent of the institution stated this problem succinctly:

. . . observe the behavior of relatives of patients to see to whom they go when they want some change effected in their loved one's environment. They may enlist the support of other team members, but the effort is all directed toward the psychiatrist.

All of these issues point to the need for students of the community mental health system to address the operational and ethical questions surrounding professional training and certification. To the degree community mental health employs individuals with little or no academic training in mental health work as case managers (e.g., psychiatric aides, liberal arts college graduates, etc.), what will be the role and value of formal academic training and professional certification in the mental health field?

SUMMARY

This report described and analyzed the problems arising in the wake of attempts to implement community mental health principles in a Midwest psychiatric institution. Data were collected during three and one-half months of participant observation in a dual hospital which operated both a traditional receiving hospital and a modern mental health center. Though the two divisions were found to differ markedly in their definition and management of the mentally ill, administrative efforts to fully implement in practice the philosophies of community mental health were met with ambivalence and dissatisfaction on the part of mental health center personnel, who revealed, in their opposition, residual characteristics of the medical model approach. A few suggestions were offered for enhancing the viability of community mental health techniques.

CHAPTER 10

Community Development as a Therapeutic Force: A Case Study with Measurements

DOROTHEA C. LEIGHTON
AND IRVING THOMAS STONE

Recent generations of sociologists have become increasingly reluctant to participate in community development programs; psychiatrists have never participated. Each discipline studies communities or individuals to learn more about human behavior and to derive theories, yet neither has been very willing to put knowledge thus gathered to a practical test in the hurly burly of the "real" world. There is little interest or feeling of responsibility in either discipline for combining respective areas of expertise in a way that would be useful for planning social change or for the amelioration of change that is clearly upsetting to the groups most involved. These are seen as jobs for "planners" or the government. Sociologists claim ignorance in detecting clinical evidence of human damage concomitant with intolerable social conditions. It is likewise common for psychiatrists to be sadly lacking in adequate acquaintance with principles of social organization. While there is now in evidence a slight tendency for some cross-disciplinary activity, the approach by both sides is still very tentative.

The senior author of this paper had the good fortune to interrupt a psychiatric residency for a year spent (with her husband) trying to find out what the anthropological way of investigating humanity had to offer to psychiatry. Living with Navajos for a winter, we frequently drove past the town dump and noted a small group of Navajo families encamped there. Conversations with other Navajos indicated that this group of tribesmen were regarded as useless, lazy, corrupt, and altogether despicable. Intimate association with non-dump Navajos and comparison of them with the dump group highlighted the fact that poverty was not the differentiating factor; almost all Navajos were extremely poor by white standards. My subsequent encounters with Eskimos, Japanese in a World War II relocation center, Zuni and Hopi Indians, plus previous intimate knowledge of various subgroups within Western culture, started cerebrations and resonances. These eventually developed into an effort to try to pin down what aspects of the social experience effect, for better or worse, human adaptation as reflected in the presence or absence of psychiatric symptoms. This in turn led to conceptualizing and operationalizing the Stirling County Study which began tentatively in 1948 (with the help of many others) and which, in a limited way, still continues.[2,3]

The Frame of Reference

This chapter describes the research and the philosophy of the Stirling County Study of psychiatric disorder and sociocultural environment, in which both authors participated. The study grew out of Adolf Meyer's psychobiology,[29] with additions from physiology, psychology, anthropology, sociology, statistics, history, and so on. The frame of reference for the study, as set forth by A. H. Leighton,[11] can be outlined very briefly:

Man exists in a state of continually striving to satisfy basic physical, psychological, and social needs. The needs, expressed abstractly, can be listed as:

I. Biological
   a. Physical security (food, shelter, health)
   b. Sexual satisfaction
II. Psychological
   a. Opportunity to express hostility (without reprisal)
   b. Opportunity to express love
   c. Opportunity to secure love
   d. Opportunity to secure recognition
   e. Opportunity to express spontaneity, creativity, volition, etc.
III. Social
   a. Orientation in terms of one's own place and the places of others in society
   b. Securing and maintaining membership in a definite human group
   c. Sense of belonging to a moral order (a system of values) and of being right in what one does

Interference with achievement of these needs, either from within or from outside the person, may produce a number of results, *one* of which is the possibility of developing symptoms that reflect the person's frustration, dissatisfaction, or actual suffering. The particular result of a given interference to need achievement is strongly influenced by the person's sentiment system, derived from his culture and quite similar to what other writers speak of as a "value system."

The Stirling County Study

On the basis of this frame of reference, the Stirling County study was designed as an investigation of the epidemiology of psychiatric disorder in a general population. Its basic hypothesis was that in a social setting where achievement of need satisfaction is most faulty, one will find the most psychiatric symptoms. An elaboration and specification of this hypothesis was that there would be many people with symptoms of psychiatric disorder living in local settlements characterized by "social disintegration."[11, 8] Such localities are deficient in social and cultural patterns that provide for the achievement of significant needs. It was expected, conversely, that there would be fewer persons with such symptoms in communities which could be characterized as relatively well integrated by these same indicators.

"Stirling County," located in a Canadian Maritime Province, was selected in 1950 as the study site. One of the first steps taken was to designate five rural "focus areas" in the county for intensive studies of both sociocultural patterns and the prevalence of psychiatric disorder. Two of these were relatively affluent, well integrated communities, and three were examples of the most economically depressed, socially disintegrated settlements to be found in the county. In addition to detailed studies of the focus areas, a survey of remaining sections of the county was also conducted to provide estimates of the overall prevalence of psychiatric symptoms and of selected sociocultural patterns.

A great effort was made to keep the study of the social setting separate from the determination of which people had psychiatric symptoms. Although in the end a single structured interview (supplemented in various ways[17]) provided material for both sides of the investigation, the major attempt to avoid contamination and prevent circularity took the form of carefully abstracting and editing the parts of the schedule to be evaluated by psychiatrists. Consequently, psychiatric evaluations were blind insofar as any identification of person or sociocultural setting was concerned, including clues to socioeconomic status, ethnicity, religiosity, etc.

The definition of "psychiatric" symptoms was taken from the first version of the *Diagnostic and Statistical Manual, Mental Disorders* (American Psychiatric Association, 1952). Since most people assume psychiatric symptoms to mean "mental illness" or at least "something serious," the quotation marks indicate that these were, in many of the individuals studied, mild and only slightly (if at all) impairing. The researchers' interest lay in identifying even slight reflections of inadequate need achievement so as to study associations between conditions of living and personal reactions as delicately as possible. It seemed desirable to count all such symptoms in each subject rather than to limit the estimate to some clinical level of "illness" or "seriousness" or to a single descriptive "diagnosis." We hoped to relate particular kinds of symptoms to particular kinds of sociocultural situations (like peptic ulcers in London bus drivers), and it was decided that the chance for this should be preserved.

As has been reported in considerable detail,[17] the basic hypothesis was confirmed. Communities at opposite ends of the integration-disintegration continuum stood in strong contrast with regard to the amount and intensity of psychiatric disorder which could be identified in individual residents.

The Focus

In this chapter we confine ourselves to discussing certain aspects of the unorganized and socioeconomically depressed communities in which we could find very few people who could be considered free of any signs of psychiatric disorder. It is worth noting that there was no evidence of a high number of psychotics in these communities. Rather, there were increased numbers of symptoms of other psychiatric categories, and these were commonly associated with a significant degree of impairment of functioning. This point is made because of the widely held opinion that poor people have psychosis (especially schizophrenia) while rich people have neurosis, a conclusion derived from studies of *treated* populations where such a relationship has been clearly demonstrated.[7] In the depressed communities studied in Stirling County, individuals had numbers of psychophysiologic and psychoneurotic symptoms, sociopathic behavior, personality disorder, and the usual small percentages of brain syndrome, mental retardation, and psychosis. It seemed to be a circular relationship where unfavorable, unsatisfactory living circumstances led to symptom development, which in turn increased the difficulty of doing anything to improve the living circumstances.

Once it was demonstrated that there was a strong relationship between unfavorable social and economic conditions and a relatively high prevalence of psychiatric symptoms, it was a natural intellectual progression to wonder if the symptoms could be diminished by intentionally improving the living conditions. The latter, of course, has been the avowed aim of many community development programs, but rarely have such programs held specific expectations of mental health consequences. Improvement of living conditions has usually been seen as a sufficient good in itself. However, with the study's commitment to the interrelationship of life circumstances and psychiatric symptoms, it seemed imperative to further test the hypothesis by seeing if changes in the mental health level might be achieved by stimulating social, educational, and economic changes of a sort that could be expected to enhance individuals' skills, interpersonal competence, and possibilities for choices.

Recent history has seen the rise of community organization and action programs in many parts of the United States and other countries, where much effort has been invested in helping the local people to identify their problems, set their priorities, and then learn how to go about improving their living circumstances. Some of these have been quite successful in ways comparable to the events to be described below which took place in the Stirling County community. To the best of our knowledge, however, no attempt has been made to estimate the mental health level of the people involved in other community-change programs, either before or after the effort. This is not surprising in view of the compelling socioeconomic needs of the people and the slow development of an understanding of the implications of sociocultural change for mental health. This has been further hindered by the impression that the estimation of mental health level can only be done by psychiatrists, who are in short supply and not trained for this kind of research. Alternative means of such measurement are discussed later in this chapter.

We first describe the series of events which took place in one of the three depressed communities studied which transformed the settlement from a depressed to an ordinary community in the space of only a few years. Whereas in 1952, at the time of the first survey, this community had all the unfavorable characteristics of a slum (wherever it is found), ten years later most of its characteristics, including its mental health rating, had become indistinguishable from those of average communities in the county. There follows, then an account of "The Road," one of the depressed focus communities, where certain intentional inputs were supplemented by spontaneous and chance events to produce significant social and economic change and a concomitant rise in the level of community mental health.

A CASE STUDY

At the beginning of the 1950s, The Road incorporated a population of 118 persons, occupying 29 households scattered along a two mile dirt road that extended from the coast to the sparsely populated interior of the county. It stood out clearly among neighboring settlements as a rural slum: a string of ramshackle, crudely patched, tar-papered and unkempt homes, situated on scrubby and rocky land which was largely untended and grown up in undersized trees among a general cover of weeds and bushes. The Road had first been settled in the 1850s, but never in its history had it constituted a highly developed, exclusive, and self-sufficient community like many in the region. From the beginning, its social life was very much a product of the character of its relations with surrounding populations.

The first settlers were families of French background, who had migrated to a predominantly English area of the county, attracted by employment in shipyards at the coast and the opportunity for hauling timber from woodlots further inland. Not being concerned with farming, these early migrants settled on poor, cheap land strategically located for both employment on the shore and the profitable timber trade.

In time, ties between the inhabitants of The Road and their natal French communities weakened. Intermarriage with surrounding English populations began to take place, the French language began to drop out of use, and significant economic bonds to the English Protestants of the area increased. Efforts by local Protestants to establish a Baptist mission on The Road proved generally ill-fated, but some converts were won and some weakening of commitment to the Catholic faith occurred. The failure of missionization, however, coupled with the incomplete assimilation of English cultural characteristics, served to perpetuate cool feelings on the part of the English in the local area toward the French. Prior

213

to the turn of the century, The Road nevertheless remained economically viable, enjoying the fruits of a booming shipbuilding industry at the coast and an active lumber trade between the coast and the interior.

At the beginning of the present century, the shipbuilding industry collapsed, and with it, the trade in lumber. This resulted in the precipitous loss of the economic resources upon which people on The Road had depended. Although the change in the economic situation also wrought hardship upon surrounding English populations, their greater education, fluency in English, social connections, and capital resources facilitated their adaptation to the economic crisis. The Road, on the other hand, had few resources to fall back upon: its inhabitants formed a small population, situated on poor land, with little capital or education, isolated from their French homeland, and socially peripheral to the neighboring English. In difficult circumstances themselves, the neighboring English were ill disposed toward supporting the people of The Road economically or otherwise, and the social boundaries between the two groups became firmer.

In the years that followed, as surrounding communities managed to recover their economic position in some measure, the people of The Road were forced to resort to arduous, low paying forms of labor which did not afford the margin of surplus that might have permitted them to break out of their economic straits. The settlement thus gradually acquired the appearance of a rural slum, with a distinctive economic position and life style which set it clearly apart from its milieu and rendered its inhabitants easy targets for disparagement as an inferior breed. With no traditional image of themselves as constituents of a cohesive and prideworthy community, the people of The Road appear to have promptly acquired the social and psychological characteristics which typified the settlement in 1950 when studies of it were begun.

Intergroup Relations

Known pejoratively throughout the county as "monkeys," Road inhabitants were found in 1950 to share a widespread reputation for laziness, drunkenness, fighting, thievery, illicit sexual indulgence, and a variety of other traits deemed indicative of amorality and mental inferiority. These characteristics were attributed, in the popular stereotype, to excessive inbreeding. Repeatedly, "Monkeytown" was singled out by informants elsewhere in Stirling as "the worst place in the county."

For their part, people on The Road did not hold a benign opinion of outsiders. While it was widely recognized that respect should be shown to the faces of people from neighboring communities, particularly those in some position of authority, it was felt that outsiders were not to be trusted, and they were conventionally regarded as hypocritical, hostile, and exploitative in their dealings with people from the settlement. Social contact with outsiders was thus avoided when possible, crude but subtle jokes at their expense were a source of much amusement, and accusations and stories concerning the outsiders' immoral activities were common conversational topics among Road residents.

However, this did not generate ingroup solidarity. Even more striking than the negative stereotype of The Road held by outsiders was the frequency and intensity with which its inhabitants themselves expressed negative conceptions of one another. A fieldworker's first contact within the settlement often stimulated remarks about The Road which matched the most extreme disparagement voiced by outsiders. Chronic animosities supported by disparaging stereotypes divided the residents along kin group lines, and even normally friendly or benign relations between close kinsmen and others were often breached by public accusations. Hostilities of this temporary sort tended to erupt with only minor provocation, coming to public view in a fight or, more commonly, in the form of character assassination on one side and response in kind. These conflicts were coupled with accusations of "putting on airs." Taken altogether, these patterns left few individuals safe from being targets of publicly expressed hostile feelings and public avowals of their untrustworthiness.

These sentiments found concrete expression in the limited and transient character of the voluntary, leisure time, social contacts among inhabitants of the settlement.[1] Such contacts were limited to occasional visits between close kinsmen for the women and to gatherings of men at a nearby dance hall, filling station, or the home of one of the local bachelors, where there would be drinking, swapping stories, and often, fighting. Aside from these activities and from contacts with one another in the course of work, a pattern of guarded, mutual social isolation was the normal state of interpersonal relations. The pattern here stood in sharp contrast to the relations sustained through a variety of regularly organized community activities among members of most other communities in the county.

Residents of the settlement thus shared an identification by outsiders as being fundamentally amoral and untrustworthy, which they reciprocated with sentiments in kind. These stereotypes appeared to guide behavior in interactions between The Road and surrounding communities. Within the settlement, even if individuals denied that such stereotypes applied to themselves, there was little support for their viewing one another as more trustworthy or deserving of social commitments than the stereotype would justify. The frequent and pervasive allegations to the contrary and the readiness to disparage one another served to continually reinforce a conception of their relations as normally mistrustful and hostile and to further the adoption of this concept as the basis of all their social dealings.

The economic position of the people of The Road in the early 1950s afforded a material standard of living far below the norm for the county as a whole. Occupationally, 74 per cent of the household heads either relied on work of the lowest category on the scale of occupational advantage-disadvantage constructed for the county or were drawing only unearned incomes. No household derived income from farms or woodlots of its own nor from fishing on its own account, both of which were typical occupations in most other rural parts of the county.

The bulk of The Road's wage earners made their living by contracting for farm labor in neighboring settlements, by hiring-on temporarily to cut timber with woodlot owners in the vicinity, or by digging clams. In any given year, a man typically engaged in some combination of these activities, since none by itself could provide a steady income. Most men supplemented these earnings by occasional day labor at various odd jobs in surrounding communities.

Farming served as a source of day labor only during the summer months. Lumbering, on the other hand, while less seasonal was nevertheless an irregular form of employment, being only occasional and for relatively short periods. The men who worked in the woods did so as employees of local lumbermen or farmers who needed extra hands for cutting wood on their own lots. The nearest clam flats, located at a distance of some 25 miles from The Road, were the scene of the most widely practiced single form of subsistence activity. Diggers were paid by the barrel by companies located in Bristol, the county seat, and clamming offered a year-round opportunity for income. Given the distance to the clamming grounds, however, daily travel back and forth to the flats was impossible. Accordingly, men from The Road established camp on the flats in crude brush or tarpaulin shelters for a week or two at a time, returning home to seek other types of work between trips. These extended sojourns and the high level of activity in clamming were characteristic of only the summer months. In the winter, the freezing rain, ice, and snow precluded camping for any extended period, and clamming was generally undertaken only as a last resort.

All these occupations represented the bottom of the county hierarchy of occupational status, and the resulting negative evaluation of their occupational roles was fully recognized by people on The Road. To outsiders, their position simply indicated their inferiority and genetic incompetence; on The Road, the low occupational position was ascribed to the exploitation and hostility of outsiders.

Social Organization

It is clear, however, that the economic history of The Road as outlined above was primarily responsible for the plight of its inhabitants. The settlement had never had the resources—the woodlots, farmland, or other capital—to produce anything of economic value locally. The one commodity it had ever offered on the local market was labor, and in this respect alone it differed from most other settlements in the county. Secondly, from the time of the decline in shipbuilding and the lumber trade, The Road had no marketable skills and no monopoly upon the type of marketable labor it was able to supply. The educational and skill level of its workers could be matched or surpassed almost anywhere in the county. The labor force was clearly unsuited to either professional roles or to other economically rewarding and respectable forms of employment. Among the opportu-

216

nities for unskilled work available, the types which could absorb the greatest numbers were those which brought the least compensation, both in status and in the amount and steadiness of income.

In 1952, nearly 80 per cent of the adults on The Road continued to identify themselves as Catholic in the French tradition, with the remainder indicating Baptist affiliation. These religious affiliations were almost entirely nominal, however. There was no local church, and people who attended services at all did so in neighboring communities. Residents attended church two or three times at most in the course of a year. Participation in church sponsored activities of a more secular nature was equally rare and peripheral. This contrasted markedly with church-related activity in a Catholic community in the French section of the county, also studied as a focus area in 1952. In the latter community, 90 per cent of the population reported attending all or most services of the church in the course of a year.[8] On a scale of public religious participation constructed for the county as a whole, The Road registered very low compared to county norms. But this low level was not reflected in private religious alienation. On the contrary, a scale of private religious participation (including such items as the personal importance of religion, prayers, grace at meals) showed The Road to be substantially closer to county norms than in the public sphere. Thus, a striking discrepancy between the levels of religious involvement was registered by the settlement on these two measures.

The typical rationale expressed for the minimal participation in public religious activities was, first, that the clergy took little interest in them and generally harbored unfriendly attitudes toward them. Secondly, Road residents felt self-conscious and uncomfortable in associating with outsiders who looked down upon them. Although persons from The Road were permitted to join in the activities of churches outside the settlement, they felt that they were accorded inferior status, and that their presence was tolerated only with obvious distaste and condescension. No alternative was afforded through indigenously organized religious activities, with the result that they completely lacked one of the institutions which served as a major focus for social activities in other communities in the county.

A small one-room school at the inland end of The Road served most families in the settlement and a few other scattered homes. Up to eight grades of formal schooling were offered here. In order to go beyond this level, a youngster would be required to board in Bristol, a financial impossibility for virtually every family.

For years, The Road school had been poorly staffed. In all but one of the ten years prior to the study, it had had no fully qualified teacher, with the post consequently occupied by a succession of individuals who had been granted temporary "permissive" teaching licenses. Understandably, there was a widespread opinion that there was little use in sending children to the school. In particular, some were encouraged to drop out and work for the family by finding odd jobs or going clamming, because the teachers "didn't know anything anyway."

Resentment was also expressed toward paying tax money to support teachers who were "no damn good."

There was no formal parents' organization associated with The Road school, while such organizations flourished in other districts in the immediate area. Furthermore, no one from The Road held a position on the locally elected Board of Trustees responsible for the management of school affairs. Little attention was paid to Board elections in the settlement, and the long standing incumbencies of the outside Board members were never challenged. Similarly, Road adults virtually never made contact with the teacher or trustees concerning such matters as the progress of children in school, the maintenance of school facilities, or the quality and selection of teachers. The local school represented the one formal institution which The Road might have claimed as its own and which afforded a potential focus for community activity. In spite of this, collective involvement related to school matters remained negligible.

Seeds of Change

An immediate outgrowth of the first study of The Road was a program for improvement drawn up by the researcher who had conducted the initial fieldwork there, Allister M. Macmillan. Macmillan succeeded in interesting school authorities to give special attention to the settlement, with the result that a man responsible for adult education in the area was encouraged to attempt an experimental program. This educator defined his objective as that of improving the skills of The Road people so as to make them more employable, and he planned to accomplish this long range goal by establishing regular adult education classes at the settlement's school. His initial tactic, however, was to attract adults to regular evening gatherings at the school by showing free movies. With the collaboration of the schoolteacher, he began by showing movies during school hours to the children, then sending them home with the news that there would be movies again in the evening for anyone who wished to attend. Attendance at the first showings was reasonably good, and the first attempt toward community organization was the suggestion by the educator that The Road people elect a committee to select subsequent programs from the list of available films. He also gradually encouraged the showing of films with educational content, and began suggesting the possibility of adult classes in the school.

Since there was no electricity in the school, the first showings required that the educator bring along a portable generator. He pointed out at a suitable time that the school ought to be electrified if the evening programs were to be carried on properly and, further, that the Department of Education was prepared to meet half the cost if the rest were raised in the neighborhood. This suggestion was made partly because of the immediate practicalities, but was also influenced by his recognition that local organization and involvement in support of the project was a necessary preliminary to success in any more ambitious program. The risk was, of course, that the wiring project might fail from lack of interest. Fortunately, it proved a success: enough money was raised to finance half the wiring and to pay the electrical bill for the succeeding year—the first voluntary contribution of Road residents to any public cause.

At this juncture, however, the project came to an abrupt halt because the adult-educator was transferred to a different district. Such a collapse was thoroughly in keeping with The Road's attitudes of suspicion, apathy, and disparagement, and completely matched the predictions of the project's opponents on The Road. Recovery seemed unlikely and the prospects for any further activities of this kind looked bleak.

In the meantime, however, county school officials had managed to secure the services of a fully qualified and interested teacher, and she continued as a catalyst for activity and involvement where the adult-educator had left off. She maintained frequent contacts with the women and encouraged them to seek improved educational conditions.* Evening bingo games were organized at the school as a means of raising money to purchase new desks, with prizes provided by the women. However, one of the teacher's most important moves was to stir up (at the suggestion of school authorities) the question of having the local school admitted to the consolidated school district of the region. Such admission meant transportation to Bristol by daily bus for all children above the sixth grade. There, educational opportunities were considerably richer and the way would be clear for going on through high school. It also meant increased taxes for the school district of which The Road was a part.

In spite of opposition on and near The Road stemming from the necessity for increased taxes, the women in favor of the move, urged on by the teacher, campaigned in its behalf through the whole school district with success. Supporters in sufficient numbers were brought out to a meeting of the district rate-payers to vote the measure through. Among those in opposition were the school Trustees, who resigned as a result of the vote. For the first time in history they were replaced by three men elected from The Road. Thus, a partial end to social isolation was achieved, along with a need for citizen participation.

Another development of major importance, beginning around 1950, was the establishment of a work circuit that linked the settlement to a major city in Ontario. Before this time, many individuals had left The Road to seek their fortune in large cities. Their lack of interpersonal skills and of previous close contact with people different from themselves, however, induced an overwhelming loneliness which soon drove them home, empty handed. Thus, the work circuit's survival might be taken as evidence of some sort of renaissance. It is impossible to trace back contributory forces to ascertain whether the early steps in community organization had played any part. Possibly the original investigation by Macmillan had begun a subtle change in self-perception—if that

---

*Although the teacher's work with women was doubtless partly motivated by her feeling at home with them, it has usually been found in depressed, disintegrated communities that the women can be motivated to move sooner and more easily than the men.

college man would spend time to come and talk to Road inhabitants again and again, perhaps they weren't really so no-account as they had thought. It seems quite clear that the women would never have had the courage to tackle the larger community on the school issue without the practice afforded by the movie program and the bingo games.

The work circuit's initiation had taken place when a family originally from The Road, who had settled in Ontario, wrote home inviting some of their relatives to join them for a time to take advantage of the comparatively lucrative employment opportunities in the city. By 1952, four people had responded and were living close to one another in the city, engaged in the same type of unskilled industrial work. With this start, a pattern developed whereby people from The Road would go to work in Ontario for six months or a year and then return home. The arrangement was such that before leaving The Road they had assurance from those in the city that jobs would be available and that they would be moving in among people whom they knew. They apparently made a good impression as workers, for when they left the city their employers were glad to accept a friend or a relative as a replacement. The returnees to The Road expended their accumulated savings on paint, furniture, house construction, cars, and investment in a variety of new economic enterprises.

It has often been a cause for astonishment to those unfamiliar with the Maritime Provinces that successful emigrants from such a community would have any wish to return. An extremely common pattern, however, is for young adults of all stations in this society to go away to the States or to upper Canada to accumulate enough money so that they can afford to "retire" to the old homestead. This may take many years, during which taxes are scrupulously paid and occasional visits made to mend the roof or to ready the home for later occupancy. No doubt the Road people were familiar with this pattern even though it had not worked well for them previously. The pattern is probably more widespread than the Maritimes—common, very likely, in many rural areas. In the States, the pressure is great to move permanently to the city, but it seems there could be many emotional gains in maintaining a foothold somewhere while undertaking new, perhaps dangerous, ventures.

In 1957 the movement reached a peak with 21 people from The Road (about 18 per cent of the total population) at the Ontario location. By 1962 some individuals had made the circuit four or five times. Both men and women and married couples as well as single people made the trip. Some newly married couples chose this adventure as a means of acquiring a sum of money to start a new home. It is clear that the circuit served as an economic pump, not only temporarily raising the income level of migrants, but resulting in significant improvement in material living conditions and capital on The Road itself. Factors important in its success seem to have been the receiving friends at the Ontario end, the arranged job, and a prepared place to live. Anxieties about being stranded among strangers in a strange place were thus reduced, while confidence in finding an acceptable job and getting fair treatment from employers was established. Far from home, the migrants had escaped the curse of their local reputation as unreliable workers.

People on The Road (and others in the vicinity who know the neighborhood well) claimed that the old habits of speech, dress, and deportment that had characterized those who made the circuit had dropped away by the time they returned. The migrants arrived back home with a confidence in their ability to do more respected forms of work and a marked unwillingness to take part in the traditional, low-status occupations of the neighborhood. They also displayed confidence in their ability to deal with outsiders on an equal footing and a desire for living down the neighborhood's unsavory reputation. It is worth noting that the same kind of change took place in the children who began to attend the consolidated school.

Coincident witn these developments, a public works project in the county, employing between 300 and 400 men over a three year period, had afforded a new (albeit temporary) source of employment for unskilled laborers at wages substantially higher than they could otherwise secure. The Road, of course, provided a ready supply of labor recruits for the project, and those employed mostly conformed to the pattern which had been established with the work circuit to Ontario: new earnings were invested in various home improvements and applied to the development of new economic enterprises of their own.

The Consequences of Social Change

By 1962, when a re-study of the focus areas of the county was undertaken, changes on The Road were evident to even the most casual observer. The population of the settlement had remained largely stable: only 11 per cent of the 1962 adult population had arrived as immigrants since 1952, virtually all of these in-marrying women. The most striking change was in the appearance of the area. Freshly painted and newly constructed or refurbished homes, surrounded by cultivated shrubbery and well tended lawns largely indistinguishable from those in neighboring, more affluent communities, had replaced the tar-paper shacks and dilapidated larger dwellings of a decade before.

Economic measures of the material standard of living of Road families also showed a marked improvement, a change not even remotely approached by the other depressed settlements in the county in the same period. Furthermore, the new economic roles and resources now evident were very similar to what could be found elsewhere in the county. For example, clamming was no longer practiced. Only one man still worked as a farm laborer, but he did so year-round on an annual salary rather than in the earlier pattern of occasional day labor. For those relatively few men who continued to rely on wage work in lumbering, the work had become steady during the season, was for major contractors, and was sufficient to enable workers to draw unemployment compensation during the slack months. Only 36 per cent of the families on The Road in 1962 gained their subsistence from traditionally low-status occupations or were dependent upon unearned income, as compared to the figure of 74 per cent a decade earlier.

Capital accumulated during the decade had led to several new economic ventures and cooperative patterns. Several men, for example, had jointly invested in the operation of a fish weir; another had acquired a lobster boat; a dairy farm and mink ranch had been established and were being operated by a group of closely related families; two men had acquired tractors and other equipment and had gone into business with their sons, hauling lumber in the winter and hiring out their services to local farmers during planting season; woodlots had been purchased and were being cut by men from several families in the settlement. Other new forms of employment included fulltime jobs at fish processing firms in the county and a variety of occupations ranging from electrical repair and maintenance work at a local resort to clerking in the department stores in Bristol.

Aside from these changes, participation in the activities of churches increased during the decade, particularly among the women. Church services were now regularly attended by almost half the women on The Road. Sisters from the nearby Catholic church were making frequent visits in a generally successful effort to encourage Sunday school attendance on the part of the children. They were also holding regular catechism classes at a home in the settlement. Church suppers and church sponsored bingo games had become a regular activity for many Road couples.

Consolidation of the primary schools in the area had taken place in 1961, when The Road had been combined with six small neighboring districts to form a single larger district. The consolidation, however, had not lessened interest and involvement of Road people in local school affairs. Women in the settlement had played an important role in the formation of the new Home and School Association which served all the communities included in the new district, and they represented The Road at its meetings.

Queried about The Road in 1962, people elsewhere in the county were likely to immediately remark on the changes they had noticed, especially their undisguised surprise at its "new look."[27] The familiar stereotypes attributing genetic inferiority and amorality to the inhabitants were no longer voiced. On a workaday level, the change in the self and public image of The Road was clearly evidenced by the greatly improved acceptance of its people by outsiders in various institutional contexts. The decade had also marked a changed outlook on The Road toward residents of neighboring communities, who were no longer warily viewed as hypocritical, hostile, and exploitative. Gone, too, were the allegations and public displays of antipathy that had previously divided both kin groups and individuals from one another. The current image of the settlement and of those within it now accentuated the positive character of intracommunity relations.

These changes were reflected in new forms of leisure-time associations. Many couples gathered regularly for card games, usually on a weekly basis, with nearly half the households in the settlement represented in such activity. The several groups meeting together for entertainment consistently included a cross section of the settlement's major kin groups. On a larger scale, although less often, "rappie pie" parties were being hosted on a rotating basis by a number of families, and attendance at these affairs also drew a substantial proportion of the population.

Perhaps the most notable development was the inauguration of the first genuine community celebrations that the settlement had witnessed in many years. Any birth or wedding had become the occasion for a "shower," held at the home of a close friend or relative of one of the principals, to which every family in the settlement was extended a formal invitation. These gatherings were not only frequent and large, but were festive affairs with both men and women in attendance. Everyone taking part donned their best attire for the event which, in addition to the usual presentation of gifts to the guests of honor, provided the occasion for a night of community singing, dancing, and card games.

Taking into account all the changes evident in 1962, developments during the decade of the '50s had clearly served to foster increased access to conventionally recognized relationships of trust and solidarity for Road inhabitants. The same factors had promoted participation in social activities where individuals were accorded a status which provided some measure of self and public respect. This signaled not only a significant transformation of social relationships among inhabitants of the settlement themselves, but an equally striking alteration of the previous state of their relations with other residents of the county.

Better Mental Health

As was noted earlier, the mental health rating of The Road population in 1952 was substantially poorer than that of the county as a whole, the latter figure being based on a survey of a sample of residents throughout the county at large in addition to data from the five focus communities. The other two depressed focus areas were also worse than the county norm, but The Road had received the poorest mental health rating of all five focus areas.[17]

In the 1962 re-survey (carried out according to previous Stirling County techniques[17]), psychiatric as well as sociocultural data were again collected from all five focus areas to determine what changes, if any, had occurred in their mental health level during the decade. Analysis of the psychiatric data from The Road revealed a significant change in a positive direction so that its mental health rating had shifted to a position virtually equivalent to the mean for the county as a whole.[14]

The re-survey also indicated that no social changes comparable to those which had taken place on The Road had occurred in the remaining two depressed settlements. Some less dramatic improvements in one of these could be noted in the

223

way of lessened inter- and intracommunity social isolation and hostility[27] and better material style of life. In neither of these settlements was there such a positive change in mental health as was found on The Road, although some improvement was registered in the one that had also experienced some social improvement.

Finally, one of the two well integrated communities that had registered a high level of mental health in 1952 showed decline in its mental health rating in 1962, even sharper than the rise on The Road. The decline in its mental health paralleled evident social change in a direction opposite to that observed on The Road, namely, a marked decrease in the level of intracommunity solidarity and organization.[14]

These findings clearly suggest the potential significance of community development programs for improving mental health in psychiatrically impaired, economically and socially depressed local groups. Individuals depend upon the support of others for carrying out the activities and winning the recognition necessary to satisfy the needs, values, and goals upon which their psychological well-being and mental health depend. Their capacity to secure such support can suffer significant impairment where prevailing social patterns deny some persons access to interpersonal bonds of solidarity and trust or when access is denied to collectively organized and performed activities which would provide roles accorded social value and respect. Insofar as programs for community development include successful efforts to alter such social consequences of membership in a socioeconomically depressed local group, benefits in the form of improved mental health for the population are likely to result.

FURTHER RESEARCH

Beginning in 1964 and presently nearing completion, a program and a series of studies in a second of Stirling's three depressed settlements has been under way, designed both as an experiment to evaluate means for intentionally stimulating change of the types which took place on The Road, and as a further test of the effects of such change on mental health.[10] One of the major aims of this research has been to experiment with techniques for achieving change that can be implemented by local people willing to organize and devote time and effort to such an undertaking.

Kern[10] says, "The specific goals of the action program were to foster cooperation, to build a positive self and community image, to promote community power, and to increase ability to plan on a long term basis." To this end, three main activities were undertaken. The first was to make several movies of successful events in the community with much citizen participation. These were shown not only to residents, but also to outside opinion leaders, especially in Bristol, which sets the standard for the area. A second effort was to solicit the participation of two men with the investigator in a cooperative garden. In spite of doubts and bad weather, a good crop was realized, and the venture stimulated

224

a request by several men for some adult agricultural education. The third undertaking was the organization of a baseball league for men and boys that included a number of teams from other communities. This provided some of the same opportunities for dispelling stereotypes and promoting communication as have been noted in some school desegregation experiences. The report does not quote figures measuring outcome, but if the major hypothesis of the Stirling County study is supported by measurements, this experiment can provide a model or useful guidelines for similar programs elsewhere which involve members of a local citizenry as the principal agents of change.

The currently widespread efforts to encourage community development noted earlier, both in this country and elsewhere, could obviously provide opportunities for further evaluation and refinement of such a sociotherapeutic approach to the improvement of mental health. The contributions of present and future development activities will depend a great deal not only on attentiveness to the social consequences and the effectiveness of techniques in terms of socioeconomic program goals, but also on techniques for adequately assessing the consequences of various types of community development activities for mental health.

As stated in the introduction, one reason for the lack of efforts to determine the mental health consequences of development programs has doubtless been the anticipated difficulty of measuring mental health or illness. The investigators planning the Stirling County Study were plagued with this problem and tried several indirect and (it turned out) unsystematic means such as collecting hospital records, interviewing key informants, and setting up an outpatient clinic. Fortunately it also planned to include a set of psychological screening questions in the structured questionnaire interview, along with a health history. These two sections, supplemented by comments from as many local doctors as knew the subject and by a hospital record where one had been found, eventually provided the material which was carefully edited and given to psychiatrists to evaluate.

In addition to the psychiatric evaluation, which was done from a base of clinical experience by a method developed to achieve reliability between raters, the screening questions could be scored independently and compared with the psychiatrists' ratings. Comparisons of the age/sex distributions of psychiatrists' ratings with the mean score of the screening questions[17] indicated that the two ways of assessing the data give very similar results. At the same time, there is the interesting fact that psychiatrists judged people 70 years of age or over to be "healthier" than the next younger age group, while the screening test score continues to rise with age. Which view of the oldest group is "right" remains to be settled.

The method of making a rating by using psychiatrists' judgments has proved stable, reliable, and teachable,[30] and it yields a list of symptom patterns, an estimate of confidence that the person has or has not any psychiatric condition, and an estimate of how much his functioning has been impaired by such a condition. A computer program has been prepared which provides ratings that are quite as reliable as those of any pair of evaluating psychiatrists.[26,5] The questionnaire has also been shown to discriminate validly between groups of known psychiatric patients[20] and community groups.

The full scale method has, however, two principal drawbacks: it is a time consuming data gathering technique and without a computer it is a psychiatrist consuming analytic technique. Once the 1952 survey had been completed and reported, it appeared highly desirable that some briefer means of achieving an approximate mental health estimate be developed for use in less painstaking and less well financed research efforts, in order to expand understanding of the dimensions of the mental health/sociocultural environment relationships under many diverse circumstances.

A Brief Mental Health Assessment Instrument

Naturally enough, thoughts turned to the psychological screening questions for this purpose. The set that had been used in the questionnaire had been selected and standardized by Allister M. Macmillan, beginning with such sources as the Armed Forces' Neuropsychiatric Screening Adjunct and the Cornell Medical Index and encompassing eventually most of the sets of psychiatric screening questions that had been devised in the post-World War II years up to about 1950. Macmillan tried out 75 such questions in a area quite similar to Stirling County, eliminated duplicates in various sets, standardized them against a group of neurotic patients in metropolitan hospitals, and selected the most useful ones by discriminant function analysis. He also tested their reliability in re-interview, and had a psychiatrist examine a sample of his subjects.[18] All indications were that the screening questions, labeled the Health Opinion Survey (HOS),* did a reasonably competent job in distinguishing various levels of psychiatric involvement by means of a numerical score. The refinements of the psychiatrists' rating described above were not, of course, available.

When the opportunity arose in some Nigerian villages to conduct a study modelled on the Stirling County Study, the screening questions were, of course, included.[13] The necessity to translate the entire questionnaire into the Yoruba language brought to attention some aspects of the screening questions that had not been particularly noticed before. One of these was the impossibility of translating some of the questions which had been found highly discriminating in English. One of these, "Have you ever felt as if you would have a nervous breakdown?" presents obvious problems of imprecision in spite of the fact that it had been used successfully with English speakers and can be translated into Spanish without difficulty.[22] A second point was that it seemed inadvisable to add to the complications of interviewing subjects through interpreters a variation in the answer modalities. Macmillan had experimented with several answer choice patterns and answer weights, but it seemed imperative to simplify the procedure, and so standard answers ("often," "sometimes," or "never") were used. The

---

*This is the set of questions, response categories, and scoring weights utilized in Myers and Bean[21] and in Rogler and Hollingshead.[22]

need for translation also served to improve considerably the grammatical form of some of the questions.

Once the Nigerian study was completed, statistical members of the research team identified 20 questions from all those that had been used that (1) agreed best with the overall psychiatric ratings and (2) had been usable in Nigeria. The latter point resulted from the desire to have screening questions that could be used under diverse sociocultural conditions. A final improvement, made a little later, consisted in framing all questions clearly in the present tense and eliminating the word "ever" from them. This change arose from a wish to use the screening questions to measure clinical change in psychiatric patients, where a definite time referent would be required. The present tense version is as follows:

The Health Opinion Survey for Assessing Mental Health Levels

1. Do you have any physical or health problems at the present?
2. Do your hands tremble enough to bother you?
3. Are you troubled by your hands or feet sweating so that they feel damp and clammy?
4. Are you bothered by your heart beating hard?
5. Do you tend to feel tired in the morning?
6. Do you have any trouble getting to sleep or staying asleep?
7. How often are you bothered by having an upset stomach?
8. Are you bothered by nightmares (dreams that frighten or upset you)?
9. Are you troubled by "cold sweats"?
10. Do you feel that you are bothered by all sorts (different kinds) of ailments in different parts of your body?
11. Do you smoke?
12. Do you have loss of appetitie?
13. Does ill health affect the amount of work (or housework) that you do?
14. Do you feel weak all over?
15. Do you have spells of dizziness?
16. Do you tend to lose weight when you worry?
17. Are you bothered by shortness of breath when you are not exerting yourself?
18. Do you feel healthy enough to carry out the things that you would like to do?
19. Do you feel in good spirits?
20. Do you sometimes wonder if anything is worthwhile anymore?

Except for the first question, which is answered *yes* or *no,* all answers are *often, sometimes,* or *never.* Scoring is accomplished by giving three points to the "sick" answer, one to the "well" answer, and two to the *sometimes* answer. Questions 2, 3, 4, 8, 9, and 17 can be used as a subscore for anxiety, and questions 5, 13, 16, 18, 19, and 20 for depression.

These direct, inoffensive, easily understood questions are frequently regarded as a medical history, having much in common with a brief standardized history.

No systematic attempt has yet been made to test wording changes or to scatter the questions throughout a longer interview schedule. The aim of each question is to convey its meaning to the subject, and any slight modification to assist in this is justifiable. All are matters of opinion with regard to symptoms commonly associated with reactions to stress, so that it is of no significance whether the person actually has a demonstrable basis for his opinion: *the degree of his concern is the measure of his mental health status.*

The strength of the instrument lies partly in the variety of organ systems covered, including the possibility of registering overall reactions (fatigue, sleep, mood). The answer categories offer some measure of frequency/intensity and are generally better received than the yes/no or agree/disagree pattern of some other scales. It seems quite likely that this instrument, the result of largely pragmatic experimentation, may in the end prove to be firmly founded on psycho-physiological interactions involving emotional, hormonal, and neural components. For example, Dr. Richard Udry found, in studying the outcome of pregnancy in a sample of some 2000 women, that those who had a successful outcome could be differentiated from unsuccessful on the basis of whether they chose the "often" or the "never" answer to a set of the HOS questions. A medical expert felt that the differential choice of response could be clearly associated with differential hormonal factors.

Evidence from a study focused on cardiovascular disease in which the HOS was given to two random samples of a population who also answered an extensive sociological questionnaire and health history and received a searching physical exam and laboratory tests, will soon advance our knowledge of the relationship of physical symptoms and findings to HOS responses.[4]

This screening instrument has now been used in a number of other studies, some of which have been published or will be published in the near future. The populations tested include: a sample of the patients of public health nurses in North Carolina[16]; a sample of the population of three rural counties in North Carolina and Virginia[6]; a cross-section of the patient population of four state mental hospitals; an entire university freshman class; university students who had consulted the psychiatrists in the student health service[31]; a sample of Makah Indians in Washington[32]; several small Indian groups in various sub-Arctic communities; the Pine Ridge Sioux[19]; five different types of work organizations in New York state[23,24,25]; and 1280 aged respondents in a sample of New York state communities.[28] It was also used in the followup of the New Haven Study[21] and in a study of schizophrenic families in Puerto Rico.[22] A new application that seems promising is in determining stress points in a school population, in which the version given above is used for grades seven to twelve, while a modification is used for grades three to six.[15]

Analysis can be done by comparing mean scores of various subgroups or by scrutinizing the characteristics of individuals found near the ends of the scoring range or both. In addition to the screening questions, data are usually gathered on common demographic variables and on other characteristics in which the

228

investigator is interested or which he believes to have some probable influence on mental health. The score can be thought of as a symptom count, or a stress score, or a mental health level, the lower levels being "healthy" as compared to the upper levels. Experience has indicated that the 20 to 30 range is within normal limits. A sharp dividing point between "sick" and "well" does not seem appropriate in most instances. So far the instrument has only been tested for group estimations. It remains to be seen how useful it may be in work with individuals, such as in measuring clinical change.

Generally speaking, correlation of mean group scores with such variables as age, sex, race, socioeconomic status, and so on, serves to indicate which subgroups of the population studied are under some sort of excess stress. More refined examination of the high scoring groups may indicate which characteristics are most strongly related to the score elevation. *Consistency of correlation of any given characteristic (e.g., sex) with high or low score should not be expected,* since score level will depend on the intensity of stressful forces impinging on either sex at a particular point in history and in a particular cultural setting. Rather, the score level tends to point out which groups are currently in trouble and which are adapting satisfactorily in the population studied.

SUMMARY AND DISCUSSION

This chapter has set forth a rationale for anticipating that certain kinds of social changes will diminish the amount of psychiatric disorder that a community group shows; it has further detailed a case study where this, in fact, happened; it has mentioned a study (which could not be included because of space considerations) where the rationale was intentionally implemented; and it has described and discussed an instrument for measuring mental health which can be readily applied by nonpsychiatrists.

This is obviously only a drop in the seething social bucket, but it is a beginning. Investigation needs to be continued and expanded in order to fill in the outlines suggested here and to refine our understanding of the ways in which the social and behavioral sciences can supplement each other and illuminate new pathways to better human functioning. We need to combine Meyer's ideas of the psychobiological integration of each person with the intuitive insights of Freud and the methods of modern social science (not available to either of the masters) in order to forge improved ways of thinking about the maladaptations of mankind and fresh ways of solving its problems.

It is worth emphasizing that, although there was a wealth of psychopathology apparent in residents of The Road, the ten year improvement took place without the benefit of psychiatry and with comparatively little medical input of any kind beyond symptomatic relief for such conditions as were treated by the local doctors. No one can say with certainty whether an intense effort by mental health workers to find and treat cases by conventional methods would have resulted in similar improvement. At the same time, the events and interactions described fit

229

into current notions of cause and effect quite compellingly and incline one to say of the outcome, "Why, of course!" There is a great need for further monitored experiments to clarify the forces at work.

REFERENCES

1. BARKER, R. S.: *Ecological Psychology*. Stanford: Stanford University Press, 1968.
2. BEISER, M.: "A Study of Personality Assets in a Rural Community." *Archives of General Psychiatry* 24:244-254, 1971.
3. BEISER, M.: "A Psychiatric Follow-up Study of 'Normal' Adults." *American Journal of Psychiatry* 127:1464, 1971.
4. CORNONI, J. C., WALLER, L. E., CASSEL, J. C., TYROLER, H. A., AND HAMES, C. G.: "The Incidence Study, Study Design and Method: The Evans County Study." *Archives of Internal Medicine* 34: 318-330, 1971.
5. EATON, M. L., GOLDFARB, A., DOWNING, J. J., AND MOSES, L. E.: "Automated Scoring of the Leighton Instrument: An Effort to Replace The Human Judge." Unpublished manuscript, 1971.
6. EDGERTON, J. W., BENTZ, K., AND HOLLISTER, W. G.: "Demographic Factors and Responses to Stress among Rural People." *American Journal of Public Health* 60:1065, 1970.
7. HOLLINGSHEAD, A. B., AND REDLICH, F.: *Social Class and Mental Illness*. New York: John Wiley and Sons, 1958.
8. HUGHES, C. C., TREMBLAY, M. A., RAPOPORT, R. N., AND LEIGHTON, A. H.: *People of Cove and Woodlot*. New York: Basic Books, 1960.
9. KELLERT, S., WILLIAMS, L. K., WHYTE, W. F., AND ALBERTI, G.: "Culture Change and Stress in Rural Peru." *Milbank Memorial Fund Quarterly* XLV:391, 1967.
10. KERN, J. C.: "Theory and Practice in a Program of Social Change." Mimeo RH #172, Harvard School of Public Health, 1970.
11. LEIGHTON, A. H.: *My Name Is Legion*. New York: Basic Books, 1959.
12. LEIGHTON, A. H.: "Poverty and Social Change." *Scientific American* 212:21, 1965.
13. LEIGHTON, A. H., LAMBO, T., HUGHES, C. C., LEIGHTON, D. C., MURPHY, J. M., AND MACKLIN, D. B.: *Psychiatric Disorder Among the Yoruba*. Ithaca: Cornell University Press, 1963.
14. LEIGHTON, D. C.: "The Changes Time Hath Wrought." Mimeograph, Cornell Program in Social Psychiatry, 1964.
15. LEIGHTON, D. C.: "Measuring Stress Levels in Children as a Program Monitoring Device." Paper presented at the Annual Meeting of the American Public Health Association, Minneapolis, 1971.
16. LEIGHTON, D. C., AND CLINE, N. F.: "The Public Health Nurse as a Mental Health Resource," in Thomas Weaver (ed.): *Essays on Medical Anthropology*. Athens: University of Georgia Press, 1968.
17. LEIGHTON, D. C., HARDING, J. S., MACKLIN, D. B., MACMILLAN, A. M., AND LEIGHTON, A. H.: *The Character of Danger*. New York: Basic Books, 1963.
18. MACMILLAN, A. M.: "The Health Opinion Survey: Technique for Estimating the Prevalence of Psychoneurotic and Related Types of Disorder in Communities." *Psychological Reports* 3:325-339, 1957.
19. MAYNARD, E., AND TWISS, G.: "That These People May Live." Mimeograph, Community Mental Health Program, Indian Health Service, Pine Ridge, South Dakota, 1969.
20. MOSES, L. F., GOLDFARB, A., GLOCK, C. Y., STARR, R. W., AND EATON, M. L.: "A Validity Study Using the Leighton Instrument." *American Journal of Public Health* 61:1785, 1971.
21. MYERS, J. K., AND BEAN, L. L.: *A Decade Later*. John Wiley and Sons, 1968.
22. ROGLER, L. H., AND HOLLINGSHEAD, A. B.: *Trapped: Families and Schizophrenia*. New York: John Wiley and Sons, 1965.
23. ROMAN, P.: "Occupational Role Change and Psychiatric Impairment." Unpublished Ph.D. Dissertation, Cornell University, 1968.
24. ROMAN, P., AND TRICE, H.: "Change and Mental Health: The Industrial Case." Paper presented to the American Sociological Association, San Francisco, 1969.

25. ROMAN, P., AND TRICE, H.: "Psychiatric Impairment Among 'Middle Americans.' " *Social Psychiatry* 9:351, 1972.
26. SMITH, W. G., TAINTOR, Z. C., AND KAPLAN, E. B.: "Computer Evaluations in Psychiatric Epidemiology." *Social Psychiatry* 1:174-181, 1967.
27. STONE, I. T.: "The Dynamics of Atomistic Organization: A Study of Social Change in Two Depressed Rural Settlements." Unpublished Ph.D. Dissertation, Cornell University, 1966.
28. TAIETZ, P.: *Community Structure and Aging.* Ithaca: New York State College of Agriculture at Cornell University, 1970.
29. WINTERS, E. (ed.): *The Collected Papers of Adolf Meyer, Vol. IV: Mental Hygiene.* Baltimore: The Johns Hopkins Press, 1952.
30. GOLDFARB, A., MOSES, L., DOWNING, J. J., AND LEIGHTON, D. C.: "Reliability of Newly Trained Raters in Community Case Findings." *American Journal of Public Health* 57:2149, 1967.
31. MATTHEWS, M. R.: "A Preliminary Descriptive Survey of HOS Responses in College Students and An Attempt at Validation." Unpublished MPH thesis, School of Public Health, University of North Carolina, 1966.
32. SHORE, J. H., KINZIE, J. D., HAMPSON, J. L., AND PATTISON, E. M.: "Psychiatric Epidemiology of an Indian Village." *Psychiatry* 36:70, 1973.

CHAPTER 11

Home Care for Psychiatric Disorders: Assessment of Effectiveness

SHIRLEY ANGRIST and SIMON DINITZ

The prolonged care mental hospital has been increasingly under critical attack. For at least 75 years, one or another critic has castigated the mental hospital as a human warehouse. Eloquent documentation by Dix, Beers, and Deutsch testified to the mental hospital as antitherapeutic. Goffman[20] scathingly indicted the mental hospital as a "total institution" characterized by disculturation, role dispossession, ceremonial degradation, and "stripping" of the self as part of the patient socialization process.

Despite the prolonged and impassioned history of criticism, we are only now engaged in dismantling the mental hospital and sending its patients to all manner of settings—even home—with deliberate and even unseemly haste. Where once there was only the alternative between tolerance and forebearance at home or hospital commitment (often for life), there is now an embarrassingly wide range of alternatives: foster homes, halfway houses, work-living arrangements, autonomous group living centers, day, night, and weekend outpatient centers, and acute treatment centers, each competing with each other and with the state mental hospitals for the scarce mental health dollar and the even scarcer qualified personnel needed. The prolonged care facility is now being transformed from a human warehouse to a revolving door institution. Patients come and go so fast that there is hardly time to socialize them to institutional life. Superintendents, who used to compete with one another on the decorousness of their "houses," then on the openness of their wards, more recently still on their success in creating therapeutic community settings, now vie with one another on how quickly they can process, treat, and return their patients home.[4,19,27] Even more enlightened superintendents compete vigorously to send their staff, singly or in teams, to render care via home visits in lieu of hospitalization.[44] It is not surprising, of course, that as release rates increase (85 per cent of all admissions to California state hospitals, for example, are released to the community in six months or less), so do readmission rates.[35] Worse still, the prolonged care hospital is becoming a permanent home to the regressed, organic, geriatric, and least tractable patients. Thus, as the state hospital becomes better, it becomes worse.

How did this impetus for home and, more broadly, community care suddenly take on all the characteristics of a religious crusade? The answer is clear but clearly not simple. First, the mounting pressure to humanize the hospital and to create a therapeutic setting is a tribute to the profound influence of psychodynamic theories that helped redefine mental illness and suggested an etiological perspective and a treatment modality (some form of psychotherapy) for dealing with psychiatric disorders. Second, revulsion with the concentration camp and its horrors led reformers of all persuasions to look anew at our own total institutions, especially the prison and the mental hospital. Third, the undisputed success in dealing with psychiatrically impaired soldiers in field hospitals and their rapid return to the front lines during World War II provided a concrete model for civilian practice. Fourth, state hospital admissions, voluntary and by court commitment, were proportionately exceeding population growth to such an extent that it was only a matter of time until the entire system would be overwhelmed.[28] At a cost of approximately $1500 to $2000 per patient per year and over $10,000 per new bed, states could no longer afford such warehouses. In contrast, minimal home care for the psychiatric patient (on the order of probation or parole in the criminal system) is only a tenth as costly and involves no major outlays for a physical plant. Material necessity obviously conditioned operational decisions. Even without the appropriate ideology, it is likely that home and community care would have emerged. New treatment ideologies speeded the trend. Fifth, and by far most significant, the unexpected appearance of psychotropic drugs revolutionized mental illness care. Ward noise was reduced, families could tolerate tranquilized or energized members, and the more bizarre behavioral manifestations of many chronic disorders could be controlled. The stampede to home, outpatient, noninstitutional care was on. The age of "intermittent patienthood" had arrived.

Home care of the mentally ill is not, of course, an entirely new concept. In other societies and in earlier periods of our own history, relatives, friends, and communities have looked after their disturbed members. Without hospitals, clinics, or psychiatrists, the sick person remained in the fabric of everyday life functioning as best he could, pardoned for what he could not do, sustained by those around him. In this sense, home care is historically and cross-culturally documented as feasible.[11]

Keeping the mentally ill at home when there were no alternatives was workable by necessity. But keeping them at home when there are chemotherapies, hospitals, clinics, therapists of many types, halfway houses, and rehabilitation programs is quite another matter. The issue now centers on the efficacy of systematic care that utilizes the whole range of treatment modes for the patient's benefit without institutionalization.

Home care of patients was studied indirectly before it surfaced as a separate concern. Several studies[2, 5, 38, 40, 43] have been done on how patients fare in the community after, between, or without hospitalization, focusing on the calibre of the individual's functioning and ability to avoid readmission to a hospital and employing such categories as psychiatric impairment, performance, outcome of hospitalization, outpatient care, "family care," and community tenure.

Noting that urban communities contain many disturbed persons who do not appear for treatment, post-World War II researchers made careful attempts to estimate the prevalence of psychiatric illness. From these epidemiological studies, it became clear that substantial proportions of urban populations provide home care for their emotionally disturbed kin, many without any professional or institutional psychiatric contact or assistance. A psychiatric census in Baltimore found 1 per cent of that city's population to be psychotic; of these, half resided in the community.[38] Even higher estimates of psychiatric impairment came from the Midtown Manhattan Study.[43] From a self-reported psychological evaluation of symptoms, nearly one quarter of respondents were rated as previously or presently impaired. Such studies[24, 40] also yield clues about the huge burden borne by households containing an emotionally impaired person.

More direct efforts to assess how the psychiatrically ill fare in the community stem from "outcome" studies.[1, 18, 32] These represent various evaluations of hospitalization focusing on the patient's post-hospital situation. Evidence from the many outcome studies conducted during the 1950s and 1960s (both before and after the widespread use of psychotropic drugs), point to continuing difficulties for both expatient and family and the great risk of relapse and rehospitalization. Some patient characteristics and situations favor adequate community functioning, while others are linked with problematic performance and frequent hospitalization.

EXPATIENTS IN THE COMMUNITY

The pioneer outcome research on lower social class patients admitted to state hospitals between 1930 and 1948 in two Arkansas counties showed that the major factor associated with good community adjustment was marital status.[1] Prompt hospitalization after the onset of illness was also linked to good post-hospital adjustment. Two thirds of the patients studied were getting along well with their families and their social participation was similar to the general population. But patients were less likely than the general population to marry or, if married, to stay that way. Patients continued to have problems getting and keeping regular work both before and after hospitalization. Most telling of all, their death rate far exceeded that of the general population.

Social class itself influences community adjustment. In one long term study, lower class status was clearly connected with negative adjustment outcome.[37] Confirming the 1950 finding that social class and mental illness are inextricably connected, the 10 year followup indicated that lower social class is highly related to a greater likelihood of being in the hospital, a lesser likelihood of being in outpatient care, a greater risk of readmission, and a lesser chance for discharge. While psychiatric impairment and employment status did not neatly single out particular class levels, social isolation was more characteristic of lower class patients. Overall, compared with nonpatients, the employment problems, also noted by other investigators,[29] and social isolation of the patients were striking.

However, social isolation may have some positive valence for patient functioning. In an English study, male schizophrenics living with siblings and in their own lodgings did better during their first post-hospital year than those who returned to spouses or parents.[5] Although complete isolation may be harmful, reduced family pressures may aid patient adjustment.

In one innovative social experiment,[16] nonfamilial living and working arrangements were highly potent factors in favorable outcomes for participating expatients. Those chronic mental patients who volunteered to enter a lodge society providing residence and an autonomous business fared far better than comparable patient volunteers in traditional aftercare programs. After initial help from professionals and consultants, the lodge became a small society of male expatients who lived together, helped look after each other, and ran a janitorial and gardening business. The lodge members had significantly longer community tenure and employment and an enhanced self-esteem. Thus community care outside the usual home context became a viable alternative. By means of a supportive, productive, and participative social situation, the expatients found their highest possible functioning level. This does not mean they were "cured" in the medical sense. Both the lodge members and the control group continued to lead rather limited, isolated social lives and to manifest psychiatric symptoms. While the lodge could reduce readmissions and foster work roles, it could not push psychosocial adjustment above the ceiling for such chronic cases.

The effects of familial context on patient performance were highlighted by an American study.[18] Patients living with spouses performed better socially and psychiatrically than those living in parental households. The hypothesized explanation of this finding, that spouses are intolerant of deviant behavior, did not hold up under scrutiny. While expectations of married patients are higher, they are also better able to proform at a higher level. In addition, relatives evidently accommodate their expectations to suit the patient's condition. Thus, the causal factor is not obvious among the several factors: patient performance, familial expectations, tolerance of deviant behavior, and the patient's ability to perform.[2] Furthermore, ability to avoid rehospitalization was found to be a function of patient symptom manifestation, not the family's willingness to tolerate his inadequate performance.

236

Other studies repeatedly confirm the poor prognosis for patients with more active and bizarre symptoms and with longer histories of illness, prior hospitalizations, and leaves of absence rather than outright release from the hospital. The sicker the patient in these ways, the worse the post-hospital adjustment and the greater the chances of readmission.[2, 6, 18, 32, 33] In fact, most of those patients who return to the hospital typically do so within the first year after release. Readmission estimates vary according to types of patients studied and the methods of estimation; one report says nearly all leave of absence patients returned within five years.[33] By contrast, only about one quarter of patients from a short term treatment hospital returned the first year.[2] For schizophrenics, readmission rates are estimated at about one third within one year.[5, 18]

Despite these rather high readmission rates and the common pattern of multiple hospitalizations, this "intermittent patienthood"[19] is not easily explained. Patients, relatives, and psychiatric professionals concur only minimally on the specific precipitants of readmission. What goes wrong? Are the problems psychiatric, physical, environmental? Congruence on these matters is low and leads to the hypothesis that situational factors may play a large part in readmission.[12, 15, 16, 35] What is clear about rehospitalization, however, is that it occurs for the more severely impaired. This holds true regardless of differences in treatment or rehabilitation programs.[31] Household members cope with the patient until the behaviors become extreme, unmanageable, and bizarre. Relatives accept the burden of housing a psychiatric patient as long as possible—hospitalization is the last resort.[2]

Instead of merely judging patient functioning by criteria such as readmission and symptom manifestation, one study compared expatients with a group of normal neighbors.[2] The comparison group of women who had never been psychiatrically treated was closely matched with the expatient group. Only white married women living with their husbands were included in the comparison group. Only patients diagnosed as functionally rather than organically impaired at the time of hospitalization and free from alcohol and drug problems were included in the expatient group. The two groups were also matched for comparable distributions of age and social class. By means of this matching procedure, the two groups of women were made equivalent in familial and demographic characteristics. Comparison of these groups in their performance of domestic tasks and in their leisure activities revealed few differences. It seemed that the very matching of background characteristics resulted in eliminating the differences in instrumental role performance. But the two groups remained significantly different in psychiatric functioning: the expatients were functioning at a substantially lower level than the controls.

An assessment of the same two groups 10 years later documented the continued psychiatric impairment of the expatients compared with the control group members.[36] Thirty-three per cent of the expatients were rehospitalized during the 10 year period, and 11 per cent were receiving outpatient clinic or private care. In contrast, only *one* control group member required hospitalization and only 11 per cent needed or received psychiatric attention of any kind during the 10 years. These patients are strikingly different from the general population: they tend to have lower occupational and educational levels, to be single, widowed, separated, or divorced, and to be living in unusual household configurations. But even when the patients had been demographically matched with normals, the same pattern continued over the 10 years. In addition to inferior marital adjustment, the expatients lost ground to the controls in various other respects, such as having more employment difficulties and problems with children.[36] There is good reason to suspect that patients who have been hospitalized are not only handicapped in their societal participation, but that their social characteristics (lower educational attainment, lower socioeconomic status, and unmarried or no longer married status) increase their risk for becoming mentally ill.[2] Once they become defined as mentally ill, especially through contact with treatment agencies, the label sticks and the condition is self-perpetuating.[3,8,30]

The outcome studies thus yield many clues about the post-hospital career of the mental patient and his family and suggest both the positive and negative aspects of maintaining psychiatric patients at home. The recent more direct evaluations of home care clarify and confirm these earlier findings.

THE PREVENTION OF HOSPITALIZATION

As noted earlier, during the late 1950s there was a growing interest in treating psychiatric patients at home. Widespread use of psychoactive drugs led to shorter hospitalizations and more extended community tenure for mental patients. Inevitably the spotlight shifted to the community. How would patients who were ordinarily hospitalized for treatment fare at home under a psychiatric treatment regimen?

Greenblatt and his associates[22] studied patients waiting for admission to a mental hospital who were offered home care. These were mainly female and unmarried; two thirds had had previous treatment and about half were diagnosed as psychotic. They received broad and eclectic treatment, including individual psychotherapy, electroshock therapy, counseling with family members, and use of a day hospital. Of these, psychotherapy was the most frequently used. Some home visits were made by psychiatrists, nurses, and social workers. The greatest success in this program was with the nonpsychotics. About half the patients had to be hospitalized.

Engelhardt and his coworkers[13] studied attempts to use drugs to prevent hospitalization of ambulatory schizophrenics seen in a clinic setting on a voluntary basis. Comparisons were made among patients receiving (1) promazine, (2) chlorpromazine, and (3) placebo. The results were mixed. In one attempt, the patients receiving medication were not hospitalized, but the study itself lost nearly two thirds of its participating patients. A second study[14] of similar patients demonstrated that the hospitalization rate increased over time. Over an extended period, the groups receiving medication did no better than the group receiving placebo. It appeared that drug treatment merely delayed hospitalization but could not prevent it in these voluntary clinic patients.

In a systematic experimental evaluation,[39] home care was compared with hospital care. Schizophrenic patients admitted consecutively to a state hospital serving Louisville, Kentucky, whose families were willing to cooperate in the program by providing supervision in the home, were randomly assigned to one of three situations: (1) home on drugs, (2) home on placebo, and (3) hospitalization. Home visits were made mainly by public health nurses. Such visits, during which medication was provided and patient functioning carefully assessed, were made weekly at first, bi-weekly after three months, and monthly after six months. Additional patients, ambulatory schizophrenics referred to the study by community practitioners, were assigned to home care on drugs or placebo. The results shed light on two criteria of outcome: readmission and patient functioning. Patients treated at home with drugs were the most successful in remaining out of the hospital continuously (77 per cent) compared with the placebo group (34 per cent). After an initial hospitalization averaging 83 days, the hospitalized group had a higher failure rate (readmission) than home care drug patients. In all the groups, most failures occurred within six months. In terms of functioning, home care patients exceeded discharged hospital control patients and made considerable improvement, expecially within the first six months; thereafter their functioning stabilized at a pre-episodic level, which was not very high. Thus, home care patients improved more during the 30 month program and were more successful in avoiding hospitalization.

The value of home care in reducing hospital admissions is echoed in results from the home treatment service established in the English coastal community of Worthing and environs.[7] Psychiatrists made home visits. Only the sickest patients were admitted to the hospital. The treatment forms most used were electroconvulsive therapy, modified insulin therapy, group and individual psychotherapies, but no drug therapy. In two years, hospitals admissions for the area showed a net decrease of 59 per cent.

The accumulated evidence attests to quite good success from home care programs in ameliorating the patient's condition and in reducing hospital readmission rates. It appears that home care, in the sense of a community based treatment service, can serve more patients per a population of 1000 than a hospital based service.[42] Comparison of these two types of services indicated that the community service recruited more psychotics and persons with illnesses of shorter duration. It also recruited more women—the widowed, the old, the lonely, and the poor. These social factors affected the disposition of cases in both services, but in the community, old age and social isolation favored hospitalization. Candidates for home treatment more often were the married, the young, those in social class III (based on the Hollingshead index), and those living with a close relative. However, on the whole, hospitalization was an unlikely disposition in the community service and a very likely occurrence in the hospital based service.

As long as community based programs provide for *ongoing* home care, they are effective in reducing readmission rates. But home care benefits do not continue once the program terminates. In a five-year followup study of the Louisville study patients,[9] the advantage of the home care drug group disappeared. All three treatment groups had about the same readmission rates during the period between the *end* of the 30 month program in 1964 and 1969: 61 per cent of the home care drug group, 57 per cent of the home care placebo group, and 61 per cent of the hospitalized controls had been readmitted at least once. When the program ended in 1964, all patient groups were left without further treatment. Without drugs and professional support, the experimental group came to resemble the control groups. We can hypothesize that even the most modest external intervention might have kept members of the home care drug group out of the hospital.

What about the patient's family? Is home care a boon or a bane? In many respects, this question is largely academic. The increase in community facilities, the ideological commitment to home care, and the rapid release of hospitalized patients have generated different questions, namely, how to minimize the disruptive effects of having a sick person at home, and the more generic question of how to treat family, as opposed to purely personal, pathology.

In a two-year followup study[21] of patients and their families from both hospital and community based services, the hospital service was shown to be more effective in reducing both anxiety and problems in the families. The social cost of psychiatric care was higher in the community service as several factors indicate: fewer men remained employed fulltime over the two years, and more families had trouble looking after their patient at home. After some investigation of these results, the researchers found that the social help given by the hospital service was much more extensive than that of the community service. The lesson from this is that the home versus hospital care dichotomy is meaningless. Unless deliberate and complete psychiatric and social services accompany community based care, it cannot count as a treatment mode distinct from the ordinary life of an impaired person left untreated in the community.

To emphasize this point, it is useful to consider a study which specifically incorporated both hospital and home care as part of a single program.[25] Psychiatric units in two general hospitals provided comprehensive services to their areas. They succeeded in satisfying patient needs without resort to prolonged hospitalization, especially of mental patients. In the four years of the study, less than 1 per cent of their patients became long term mental hospital patients. Although the units drew recurrent admissions, patients had short stays, usually lasting a few months. Schizophrenics required hospitalization somewhat more often and for longer periods than other patients. This more seriously ill category of patients nevertheless spent about half of the four years in the community. Psychiatric hospital admissions were typically male, young, single, schizophrenic, and showed dangerous behavior and extended illness. The aged manifested no special difficulties. For all of the patients, problems of finding employment, of physical illness, and of restricted living were commonplace. Surprisingly, use of social and medical services, outpatient group therapy, and private therapy was moderate; no undue case loads developed.

This same study reveals much about the social cost for the families of psychiatric patients.[23, 25] Objective burden, as measured by patient symptom manifestation and effects on family life, was present in about half the families. Slightly over one third of the patients exhibited recurrent abnormal behavior regardless of age, sex, social class, and marital status. Over the four years, interference with domestic routine and separation from children were the greatest problems. Effects on income and on the health of other family members were comparatively small. Indication of family accommodation to housing a patient was taken from how they perceived their situation or their subjective burden. Of the households rated with objective burden nearly one quarter expressed no subjective burden. The remainder reported subjective burden, but only 20 per cent said this was severe. While household members were often relieved when the patient was hospitalized, having the patient at home did not increase expressed subjective burden.

SOME ISSUES IN HOME CARE EFFECTIVENESS

Although no firm case can be made for home care programs as the *best* overall psychiatric treatment strategy, the above studies reveal that caring for psychiatric patients at home is possible and manageable, and, furthermore, that under certain conditions it can be more effective than hospitalization. However, there are issues that require added discussion, research, and clarification. There can be various criteria for evaluating home care effectiveness and disparate views of the patient's condition according to whether patient, relative, employer, or health professional is the judge. The crucial issue is clear: what criteria should be used? We suggest the following criteria for appraising home care programs against other treatment strategies; the first two have been frequently used, but the third remains seriously neglected:

(1) What are the risks of relapse and rehospitalization?
(2) What level of functioning do patients achieve?
(3) What is the social cost to family and to society?

Readmission to Hospital

This criterion is the easiest to measure and evaluate. From the studies described earlier, substantial evidence indicates that regardless of the type of treatment, most psychiatric patients, once under the aegis of a treatment agency, remain high risks for relapse and hospitalization. In all treatment strategies— short or long term hospitalization, in a psychiatric or general hospital, in a clinic

241

or hospital, community based or hospital based care—institutionalization for some patients for some periods is inevitable. Some argue that systematic home care services can entirely prevent hospitalization, others say that hospitalization is merely delayed and its incidence reduced. By now this is a moot issue. The sicker patients, with longer illness duration and longer treatment histories, are indeed high risks for hospitalization. The high risk for these categories is aggravated when certain social factors are operative: lower social class, nonmarried status, low income, old age. Since admission usually results from the patient's bizarre or unmanageable behavior, relapse in his condition likely leads to hospitalization. Relatives do what they can. Hospitalization occurs when they cannot cope with the patient's symptoms.

A program defined as *total home care* devoid of institutionalization as an alternative is destined to be unworkable. If the goal of home care is to prevent hospitalization for all patients, that goal is untenable. If, however, the aim of home care is to avoid hospitalization for some patients and to delay hospitalization and minimize its duration for *most* patients, such an aim is indeed feasible.

The Level of Patient Functioning

This is another well documented criterion for evaluating home care effectiveness. Whether the evidence is from epidemiological, followup, or actual home care research, it is explicit in recording the low level functioning which characterizes patients in the community. Regardless of the type of treatment received, its variety, intensity, or duration, patients perform poorly compared to normal persons. Those with greater psychiatric impairment typically function worse than those with less impairment. Whatever the measure of psychiatric functioning, the sicker patient has more numerous and more severe symptoms. Still the ability to hold a job, run a household, or interact with people can vary. In general, the worse the psychiatric condition, the more problems arise in the social, domestic, and work areas. But many patients perform as well socially and domestically as nonpatients. Difficulty in getting and keeping gainful employment is common for both men and women patients. Yet this problem can be lightened by services geared to rehabilitation, occupational therapy, vocational counseling, and job placement.

Just as some social factors operate to foster readmission, there are others that foster low level functioning in the community. The single, widowed, or separated, the aged, the chronically physically ill, and the socially isolated patients tend to perform poorly.

Given the pervasive handicaps in patient performance, the goals of home care programs must be realistic. High level functioning is an unrealistic aim. If a goal of home care programs is to ameliorate the patient's condition and to maintain it in a "process" rather than a "reactive" state, that goal is feasible. The effectiveness of present treatment modalities makes restoration of the patient to a pre-episodic level viable, but return to a pre-onset condition is not yet an outcome

242

with high probability. The difficulties of managing the mentally ill in society remain despite growing acceptance of community care approaches. Persons who are marginal, deviant, subnormal, sick, yet well enough to be home, remain a problem to society and a challenge to psychiatry.

The Social Cost of Illness

Not enough is known about the precise burdens to family and society for maintaining the psychiatrically ill either at home *or* in institutions. The availability of the information required to estimate the comparative social cost of traditional and new forms of community centered care is skimpy at best. Indications are that the burdens are great under both the old and the new forms. (For estimates before the initiation of community mental health centers, see Fein.[17])

Estimates of the direct costs of psychiatric care amount to about two billion dollars annually in the United States.[2] Apart from such expenditures, care and treatment facilities and services involve perhaps a quarter million professionals and workers at all levels, serving some one and a quarter million patients, 80 per cent of whom are admitted to public mental hospitals. But substantial numbers, perhaps another million, are in private treatment or outpatient clinics. The complex mental health industry with its varied services, manpower shortage, and shifting treatment concepts has been difficult to assess. Cost of treatment and outcome effectiveness have been hardly gauged at all.

The current American model of the community mental health center authorized and funded by the Congress in 1963 specifies five essential services: inpatient, outpatient, partial hospitalization, emergency 24-hour services, and consultation and education services.[39] In addition, an adequate center would include diagnostic and rehabilitation services, pre- and after-care services, and training, research, and evaluation programs. Adequate community treatment programs must meet criteria of comprehensiveness, coordination, and continuity. This means they must offer a full range of services to all age groups and diagnostic categories, they must coordinate both psychiatric and nonpsychiatric services through a central agency, and they must provide for patients' free and easy movement through the various services.

Fulfillment of this model in all its aspects by specific centers remains to be appraised. There are dangers in expecting more than such a model provides.[10] But default in delivering the basic requisites that such a model promises is already evident.[26] From 1963 to 1969, the United States has spent a total of about $400 million on the community mental health center program—about what the State of New York Department of Mental Hygiene spends on its own programs annually. Disproportionate amounts still go to the state hospitals that the new centers were supposed to replace. In 1970, more than half the persons entering state mental hospitals were readmissions. Despite the growth of community mental health centers, most of these countless persons are pretty much on their own between hospitalizations.

Needed yet to fulfill the community mental health center model are trained home care workers. The elaborate efforts of orienting a professional staff and educating hospital administrators and psychiatrists for an experimental home care project hint of costs yet to be borne by any nationwide programs.[39] Systematic home care requires that health professionals leave their offices, hospitals, and clinics to use their expertise in the patient's community location. Examining the patient at home, talking to relatives, administering medication, referring the patient to appropriate agencies, assessing the patient's and family's conditions, arranging for periodic hospitalization, re-assessing the patient after hospitalization, and generally monitoring all such matters over time—these are the tasks home care practitioners must perform. Training of health professionals and paraprofessionals must shift its emphasis accordingly from hospital to community, from office to home, from formality to informality, from appointments to visits, and from single treatment modes to multiple treatment modes. Much pioneering remains in shaping models of home treatment. But it is likely that community based treatment will require the provision for help for families in bearing the burden of sustaining a patient, for social difficulties as well as for psychiatric problems.

In these ways, then, the economic and social costs of mental illness seem vast and unfathomable. However, advocates of the new programs would argue that social costs will continue to be high as long as financial expenditures fall so short of the amounts required and as long as minimal services and facilities exist. The aim of effective home care is not merely to avoid institutionalization; it is also to rehabilitate and to motivate the patient to function as close to normal as possible.

There is sufficient evidence to indicate that the long term costs of mental illness can be reduced in specific ways. Systematic home care programs can reduce hospitalization, thus minimizing not only institutional costs but also the patient's time away from family and work; they can also reduce wear and tear on household members unable to cope alone with their sick member. A psychiatric patient, whether at home or in the hospital, can increase family anxiety and distress, alter normal life routines and relationships with children, decrease household income, and injure the health of family members. The issue of cost must confront such sticky problems as these which no treatment program alone can overcome. Families have to and do—sometimes well, sometimes poorly—cope with the stresses and difficulties resulting from their responsibility for a psychiatrically ill person at home or in the hospital. At best, a treatment mode can alleviate the family stresses at least temporarily. As for the patient, volumes of research show that the mentally ill person may suffer as much at home as in a hospital. Remaining in the household can mean reinforcement of pathological interaction between members; in this way, the initial precipitants of the illness continue to operate, furthering the patient's deterioration. Prolonged hospitalization, however, carries the risk of inducing "institutionalism" in the patient—dependence on the hospital, withdrawal from significant others and the

244

larger society, and general deterioration. Workable home care must include innovative arrangements such as lodges and expatient "societies" or "families."[5],[16]

There are few measures of social costs so far. Hopefully, attempts to measure and reduce the social costs of mental illness will yield answers to the questions: What is the very best that can be done for the patient? What is the very best that can be done for the family? Provision of a full range of treatment modes on the highest medical, technical, and humane levels is essential. The task is to learn in what specific ways both institutions and households should carry the burden of care.

Controversies over the location, agents, and modalities of treatment of the mentally ill have obscured a much more significant social issue: the management of marginal and submarginal persons in a complex society. Reliance on institutionalization has not ameliorated that task. The problems are much the same whether the subgroup consists of the mentally ill, chronic welfare cases, chronically disabled, the aged, former prisoners, or the retarded. In the past, social scientists have focused on the differences rather than on the similarities among these categories of socially stigmatized people. But the fact is that the mentally ill share with other social deviants their common troubles of living: family problems and problem families; chronic under- or unemployment and, in general, an inability to perform satisfactorily on a job even when one is obtained; interpersonal problems expressed in withdrawal, acting out, or aggressive behavior; instrumental role performance problems; and on a more personal level, loss of self-esteem, defeatism, minimal expectations for performance, frustration, and rage.

In this chapter we have described various aspects of home care, stressing what is known about particular evaluative programs and their effects on patients and families. We have also emphasized the pervasive specific problems which beset households with a mental patient. Experimental programs are limited by the fact that they are temporary rather than ongoing. The defect of some programs is their lack of evaluative measures by which to judge effectiveness. Based on the existing evidence, we must conclude that those home care programs are effective which mobilize these indispensable requisites: a staff trained in home care; comprehensive treatment and facilities, including job training and placement and medical and social services, to maintain patient and family in a total life scheme; provision for inpatient care for acute phases of disease; sustained and adequate funding of programs; a community educated to accept and promote home care programs; and realistic goals for patient functioning.

REFERENCES

1. ADLER, L. M., CODDINGTON, J. W., AND STEWART, D. D.: *Mental Illness in Washington County, Arkansas: Incidence, Recovery and Posthospital Adjustment.* Fayetteville, Arkansas: University of Arkansas, 1952.

2. ANGRIST, S., LEFTON, M., DINITZ, S., AND PASAMANICK, B.: *Women After Treatment: A Study of Former Mental Patients and Their Normal Neighbors.* New York: Appleton-Century-Crofts, 1968.

3. BERAN, NANCY: "Competing Mental Health Ideologies: A Study of Psychiatric Transfer." Doctoral Dissertation, Department of Sociology, The Ohio State University, 1970.

4. BOCHOVEN, J. S.: "Moral Treatment in American Psychiatry." *Journal of Nervous and Mental Disease* 124: 167-194, 292-321, 1956.

5. BROWN, G. W.: "Experiences of Discharged Chronic Schizophrenic Patients in Various Types of Living Groups." *Milbank Memorial Fund Quarterly* 37: 105-131, 1959.

6. BURKE, L., DEYKIN, E., JACOBSON, S., AND HALEY, S.: "The Depressed Woman Returns." *Archives of General Psychiatry* 16: 548-553, 1967.

7. CARSE, J., PANTON, N. E., AND WATT, A.: "A District Mental Health Service: The Worthing Experiment." *Lancet* 1:39-42, 1958.

8. CLAUSEN, J., AND YARROW, M. R. (eds.): "The Impact of Mental Illness on the Family." *Journal of Social Issues* 11, 1955.

9. DAVIS, ANN E., DINITZ, S., AND PASAMANICK, BENJAMIN: "Schizophrenics in the Community: Five Years Later". Unpublished manuscript, 1970.

10. DINITZ, S., AND BERAN, N.: "The Community Mental Health Approach as a Boundaryless and Boundary "Busting" System." Paper presented at the American Orthopsychiatric Association Annual Meeting, San Francisco, 1970.

11. EATON, J. W., AND WEIL, R. J.: *Culture and Mental Disorders: A Comparative Study of the Hutterites and Other Populations.* Glencoe: The Free Press, 1955.

12. ELLSWORTH, R. B., FOSTER, L., CHILDERS, B., ARTHUR, G., AND KROEKER, D.: "Hospital and Community Adjustment as Perceived by Psychiatric Patients, Their Families and Staff." *Journal of Consulting and Clinical Psychology.* Monograph Supplement 32: Part 2, 1968.

13. ENGELHARDT, D. M., FREEDMAN, N., GLICK, B. S., HANKOFF, L. D., AND MANN, D.: "Prevention of Psychiatric Hospitalization with Use of Psychopharmacological Agents." *Journal of the American Medical Association* 173: 147-149, 1960.

14. ENGELHARDT, D. M., *et al.*: "Phenothiazines in Prevention of Psychiatric Hospitalization: II, Duration of Treatment Exposure." *Journal of the American Medical Association* 186: 981-983, 1963.

15. FAIRWEATHER, G. W. (ed.): *Social Psychology in Treating Mental Patients: An Experimental Approach.* New York: John Wiley and Sons, 1964.

16. FAIRWEATHER, G. W., SANDERS, D. H., CRESSLER, D. L., AND MAYNARD, H.: *Community Life for the Mentally Ill: An Alternative to Institutional Care.* Chicago: Aldine, 1969.

17. FEIN, RASHI: *Economics of Mental Health.* New York: Basic Books, 1958.

18. FREEMAN, H. E., AND SIMMONS, O. G.: *The Mental Patient Comes Home.* New York: John Wiley and Sons, 1963.

19. FRIEDMAN, IRA, VON MERING, O., AND HINKO, E. N.: "Intermittent Patienthood." *Archives of General Psychiatry* 14: 286-392, 1966.

20. GOFFMAN, ERVING: *Asylums.* New York: Doubleday-Anchor, 1961.

21. GRAD, J. C.: "A Two-Year Follow-Up," in R. H. Williams and L. D. Ozarin (eds.): *Community Mental Health,* pp. 430-454. San Francisco: Jossey-Bass, 1968.

22. GREENBLATT, M., MOORE, R. F., ALBERT, R. S., AND SOLOMON, M. H.: *The Prevention of Hospitalization: Treatment Without Admission for Psychiatric Patients.* New York: Grune and Stratton, 1963.

23. HAMILTON, M. W.: "The Hospital and the Household," in R. H. Williams and L. D. Ozarin (eds.): *Community Mental Health,* pp. 416-428. San Francisco: Jossey-Bass, 1968.

24. HOCH, P. S., AND ZUBIN, J. (eds.): *Comparative Epidemiology of the Mental Disorders.* New York: Grune and Stratton, 1961.

25. HOENIG, J., AND HAMILTON, M. W.: *The Desegregation of the Mentally Ill.* London: Routledge and Kegan Paul, 1969.

26. ISENBERG, B.: "Coping with Society: Care of Mentally Ill Outside Institutions Lags despite Promise." *Wall Street Journal,* July 10, 1970, pp. 1 and 8.

27. JONES, MAXWELL: *The Therapeutic Community.* New York: Basic Books, 1953.

28. KRAMER, M., POLLACK, E. S., AND REDICK, R. W.: "Mental Disorders in the United States: Current Status and Future Goals," in P. S. Hoch and J. Zubin (eds.): *Comparative Epidemiology of the Mental Disorders,* pp. 68-79. New York: Grune and Stratton, 1961.

246

29. LAMB, H. R.: "Release of Chronic Psychiatric Patients into the Community." *Archives of General Psychiatry* 9: 38-44, 1968.

30. MECHANIC, D.: *Mental Health and Social Policy.* Englewood Cliffs, New Jersey: Prentice-Hall, 1969.

31. MEYER, H. J., AND BORGATTA, E. F.: *An Experiment in Mental Patient Rehabilitation.* New York: Russell Sage Foundation, 1959.

32. MICHAUX, W. W., KATZ, M. M., KURLAND, A. A., AND GANSEREIT, K. H.: *The First Year Out: Mental Patients After Hospitalization.* Baltimore: The Johns Hopkins Press, 1969.

33. MILLER, D.: *Worlds That Fail, Part I: Retrospective Analysis of Mental Patients' Careers.* State of California, Department Of Mental Hygiene, Research Monograph No. 6, 1965.

34. MILLER, D., AND DAWSON, W.: *Worlds That Fail, Part II: Disbanded Worlds: A Study of Returns to the Mental Hospital.* State of California, Department of Mental Hygiene, Research Monograph No. 7, 1965.

35. MILLER, D.: "Retrospective Analysis of Posthospital Mental Patients' Worlds." *Journal of Health and Social Behavior* 8: 136-140, 1967

36. MOLHOLM, L. H.: *Female Mental Patients and Normal Female Controls: A Restudy Ten Years Later.* Doctoral Dissertation, Department of Sociology, The Ohio State University, 1970.

37. MYERS, J. K., AND BEAN, L. L.: *A Decade Later: A Follow-Up of Social Class and Mental Illness.* New York: John Wiley and Sons, 1968.

38. PASAMANICK, B., ROBERTS, D. W., LEMKAU, P. W., AND KREUGER, D. B.: "A Survey of Mental Disease in an Urban Population: I. Prevalence by Age, Sex and Severity of Impairment." *American Journal of Public Health* 47: 923-929, 1957.

39. PASAMANICK, B., SCARPITTI, F. R., AND DINITZ, S.: *Schizophrenics in the Community: An Experimental Study in the Prevention of Hospitalization.* New York: Appleton-Century-Crofts, 1967.

40. PLUNKETT, R. J., AND GORDON, J. E.: *Epidemiology and Mental Illness.* New York: Basic Books, 1960.

41. ROGLER, L. H., AND HOLLINGSHEAD, A. B.: *Trapped: Families and Schizophrenia.* New York: John Wiley and Sons, 1965.

42. SAINSBURY, P.: "Research Methods in Evaluation," in R. H. Williams and L. D. Ozarin (eds.): *Community Mental Health,* p. 212-236. San Francisco: Jossey-Bass, 1968.

43. SROLE, L., LANGNER, T. S., MICHAEL, S. T., OPLER, M. K., AND RENNIE, T. A. C.: *Mental Health in the Metropolis: The Manhattan Midtown Study,* Vol. 1. New York: McGraw-Hill, 1962.

44. WEINER, L., BECKER, A., AND FREEDMAN, T. T.: *Home Treatment: Spearhead of Community Psychiatry.* Pittsburgh: University of Pittsburgh Press, 1967.

247

Index

ADMINISTRATION of community mental health programs, 72-74

Alcoholism
as focus of prevention, 95-96
definition of, 103-104
etiology of, 104
strategies of prevention of, 102-103
treatment of, 106

American values and social programs, 3, 15-16, 19, 24, 108

Assumptions of community mental health programs, 136-139

BASE service unit, 184

Behavior change, means of, 105

Behavior therapy, 123-124

Brief psychotherapies, 122-123

CASE manager concept, 196, 198-200, 204-206

Catchment areas, 64

Collaboration, interprofessional, in community mental health, 74-77

Collectivities as dependent variables, 32

Community(ies)
as a social field, 56-57
as focus of treatment, 125
classification of, 52
definition of, 51-52, 71
field theory of, 56-62
interest areas and, 57-58

Community acceptance of mental health programs, 62-63

Community activities of mental health programs, 124-125

Community development
as a therapeutic force, 209-230
strategies of, 224-225

Community field(s)
community psychiatry and, 59-62
types of, 58-59
theory. See Field theory.

Community intervention, 59. See also Intervention.

Community Mental Health Centers Act of 1963, 2, 17, 24-26, 34, 69, 108-109, 179-180
assumptions of, 24
interpretation of, 70
regulations of, 74

Community mental health programs, description of, 120-127, 182-188, 196

Community needs and individual rights, 83-94

Community psychiatrist. See also Psychiatrist.
problems for, 47-49
role of, 43-45, 47-49
training of, 41-42

Community psychiatry
definition of, 181
implications of community sociology for, 62-65

Community sociology, implications of, for community psychiatry, 62-65

Community survey studies, 28-29

Community theory and research
cultural-ethnographic approach, 54-55
ecological approach, 52-53
field theory, 56-62
functional analysis, 53-54. See also Social systems theory.
monographical studies, 55
social systems perspective, 53-54
sociocultural ecological approach, 53
structural-functional approach. See Social systems theory.
traditions in, 52-55
typological tradition, 55

Comparison group strategy in evaluation, 157-159

Comparison group studies, 158-159

Concerns of community psychiatry, 69

Conflict
between evaluators and practitioners, 128-129, 132-133, 142-144
cooperation and, in community mental health, 195-207
evaluation design and, 130-134

Constructive confrontation as a prevention strategy, 98-99, 107
Constructive typology, 165
Consultation, in community mental health programs, 124-125, 184-186, 188-189
Control groups in evaluation, 146, 152, 155-157
Coordination of services in community mental health programs, 77-78, 125-126
Cultural-ethnographic theory and research, 54-55

DARWINISM, social, 15-17, 19
Data collection banks, 77-78
Data collection system, 83-84, 94
  design of, 85-86, 91-92
  initiation of, 92-93
  public acceptance of, 87-91, 93
Dependent variables
  social collectivities as, 32
  social structure as, 26-28
Differential risks as a prevention strategy, 96-97
Drugs in prevention of hospitalization, 238-239

EARLY identification as a prevention strategy, 98
Ecology, 52-53
Education as a prevention strategy, 97-98
Education and consultation, 124-125, 184-186, 188-189
Epidemiology of psychiatric disorder, 210-212
Evaluation of community mental health programs, 119, 121-130, 143
  American values and, 166-167
  as basis for program change, 134-136
  as threat to practitioners, 134-136
  assumption of success and, 139-141
  comparison group strategy in, 157-159
  control groups in, 146, 152, 155-157
  criteria of program success and, 152-153
  definition of program goals in, 147-151
  design of, 120-121
    as source of conflict, 130-134
  experimental design in, 146, 151-154
    adaptation of, 155-157
  goal attainment model in, 146-151
  focus of, 130
  Hawthorne effect of, 151, 153
  improvement of, 154-171
  indigenous model in, 166-171
    self-evaluation and, 166-167
  negative results of, 135-136
  of home care treatment, 233-245
  of program assumptions, 136-139
  overselling and exploitation in, 144-145
  professional styles and, 141-142
  purpose of, 130-134
  research compromise in, 145
  shortcomings of, 172
  systems model in, 159-165

Evaluator(s)
  practitioners and, conflict between, 128-129, 132-133, 142-144
  relationship to community mental health programs, 127-146
Expatient adjustment to community, 235-238
Experimental design in evaluation, 146, 151-154
  adaptation of, 155-157

FAMILIAL context, effect on expatient adjustment, 236, 237
Family treatment, 122
Field theory
  concepts in, 56-57
  of community, 56-62
  levels of analysis in, 58, 60-62
Functional analysis, 53-54. See also Social systems theory.
Functional substitutes, as a prevention strategy, 101-102

GEOGRAPHICAL boundaries of community mental health programs, 64, 71-74
Goal attainment model in evaluation, 146-151
Goals of community psychiatry, 21, 48
Group therapy, 124

HAWTHORNE effect, 151, 153
Health Opinion Survey (HOS), 226-229
Home care for psychiatric patients
  compared to hospitalization, 239-241
  effect on family, 240-241, 243-245
  effect on patient functioning, 242-243
  evaluation of, 233-245
  in prevention of hospitalization, 238-241
  rehospitalization and, 240, 241-242
  social cost of, 243-245
Hospital, psychiatric, 233-234
  readmission to, 237
  studies of, 29-30
Hospitalization, 79, 81, 233-234
  compared to home care, 239-241
  partial, 122, 183-184
  prevention of, 238-241
Hospitalized patients, characteristics of, 238

INDIGENOUS model, use of, in evaluation, 166-171
Individual rights and public interests, 77-81, 83-94
Inpatient service in community mental health center, 182, 187-188
Interaction field perspective, 56. See also Field theory.
Interest areas within community, 57-58
Interprofessional collaboration in community mental health, 74-77

250

Intervention, 42-45, 48-49, 59
  focus of, 80
  right of, 105-106, 107

Joint Commission on Mental Health and Mental Illness, 4, 22, 24
  report of, 22-23
Jurisdictional problems in community psychiatry,
  individual rights and public interest, 77-81
  political, 70-74
  professional, 74-77

Labeling perspective, 4, 5
Leadership in community mental health programs, 63. *See also* Treatment team leadership.
Legal issues in community psychiatry, 69-77, 78-80
  individual rights and public interest, 77-81, 83-94

Medical disease model of mental illness, 6, 10, 32-33, 195, 206
  definition of, 18
  inception of, 13
Mental health
  definition of, 76
  improvement of, 223-224
Mental health field
  sociological objectives and perspectives in, 26-28
  sociological research in, 28-31. *See also* Sociological research.
Mental Health Study Act of 1955, 22
Mental health needs
  definition of, 193
  determination of, 191-192
Mental health and illness
  measurement of, 211, 225-229
    Health Opinion Survey, 226-229
  public policy on, 10-24
  social planning and, 21-26
Mental illness
  as a social problem, 21-22
  conception of, 13, 14, 17-18, 19-21, 25
    social structure and, 11, 12
  definition of, 46-47, 78-80
  facts of, 45-47
  methods for dealing with, 11-14, 16-24
  prevention of, 44-45
  public policy towards. *See* Public policy on mental health.
  social and economic costs of, 243-245
  social class and, 236
  social disintegration and, 209-230
  social isolation and, 236

social structure and, 12, 15-17, 19, 21-23, 209-230
  sociocultural patterns and, 209-230
  symptoms of, 211
  treatment of, 14-15, 17-18, 23
  urban problems and, 25-26
  widening definition of, 46-47
Mentally ill
  legal status of, 78-80
  social control and, 80
Milieu therapy, 121-122
Monographical studies of community, 55
Multidisciplinary collaboration in community mental health, 74-77

National Institute of Mental Health, 22
National Mental Health Act of 1946, 21-22
New Haven study, 83-94
Nonmedical and paramedical personnel, 76-77, 198-205
Normative change, as a prevention strategy, 100

Operant conditioning, 123-124
Organizational adaptation to community mental health, 179-194, 195-207
Organizational analysis by systems model, 159-165
Organizational change, 204
Organizational setting of community mental health center, 181-186
Orientation of community mental health, 20-21, 35, 69
Outpatient service in community mental health center, 182-183

Paramedical and nonmedical personnel, 76-77, 198-205
Partial hospitalization, 122, 183-184
Patient population, changes in, 190-191
Patient selection, criteria for, 190, 191
Political jurisdiction in community psychiatry, 70-74
Planning of community mental health programs, 63-64, 77-78
Politics of community psychiatry, 47-49
Practitioner(s)
  evaluators and, conflict between, 128-129, 132-133, 142-143
  socialization of, 192
Prevention, 4, 8, 44-45, 125
  assumptions of, 103-108
  behavior change and, 105
  definition of, 95
  definition of target of, 103-104
  effectiveness of, 106
  evaluation of, 102-103, 106
  known etiology and, 104
  of alcoholism, 95-96, 102-103

Prevention—*Continued*
  of hospitalization, 238-241
  right to intervene and, 105-106, 107
  role of medical profession in, 108
  side effects of, 106
  social change and, 104-105
  social values and, 108
  strategies of,
    constructive confrontation, 98-99, 107
    differential risks, 96-97
    early identification, 98
    education, 97-98
    functional substitutes, 101-102
    normative change, 100
    prohibition, 100-101
    reduction of risks, 99
    replicating immune social conditions, 99-
      100
    revision of societal definitions, 102, 107-
      108
    severe sanctions, 101, 107
    social innoculation, 97
Prevention movement, supports for, 108-109
Preventive psychiatry, 95-109. *See also* Pre-
    vention.
Private rights and community needs, 83-94
Privileged information, 78, 89-90
Professional accountability in community
    mental health, 74-77
Professional jurisdiction in community psy-
    chiatry, 74-77
Professional styles and evaluation, 141-142
Program planning, 63-64, 77-78
Program success, criteria for, 152-153
Prohibition as a prevention strategy, 100-101
Psychiatric case register, 77-78
  in evaluation, 169
  systems model and, 164-165
Psychiatric symptoms, definition of, 211
Psychiatrist, role of, 3, 4, 108, 187-189, 198-
    203, 205-206. *See also* Community psy-
    chiatrist.
Psychiatry
  community. *See* Community psychiatry.
  development of, 14
  social. *See* Social psychiatry.
Psychoanalysis, 17-18
Public policy on mental health
  community oriented, implications of, 24-26
  history of, 10
    1920 to present, 17-24
    nineteenth and early twentieth centuries,
      14-17
    pre-seventeenth century, 11-12
    seventeenth and eighteenth centuries, 12-14
Public interest and individual rights, 77-81, 83-
    94

QUALITATIVE research methods, 165

REDUCTION of risks as a prevention strategy, 99
Rehospitalization, 237, 241-242
  after home care, 240
Replicating immune social conditions as a pre-
    vention strategy, 99-100
Research, sociological. *See* Sociological re-
    search; Evaluation of community mental
    health programs; Community theory
    and research.
Right to privacy, 77-78
  public interest and, 83-94
Roles, tasks, and responsibilities in community
    mental health, 186-189, 193-194, 196-
    203

SERVICES of community mental health pro-
    grams, 120-127, 180, 182-188, 196
  coordination of, 77-78, 125-126
Settings of community mental health programs,
    127
Severe sanctions as a prevention strategy, 101,
    107
Social change
  consequences of, 221-224
  initiation of, 218-221
  means of, 104-105
Social class and mental illness, 236
Social collectivities as dependent variables, 32
Social control and the mentally ill, 80
Social Darwinism, 15-17, 19
Social disintegration and mental illness, 209-230
Social innoculation as a prevention strategy, 97
Social intervention, 59. *See also* Intervention.
Social isolation and mental illness, 236
Social programs and American values, 3, 15-16,
    19, 24
Social psychiatry
  definition of, 181
  orientation of, 20-21
Social psychological perspective on community,
    56
Social structure
  as a dependent variable, 26-28
  conceptions of mental illness and, 11, 12
  mental illness and, 12, 15-17, 19, 21-23
Social systems theory, 6, 33-34, 53-54. *See also*
    Systems model.
Social welfarism, 19, 24
Societal definitions, revision of, as a prevention
    strategy, 102, 107-108
Sociocultural ecology, 53
Sociocultural patterns and mental illness, 209-
    230
Sociological influence on community mental
    health movement, 5

Sociological involvement in community mental health, 3-4, 5
  objectives and perspectives in, 26-28, 31-34
  tasks for, 10
Sociological research. *See also* Community theory and research; Evaluation of community mental health programs.
  collectivity approach, 32-35
  in mental health field
    community survey studies, 28-29
    descriptive studies of psychiatric hospitals, 29-30
    focus of, 26-28
    psychodynamically oriented studies, 30
  methodology of, 10, 27-28
  types of approaches in, 28-31
Stirling County Studies, 33, 210-213, 224-225
  frame of reference of, 210
  The Road. *See* The Road.
Structural-functional theory, 53-54. *See also* Social systems theory.
Symptoms of mental illness, definition of, 211
Systems model. *See also* Social systems theory.
  closed, 160-161
  in community psychiatry, 42-45
  in evaluation, 159-165
  open, 160-161
  organizational effectiveness and, 161-162
  organizational survival and, 161
  psychiatric case register and, 164-165
  research methods and, 165
  social engineering and, 42-43, 48-49
  studies based on, 162-165

TEAMS. *See* Treatment teams.
The Road
  case study of, 213-224

intergroup relations in, 214-216
mental health level in, improvement of, 223-224
social change in,
  consequences of, 221-224
  initiation of, 218-221
social organization of, 216-218
Therapists in community mental health programs, 126
Therapy in community mental health programs, modes of
  behavior therapy, 123-124
  brief psychotherapies, 122-123
  family treatment, 122
  group therapy, 124
  home care, 233-247
  hospitalization, partial, 122
  milieu therapy, 121-122
  operant conditioning, 123-124
  transitional communities, 122
  walk-in clinics, 123
Third Psychiatric Revolution, 2, 17
Transitional communities, 122
Treatment
  of communities, 125
  of mental illness, 14-15, 17-18, 23. *See also* Therapy, modes of, and Services of community mental health programs.
Treatment teams, 196
  leadership of, 63, 197-205
Twenty-four hour emergency service, 183, 188
Typological theory and research, 55

VALUES and social programs, 3, 15-16, 19, 24, 108

WALK-IN clinics, 123